Autism Spectrum Disorders

A Research Review for Practitioners

D0451996

Compliments of the

UCDAVIS
M.I.N.D. INSTITUTE

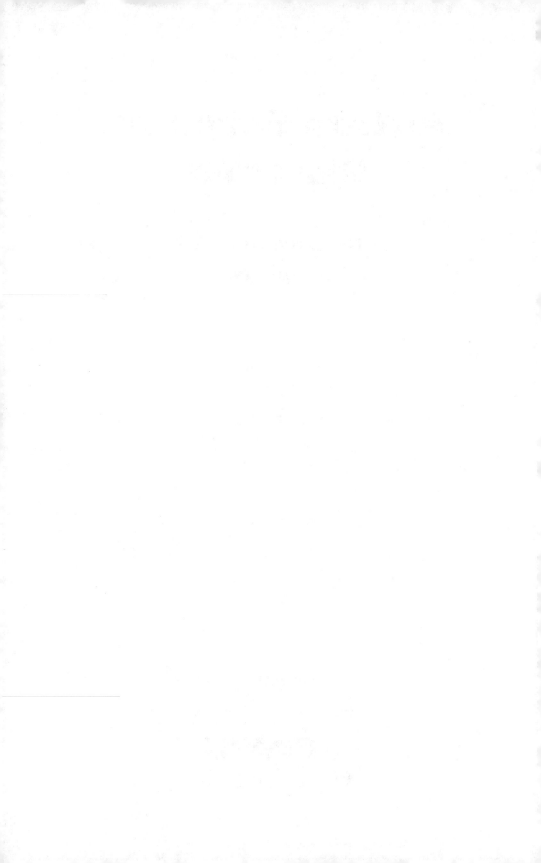

Autism Spectrum Disorders

A Research Review for Practitioners

Edited by

Sally Ozonoff, Ph.D.

Sally J. Rogers, Ph.D.

Robert L. Hendren, D.O.

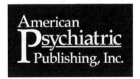

American Psychiatric Publishing, Inc.

Washington, DC
London, England

Copyright © 2003 American Psychiatric Publishing, Inc.
ALL RIGHTS RESERVED

Manufactured in the United States of America on acid-free paper
07 06 05 04 03   5 4 3 2 1
First Edition

Typeset in Adobe's Baskerville and Frutiger55 Roman

American Psychiatric Publishing, Inc.
1000 Wilson Boulevard
Arlington, VA 22209-3901
www.appi.org

Library of Congress Cataloging-in-Publication Data
Autism spectrum disorders : a research review for practitioners / edited by Sally Ozonoff, Sally J. Rogers, Robert L. Hendren.— 1st ed.
        p. ; cm.
    Includes bibliographical references and index.
    ISBN 1-58562-119-6 (alk. paper)
    1. Autism. 2. Autism—Patients—Rehabilitation. 3. Autism in children. 4. Outcome assessment (Medical care) I. Ozonoff, Sally. II. Rogers, Sally J. III. Hendren, Robert L., 1949–
    [DNLM: 1. Autistic Disorder—diagnosis. 2. Autistic Disorder—therapy. 3. Autistic Disorder—etiology. 4. Outcome and Process Assessment (Health Care) WM 203.5 A93838 2003]
    RC553.A88A8744 2003
    618.92'8982–dc21

                                                                2003043663

British Library Cataloguing in Publication Data
A CIP record is available from the British Library.

To my father, who instilled a love of editing in me.
—Sally Ozonoff, Ph.D.

To the children and families with autism who have taught me about autism.
—Sally J. Rogers, Ph.D.

To my family and to families everywhere.
—Robert L. Hendren, D.O.

Contents

Part I
Introduction

Part II
Interdisciplinary Approaches to Assessment

Part III
Treatment

Chapter 10
Professional–Parent Collaboration: The M.I.N.D. Institute
Model
Thomas F. Anders, M.D.
Charles R. Gardner Jr.
Sarah E. Gardner

Appendix
Resources

Index

Contributors

Thomas F. Anders, M.D.
Former Executive Associate Dean and Associate Dean of Academic Affairs, University of California–Davis School of Medicine, M.I.N.D. Institute, and Professor, Department of Psychiatry, M.I.N.D. Institute, University of California–Davis Medical Center, Sacramento, California

John R. Brown, Ph.D.
Education and Outreach Coordinator, M.I.N.D. Institute, and Assistant Clinical Professor, Department of Psychiatry, M.I.N.D. Institute, University of California–Davis Medical Center, Sacramento, California

Blythe A. Corbett, Ph.D.
Assistant Clinical Professor, Department of Psychiatry, M.I.N.D. Institute, University of California–Davis Medical Center, Sacramento, California

Vincent des Portes, M.D., Ph.D.
Child Neurologist, Centre Hospitalier Lyon Sud, France; former Visiting Scholar, M.I.N.D. Institute

Charles R. Gardner Jr.
Founding Family of the M.I.N.D. Institute, University of California–Davis Medical Center, Sacramento, California

Sarah E. Gardner
Founding Family of the M.I.N.D. Institute, University of California–Davis Medical Center, Sacramento, California

Beth L. Goodlin-Jones, Ph.D.
Clinical Associate Professor, Department of Psychiatry, M.I.N.D. Institute, Universtiy of California–Davis Medical Center, Sacramento, California

Randi J. Hagerman, M.D.
Medical Director, M.I.N.D. Institute, and Professor and Tsakopoulos-Vismara Chair of Pediatrics, M.I.N.D. Institute, University of California–Davis Medical Center, Sacramento, California

Robin L. Hansen, M.D.
Clinical Associate Professor, Department of Pediatrics, M.I.N.D. Institute, University of California–Davis Medical Center, Sacramento, California

Robert L. Hendren, D.O.
Executive Director, M.I.N.D. Institute, and Professor, Department of Psychiatry, University of California–Davis Medical Center, Sacramento, California

Peter S. Jensen, M.D.
Ruane Professor of Child Psychiatry and Director, Center for Advancing Children's Mental Health, Columbia University/New York State Psychiatric Institute, New York, New York

Ann M. Mastergeorge, Ph.D.
Assistant Research Professor, Department of Human & Community Development, M.I.N.D. Institute, University of California–Davis Medical Center, Sacramento, California

Sally Ozonoff, Ph.D.
Associate Professor, Department of Psychiatry, M.I.N.D. Institute, University of California–Davis Medical Center, Sacramento, California

Sally J. Rogers, Ph.D.
Professor, Department of Psychiatry, M.I.N.D. Institute, University of California–Davis Medical Center, Sacramento, California

Marjorie Solomon, Ph.D.
Postgraduate Researcher and M.I.N.D. Institute Scholar, M.I.N.D. Institute, University of California–Davis Medical Center, Sacramento, California

Barry R. Tharp, M.D.
Director of M.I.N.D. Institute Clinic and Clinical Professor, Departments of Neurology and Pediatrics, M.I.N.D. Institute, University of California–Davis Medical Center, Sacramento, California

Acknowledgments

This book would not have been possible without the contributions of my colleagues, the clinicians and researchers of the M.I.N.D. Institute. Someone told me that editing a book was the quickest way to make enemies, but the editing of this book was a wonderfully satisfying experience. Thank you to all my colleagues who worked tirelessly to turn out draft after draft of their chapters with nary a complaint. Thank you also to Dr. Robert Hales and the professionals at American Psychiatric Publishing, Inc., who did everything within their power to make the vision of this book become a reality in record time. Much appreciation goes to Debie Schilling for her expertise in manuscript preparation. Thank you to all the families who allowed us to learn about autism through them. Finally, thank you to my family for your support and love every day.

—Sally Ozonoff, Ph.D.

If it were not for the energy and commitment of my new colleagues at the UC Davis M.I.N.D. Institute, this book would not have been written. I appreciate the encouragement of our director, the incredible organization of the first author, and the support of friends and family during the writing process. I am especially grateful to Debie Schilling and Oanh Meyer for all their hard work in preparing the manuscript.

—Sally J. Rogers, Ph.D.

Working with the diverse group of clinicians, researchers, educators, and others sharing the mission of the M.I.N.D. Institute has been a wonderful opportunity to think broadly and deeply about autism and about neurodevelopment. We feel especially appreciative of the parent activists who were inspired to create the principles that founded the M.I.N.D. Institute and the donors, legislators, and citizens of California who have made this dream a reality. Being inspired to try to live up to their dreams has and will continue to move us beyond what any of could do individually. This book represents an early step in interdisciplinary collaboration to create better treatments and ultimately cure(s) for autism and other neurodevelopmental disorders.

—Robert L. Hendren, D.O.

Foreword

Peter S. Jensen, M.D.

There is increasing recognition that many neurodevelopmental disorders are best characterized as falling along a spectrum. In essence, what is meant by "spectrum disorders" is that there are multiple variants and partial expressions of a given disorder in persons with similar biologic and family risk. These considerations are now being increasingly applied to autism (e.g., Murphy et al. 2000)—hence the term *autism spectrum disorders* (ASD), the focus of this most welcome book.

But why is this book needed? Autism is a devastating condition and when fully manifested, is generally not difficult to spot, though ASD variants may necessitate greater diagnostic expertise. Yet even when a child manifests classic forms of autism, diagnosis and intervention are often delayed—a tragic but common occurrence that bespeaks the need for a volume such as this to assist practitioners in earlier and more accurate diagnosis.

Moreover, as the chapters on assessment and diagnosis show, there are new possibilities for diagnosing autism at an earlier age, well before the classic symptoms become apparent at age 2 or 3 (e.g., Stone et al. 1999; Teitelbaum et al. 1998). Although psychiatric diagnoses in very young children historically have been quite problematic, with autism the story has been somewhat different. This area of diagnosis has made rapid strides over the last decade, principally due to the development of structured diagnostic interviews and sophisticated observational methods. Thus, early and accurate diagnosis *should* be within the practitioner's reach. Early diagnosis in this disorder seems especially important, given the apparent effectiveness of intensive behavioral and educational interventions.

As you will soon see, this is an outstanding volume, both in its scholarship and in its breadth of coverage. Not just another text on an important childhood disorder, this book manages three remarkable accomplishments for its readers specifically and for the autism field generally. First, to my best knowledge, this is the only major volume produced to date that focuses specifically on bringing the latest research findings to the gamut of relevant *practitioners* in such a fashion as to best serve their needs for information concerning 1) early and accurate diagnosis, 2) up-to-date understanding of etiologic theories and contributory causes, 3) the juxtaposition of these scientifically based facts with the various autism myths and misunderstandings, and 4) the explication of the roles that each major professional discipline must play in a comprehensive assessment, diagnosis, and intervention plan for a child with ASD. On these grounds alone, this book, produced by a "who's who" list of leaders and expert investigators in the field of autism, should serve as a template to all of us—regardless of whether we are early educational, pediatric, developmental, psychiatric, or neurologic practitioners—on "how it's done," or at the very least, how it *should* be done.

Second, perhaps by virtue of the task the authors and editors have set for themselves in addressing the needs of the array of "need-to-be-involved" practitioners, the volume is extraordinary in its multidisciplinary input: its contributors come from the fields of pediatrics, psychology, psychiatry, neurology, genetics, education, and early childhood development. Of course, this range of contributors is as it must be: children with ASD may first present in a wide variety of settings, where early diagnosis and intervention *may* be possible, if only one knew what to look for and what then to do. And regardless of the child's service system entry portal, he or she needs the same range of professional expertise to enable a complete workup to rule out mimicking conditions, explore various mutable contributory causes, and develop and implement a comprehensive intervention program. Without this range of multidisciplinary expertise—unfortunately, usually available only in ASD-focused specialty settings—intervention programs will be nonproficient, incomplete, insufficiently intense, or worst of all, simply unavailable. The need to build this kind of infrastructure for the ASD field is the subtext running throughout the entire volume.

Third, and most remarkable of all, this volume articulates—as does the M.I.N.D. Institute, from which all of the book's contributors are drawn—the necessity of stakeholder/parent perspectives and partnerships in understanding and working with the disorder. The M.I.N.D. Institute represents not just the finest input from experts in the assessment, diagnosis, and treatment of ASD; it also epitomizes the critical partnerships between these professionals and those stakeholders that taxpayer-supported science is supposed to serve: children and families struggling with the enormous burden of ASD. In fact, to my knowledge, the M.I.N.D. Institute constitutes the first parent-initiated and consumer/taxpayer-supported institute focused on meeting the challenges of ASD, not just in terms of a promissory note for future research results, but also in ensuring that current research results are fully applied to children *today*—the focus of this volume.

And while on the topic of families, I note that this extraordinary coming together of investigator talent and motivated stakeholder families demarcates an important new phenomenon not just in the ASD field, but in all areas of neurodevelopmental disorders. Empowered stakeholder-parents are stepping forth not only to articulate their children's needs, but to dispute such assumptions as "one can't change the system" or "autism is incurable," as well as refuse to silently accept the shame and stigma long associated with such conditions. Remarkably also, such impassioned parents have become the most effective champions of securing additional research funds needed to remove autism and related conditions from their long-standing position of "benign neglect" in the fields of pediatrics, education, psychology, and psychiatry. Such changes were unforeseen even as recently as 10 to 15 years ago, when theories still abounded concerning parents' supposed etiologic roles in the onset of the disorder through nonempathic parenting styles.

Fortunately, improved understanding of the causes and correlates of specific disorders such as autism is increasingly possible through the advent of new technologies that are providing information heretofore unavailable. Using techniques such as post mortem histologic studies, in vivo magnetic resonance imaging (MRI), positron emission tomography (PET), and functional magnetic resonance imaging (fMRI), autism investigators are able to demonstrate a whole array of complex etiologic underpinnings of ASD, such as perturbations in the interconnected circuits with both facilitory and inhibitory functions that can lead to varying changes in widely separated areas of the brain, sometimes far from the presumed "lesions" associated with autism (Bailey et al. 1998; Chugani et al. 1997). Such changes also may include abnormalities in neuronal migration in the brain stem and cerebellum, as well as disturbances in other parameters, including neuronal number, survival, and orientation in the cerebral cortex. These same neuroimaging technologies are now offering major prospects for understanding specific brain regions that might be disturbed in children with ASD and which functions those brain regions subserve. Again, in keeping with one of the major themes of the book, this type of research typically requires the input of multiple disciplines, such as experts from neuropsychology (who are adept at devising strategic tests to elucidate functions specific to particular brain regions, such as face-recognition and inanimate object-recognition capacities [Schultz et al. 2000]), neuroscience, neuroimaging, and clinical psychiatry. These types of studies are not of intellectual interest only, because they may presage new therapeutic methods that couple such brain activation tasks with strategies to teach subjects how to develop "workarounds" to strengthen other areas of the brain as a part of their rehabilitation—a new approach to intervention altogether! As is quite clear from reading the book's chapters on etiology, assessments, and treatments, we have come quite a ways from the old notions of "refrigerator parenting"!

This volume shows readers not only where science is being "put to work" to yield new understanding, but also where science can be used to dispute notions that may be popular but are probably incorrect, such as the concerns raised in the last 3 years about possible linkages between immunization (MMR, measles-mumps-rubella) and autism. A number of studies have shown that immunization rates and rates of the diagnosis of autism do not appear to be linked (e.g., Dales et al. 2001). Similarly, science has tackled fads about supposedly powerful new treatments, such as secretin. When negative results have been produced, the findings have likely saved many families and children from exposure to ineffective and possibly harmful treatments (Sandler et al. 1999).

One lesson from such studies is clear: practitioners and investigators alike need to understand the extent of the human tragedy that illnesses such as autism impose on children and their families. Under desperate conditions, families understandably search for answers, particularly in view of the historically pessimistic outlook among medical professionals concerning this disorder and its treatments. Yet a second lesson is also apparent: anecdotal data coupled with passion, desperation, and determination, applied without careful scientific rigor such as comparisons involving placebos or appropriate contrast groups, often leads to incorrect conclusions, with the result that children may be exposed to nontherapeutic, even dangerous, treatments or be deprived of other therapeutic interventions (e.g., immunizations).

But there is hope on the horizon. Parent groups have recently become energized in supporting, even insisting on, a program of research to change the current state of affairs. Even the name of one of the groups— Cure Autism Now—reflects a commitment to increase the pace and level of scientific efforts to find empirically supported treatments, prevention strategies, and eventually cures.

In sum, this volume offers new hope—hope for practitioners that we can make a difference by applying the scientific findings in the pages of this volume, hope for parents and families that new opportunities for early diagnosis and intervention will yield improved outcomes for their children, and hope for us all that a new era of parent–professional science-based partnerships is at hand, and that by working together we can change the course of the lives of children with autism spectrum disorders. The editors and authors have done all of us a great service.

References

Bailey A, Luthert P, Dean A, et al: A clinicopathologic study of autism. Brain 121:889–905, 1998

Chugani DC, Muzik O, Rothermel R, et al: Altered serotonin synthesis in the dentatothalamocortical pathway in autistic boys. Ann Neurol 42:666–669, 1997

Dales L, Hammer SJ, Smith NJ: Time trends in autism and in MMR immunization coverage in California. JAMA 285:1183–1185, 2001

Murphy M, Bolton PF, Pickles A, et al: Personality traits of the relatives of autistic probands. Psychol Med 30:1411–1424, 2000

Sandler AD, Sutton KA, DeWeese J, et al: Lack of benefit of a single dose of synthetic human secretin in the treatment of autism and pervasive developmental disorder. N Engl J Med 41:1801–1806, 1999

Schultz RT, Gauthier I, Klin A, et al: Abnormal ventral temporal cortical activity during face discrimination among individuals with autism and Asperger's syndrome. Arch Gen Psychiatry 57:331–340, 2000

Stone WL, Lee EB, Ashford L, et al: Can autism be diagnosed accurately in children under 3 years? J Child Psychol Psychiatry 40:219–226, 1999

Teitelbaum P, Teitelbaum O, Nye J, et al: Movement analysis in infancy may be useful for early diagnosis of autism. Proc Natl Acad Sci U S A 95:13982–13987, 1998

Part I

Introduction

Chapter 1

From Kanner to the Millennium

Scientific Advances That Have Shaped Clinical Practice

Sally Ozonoff, Ph.D.
Sally J. Rogers, Ph.D.

Introduction

Autism was once thought to be a rare disorder. Knowledge of the condition, its diagnosis and management, and its causes, course, and outcome was not considered necessary for most mental health practitioners and was not routinely covered in professional training. In many communities, evaluation of autism was done by a small group of specialists, and treatment programs were not readily accessible. Now, however, with the number of children identified with autism spectrum disorders skyrocketing and a wide range of treatment options available, the responsibility of practitioners to engage in screening, diagnosis, evaluation, and referral for appropriate intervention is high. There is much greater awareness of autism spectrum disorders on the part of both professionals and the general public. Stories related to autism appear often in the media. Practitioners must work hard to stay up to date in their knowledge of autism spectrum disorders.

This book synthesizes the most recent research on the etiology, assessment, and treatment of autism spectrum disorders for practitioners.

3

Reviews of the scientific literature and practical implications for clinical care are provided. In this era of evidence-based medicine, this book provides empirically supported guidelines for evaluation and treatment, outlined in subsequent chapters that highlight the role of various professional disciplines. It is the goal of this book to help the nonspecialist provide state-of-the-art care, with a foundation in solid empirical research, for patients presenting with social, communication, and developmental problems indicative of an autism spectrum disorder. In this chapter, we provide a historical perspective tracing the major scientific advances, debates, and hypotheses that have informed clinical practice since autism was first described by Kanner in 1943. We close the chapter with some thoughts about ways to use these advances in work with patients and families.

This chapter introduces a series of chapters on interdisciplinary assessment and treatment issues. Any discipline can assume the primary role in coordinating evaluation and care for patients with autism, but this work is best done in collaboration with other professionals. In subsequent chapters, we present a model of team building and cross-disciplinary collaboration that is practiced at the institution with which most of the authors are associated, the M.I.N.D. Institute at the University of California–Davis. Each chapter reviews the important theories, research findings, and scientific debates relevant to a particular discipline and applies them to clinical care.

Kanner's Description

In an incisive, clinically rich paper that has become a classic, Leo Kanner, a child psychiatrist at Johns Hopkins University, characterized 11 children with a previously undescribed syndrome (Kanner 1943). They shared a fundamental inability to relate to others, a failure to use language to convey meaning, and an obsessive desire for the maintenance of sameness. Anxiety also played a prominent role in the presentation; the children often displayed intense fears of common things (e.g., tricycles, egg beaters, running water). All the children were described as highly enthusiastic, even "ecstatic" and "manic," about certain objects or topics. Kanner felt that the children were "endowed with good cognitive potentialities," as evidenced by their "astounding vocabulary," excellent memory and visual-spatial skills, strong interest in numbers and letters, and often precocious literacy. Kanner felt that the condition was congenital, involving "from the start" an extreme aloneness, and distinguished it from schizophrenia, whose social withdrawal comes after years of mostly typical development. About half of the children Kanner described had unusually large head circumferences. He commented that all came from very intelligent and high-achieving families at the upper end of the socioeconomic scale. He described the parents as "obsessive" and detail oriented. Kanner noted that some parents and siblings had experienced language delays and symptoms of autism themselves. Repeated otitis media and other infections were noted in some children. Appetite and eating patterns were nearly universally disrupted. One of the original 11 children developed seizures.

Over 60 years ago, in only 33 pages, Kanner identified the pathognomonic features of the disorder that are still considered essential to its diagnosis, highlighting both the profound difficulties of autism but also noting the considerable talents that can be present. He identified comorbid anxiety and mood issues and, in passing, noted the physical features of macrocephaly and repeated infections. Kanner felt strongly that the condition was congenital and suggested that qualitatively similar symptoms ran in families. Many of these observations went unappreciated for many years but now have strong empirical support. Almost prophetically, Kanner noted that although autism appears to be rare, it is "probably more frequent than indicated by the paucity of observed cases" (p. 242).

We have learned a great deal about autism spectrum disorders (ASD) since Kanner's landmark paper. Major advances in understanding the biological bases of ASD have taken place. Research on the behavioral and cognitive phenotype has exploded, leading to more refined diagnostic practices and better educational and therapeutic interventions. Clinical practice, shaped by empirical research, has changed dramatically from a few decades ago. After presenting some basics about ASD, this chapter reviews the major scientific advances that have changed clinical practice.

Clinical Features

Symptoms and Diagnosis

As specified in DSM-IV-TR (American Psychiatric Association 2000), autism spectrum disorders involve limitations in social relatedness, verbal and nonverbal communication, and range of interests and behaviors. There are five specific autism spectrum diagnoses (or pervasive developmental disorders, the term used by DSM-IV-TR that is synonymous with ASD). They are autistic disorder, Asperger disorder, Rett disorder, childhood disintegrative disorder, and pervasive developmental disorder not otherwise specified.

Table 1–1 lists DSM-IV-TR criteria for autistic disorder. In the social domain, symptoms include impaired use of nonverbal behaviors (e.g., eye contact, facial expression, gestures) to regulate social interaction, failure to develop age-appropriate peer relationships, little seeking to share enjoyment or interests with other people, and limited social-emotional reciprocity. Communication deficits include delay in development of or absence of spoken language, difficulty initiating or sustaining conversation, idiosyncratic or repetitive language, and imitation and pretend play deficits. In the behaviors and interests domain, there are often encompassing, unusual interests; inflexible adherence to nonfunctional routines; stereotyped body movements; and preoccupation with parts or sensory qualities of objects (American Psychiatric Association 2000). To meet criteria for autistic disorder, an individual must demonstrate at least 6 of the 12 symptoms, with at least 2 coming from the social domain and 1 each from the communication and restricted behaviors/interests categories. At least 1 symptom must have been present before 36 months of age (American Psychiatric Association 2000).

Asperger disorder (or Asperger syndrome, as we shall call it throughout this book) shares the social disabilities and restricted, repetitive behaviors of autism, but language abilities are well developed and cognitive functioning is not impaired. Its symptoms are identical to those listed in Table 1–1 for autistic disorder, except there is no requirement that the child demonstrate difficulties in the second category, communication. Although described almost 60 years ago by Austrian pediatrician Hans Asperger (1944), the Asperger syndrome diagnosis was not included in the DSM criteria until the 4th edition. In the DSM-IV-TR diagnostic system, the main point of differentiation from autistic disorder, especially for the higher-functioning subtype, is that those with Asperger syndrome do not exhibit significant delays in the onset or early course of language. As specified in DSM-IV-TR, non-echoed, communicative use of single words must be demonstrated by age 2 and meaningful phrase speech by age 3. Most parents of children with Asperger syndrome are not concerned about early language development and may even report precocious language abilities, such as a large vocabulary and adultlike phrasing from an early age. Autistic disorder must be ruled out before a diagnosis of Asperger syndrome is made. In the DSM-IV-TR system, the diagnosis of autism always takes precedence over that of Asperger syndrome. Thus, if a child meets criteria for autistic disorder, the diagnosis must be autism even if he or she displays excellent structural language and cognitive skills and other "typical" features of Asperger syndrome.

Individuals who meet criteria for autistic disorder and are intellectually normal are considered "high functioning." Research comparing Asperger

Table 1–1. DSM-IV-TR criteria for autistic disorder

DSM-IV-TR symptom	Examples
Deficits in reciprocal social interaction	
1a) Difficulty using nonverbal behaviors to regulate social interaction	Trouble looking others in the eye
	Little use of gestures while speaking
	Few or unusual facial expressions
	Trouble knowing how close to stand to others
	Unusual intonation or voice quality
1b) Failure to develop age-appropriate peer relationships	Few or no friends
	Relationships only with those much older or younger than the child or with family members
	Relationships based primarily on special interests
	Trouble interacting in groups and following cooperative rules of games
1c) Little sharing of pleasure, achievements, or interests with others	Enjoys favorite activities, television shows, toys alone, without trying to involve other people
	Does not try to call others' attention to activities, interests, or accomplishments
	Little interest in or reaction to praise
1d) Lack of social or emotional reciprocity	Does not respond to others; "appears deaf"
	Not aware of others; "oblivious" to their existence
	Does not notice when others are hurt or upset; does not offer comfort
Deficits in communication	
2a) Delay in or total lack of development of language	No use of words to communicate by age 2
	No simple phrases (e.g., "more milk") by age 3
	After speech develops, immature grammar or repeated errors

Table 1–1. DSM-IV-TR criteria for autistic disorder (*continued*)

DSM-IV-TR symptom	Examples
2b) Difficulty holding conversations	Trouble knowing how to start, keep going, and/or end a conversation
	Little back-and-forth; may talk on and on in a monologue
	Failure to respond to the comments of others; response only to direct questions
	Difficulty talking about topics not of special interest
2c) Unusual or repetitive language	Repeating what others say to him/her (echolalia)
	Repeating from videos, books, or commercials at inappropriate times or out of context
	Using words or phrases that the child has made up or that have special meaning only to him/her
	Overly formal, pedantic style of speaking (sounds like "a little professor")
2d) Play that is not appropriate for developmental level	Little acting out scenarios with toys
	Rarely pretends an object is something else (e.g., a banana is a telephone)
	Prefers to use toys in a concrete manner (e.g., building with blocks, arranging dollhouse furniture) rather than pretending with them
	When young, little interest in social games like peek-a-boo, ring-around-the-rosie, etc.

Restricted, repetitive behaviors, interests or activities

3a) Interests that are narrow in focus, overly intense, and/or unusual	Very strong focus on particular topics to the exclusion of other topics
	Difficulty "letting go" of special topics or activities
	Interference with other activities (e.g., delays eating or toileting due to focus on activity)
	Interest in unusual topics (sprinkler systems, movie ratings, astrophysics, radio station call letters)
	Excellent memory for details of special interests

Table 1–1. DSM-IV-TR criteria for autistic disorder (*continued*)

DSM-IV-TR symptom	Examples
3b) Unreasonable insistence on sameness and following familiar routines	Wants to perform certain activities in an exact order (e.g., close car doors in specific order)
	Easily upset by minor changes in routine (e.g., taking a different route home from school)
	Need for advance warning of any changes
	Becomes highly anxious and upset if routines or rituals not followed
3c) Repetitive motor mannerisms	Flaps hands when excited or upset
	Flicks fingers in front of eyes
	Odd hand postures or other hand movements
	Spins or rocks for long periods of time
	Walks and/or runs on tiptoe
3d) Preoccupation with parts of objects	Uses objects in ways not intended (e.g., flicks doll's eyes, repeatedly opens and closes doors on toy car)
	Interest in sensory qualities of objects (e.g., likes to sniff objects or look at them closely)
	Likes objects that move (e.g., fans, running water, spinning wheels)
	Attachment to unusual objects (orange peel, string)

Source. Reprinted from Ozonoff S, Dawson G, McPartland J: *A Parent's Guide to Asperger Syndrome and High-Functioning Autism: How to Meet the Challenges and Help Your Child Thrive.* New York, Guilford, 2002. Copyright 2002, The Guilford Press. Used with permission.

syndrome and high-functioning autism (HFA) provides mixed evidence of the distinction's external validity, and a consensus is beginning to emerge that the two conditions are more similar than different. Early-history differences are evident between the disorders, with children with Asperger syndrome showing less severity and better language ability in the preschool years than children with HFA, by definition (Ozonoff et al. 2000). Follow-up studies demonstrate similar trajectories in outcome, however. Szatmari et al. (2000) demonstrated that 2 years after study enrollment, children with HFA who had developed verbal fluency were virtually indistinguishable from those with Asperger syndrome. Similarly, Ozonoff et al. (2000) found that children with Asperger syndrome required fewer years of special education and had a slightly better outcome than children with HFA, but overall found very few differences between the subtypes. Research on the neuropsychology of the conditions also suggests that they are more similar than different. Studies have found impairments in executive function, social cognition, and motor skills in both subtypes (summarized in Ozonoff and Griffith 2000). The one exception found in most research is that individuals with Asperger syndrome perform better on language tests than those with autism, a not surprising finding secondary to the requirement of normal language onset for the Asperger diagnosis. Some studies have found visual-spatial deficits in Asperger syndrome rather than the strengths typical of autism (Klin et al. 1995), but other studies have not replicated this finding (Manjiviona and Prior 1995; Ozonoff et al. 2000; Szatmari et al. 1990). We have no indication at present that different treatment approaches are required for Asperger syndrome and high-functioning autism. Thus, the jury is still out on whether the two are functionally different. Several concerns about the DSM-IV (American Psychiatric Association 1994) definition of Asperger syndrome have been raised, including the possibilities that the criteria are underinclusive, underestimate the prevalence of Asperger syndrome, and do not correspond with the spirit of Asperger's (1944) original description (Eisenmajer et al. 1996; Miller and Ozonoff 1997; Szatmari et al. 1995). The major clinical implication of this research is that it is important to convey the functional similarities between the conditions to parents. Be sure they understand that they can use resources and intervention approaches for either disorder (e.g., interventions for Asperger syndrome will likely also help children with high-functioning autism and vice versa). Counsel parents not to be concerned if their child receives the "other" diagnosis in the future, and be sure they understand that this reflects not a change in function but rather diagnostic variability among clinicians.

Two other conditions appearing in DSM-IV-TR within the pervasive developmental disorders (PDD) category are Rett disorder and childhood disintegrative disorder. As we have come to understand more about these conditions and their respective etiologies, particularly Rett disorder, their relationship to the autism spectrum has become less clear. It is likely that these conditions will not be so closely associated with autism in the future and will be considered distinct neurodegenerative disorders.

Rett disorder, in its classic and best-recognized form, is a behavioral syndrome found only in girls. The infant appears fine at birth and develops normally for at least 5 months (and often longer), attaining head control, following objects and people with her eyes, rolling over, and sitting by herself. But within 6 months to a year or two later, she begins to lose use of her hands and interest in others and in social interaction. The growth of her head slows, reflecting slowing in brain development. Depending on the age at which the regression begins, specific language, cognitive, and motor skills (e.g., pointing, playing with toys, walking, talking) either are lost or never develop. The classic symptoms of Rett disorder include unsteady gait; lack of language; lack of functional hand use; almost constant stereotyped hand movements, including repetitive wringing, "washing," twisting, clapping, or rubbing of the hands in the midline; severe cognitive deficits; and lack of typical social interaction. Recently, a gene was isolated on the X chromosome, *MECP2*, which appears responsible for most cases of Rett disorder (Amir et al. 1999). With understanding of etiology and with the genotyping technology widely available has come the realization that the phenotype is broader than originally thought. For example, boys can inherit the mutation but display an X-linked mental retardation syndrome that does not include the pathognomonic symptoms of the classic Rett phenotype (Kerr 2002).

Childhood disintegrative disorder (CDD) is a very rare condition that also involves a period of normal development followed by a loss of skills, resulting in severe impairments in cognitive, self-help, and other abilities. The pattern is very different from Rett disorder, however, and the two are easily distinguished. Childhood disintegrative disorder can occur in either boys or girls but is much more common in boys. In CDD, an abrupt and severe regression occurs after at least 2 (and up to 10) years of normal development. Prior to the regression, the child displays normal speech, social relations, intelligence, and self-help skills. There is then a catastrophic loss of skills, with the child withdrawing, no longer talking, and losing motor, cognitive, and self-care skills such as toilet-training, and other abilities (Volkmar and Rutter 1995). The period of regression lasts 4 to 8 weeks and is marked by agitation and panic on the part of the child. After the regression, the child has all the characteristics of severe autism and severe mental retardation. However, unlike typical autism, there is little developmental growth after treatment and the condition continues as a chronic, severe developmental disability. Many researchers suspect that CDD is a distinct neurodegenerative disorder with a very different etiology from that of typical autism. Children displaying this symptom pattern need a detailed medical workup, including neurological and immunological testing, to identify possible biomedical factors involved in the regression.

The fifth and final condition within the PDD category is pervasive developmental disorder not otherwise specified (PDDNOS). This label is used for children who experience difficulties in at least two of the three autism-related symptom clusters (clear difficulty relating to others, as well as either communication problems or repetitive behaviors) but who do not meet criteria for any of the other PDDs. The same list of symptoms outlined in Table 1–1 is used to diagnose PDDNOS, but only one difficulty within the "reciprocal social interaction" domain and one symptom from either the "communication deficits" or "repetitive, restricted behaviors" domain are required. Children with PDDNOS have autistic-like behaviors and difficulties, but have either too few symptoms or a different pattern of symptoms from the other conditions in the PDD category. For example, a child might be diagnosed with PDDNOS if he displayed only four of the DSM-IV symptoms (ruling out autistic disorder), displayed a delay in language onset (ruling out Asperger syndrome), and showed no regression in development (ruling out both Rett and childhood disintegrative disorders). Unfortunately, PDDNOS is often misdiagnosed, as demonstrated by the DSM-IV field trials (Volkmar et al. 1994). Approximately one-third of children in the study diagnosed with PDDNOS actually met full criteria for autism, and another third did not have any diagnosis on the autism spectrum. Children in the latter group fell into two categories: 1) those with general language or learning problems and mildly delayed social skills and 2) those with hyperactive, distractible, highly disorganized behavior. In both cases, clinicians apparently felt that other diagnoses (e.g., mental retardation, attention-deficit/hyperactivity disorder [ADHD]) underappreciated the severity and pervasiveness of the disturbance, so they used the PDDNOS diagnosis even though the child did not actually meet diagnostic criteria. Thus, it is strongly recommended that professionals take a second look at any child diagnosed with PDDNOS and apply the DSM-IV-TR criteria stringently to make sure that it is an accurate diagnosis.

Course

The onset of autism occurs before age 3, at two peak periods. The majority of children display developmental abnormalities within the first 2 years of life. Although they are not always recognized at the time, a careful retrospective developmental history typically yields evidence of abnormalities in social responsiveness and early social-communicative behaviors, such as baby games and communicative gestures. A smaller group of children with autism display a period of normal or mostly normal development, followed by a loss of communication and social skills and onset of autism (Kurita 1985). The regression occurs most commonly between 12 and 24 months of age (thus distinguishing it from CDD); in rare cases it occurs after age 2 but before the third birthday. Although the existence of regression was questioned many years ago and at times ascribed to poor parental recall or parental denial (Short and Schopler 1988), the availability of home videotapes has now provided empirical validation of the regression phenomenon (Werner and Munson 2001). No epidemiologic study has conclusively defined the prevalence of autistic regression, but it has been found to be as low as 20% (Lord 1995) and as high as 50% (DeMyer 1979) of study samples, with two of the larger studies finding rates around 30% (Kurita 1985; Tuchman and Rapin 1997). The causes of regression are not yet understood. One hypothesis is that regression is due to complications of early infection, vaccination, or other environmentally mediated biologic exposures, as discussed in more detail in Chapter 8. A competing theory is that regression, like early-onset autism, is largely genetically influenced, but the genes have a later onset of action (Lainhart et al. 2002).

Most individuals with ASD improve with time and age. Symptoms of autism, particularly the repetitive and stereotypic behaviors, appear to increase for a few years after onset, usually peaking in the preschool period, but then begin to level off or decline in the school-age years. Most individuals continue to meet diagnostic criteria for ASD as teenagers and adults (Gonzalez et al. 1993; Piven et al. 1996a), however, and outcome studies suggest that long-term morbidity is significant. There has been one empirical report of normal functioning achieved in close to 50% of children who received early intensive behavioral intervention (Lovaas 1987; McEachin et al. 1993), as discussed more fully in Chapter 6. However, replications of that work have not reported the same level of "recovery," though they have demonstrated positive effects of the treatment. Books written by adults with autism spectrum disorders who have gone to college, developed successful careers, and/or married provide examples of "best outcomes" (Grandin 1996; Willey 1999). But the majority of studies find a variety of residual social difficulties and low rates of independent living, full-time, unsupported employment, and marriage even in relatively high-functioning adults (Gillberg 1991; Howlin and Goode 1998; Rumsey et al. 1985). Across all the studies conducted so far, the most powerful predictors of adult outcome are IQ scores and verbal ability at age 5 (Lotter 1974; Rutter 1984).

Kanner predicted that outcome might improve in the future as the disorder became better recognized and new treatments were developed. Recent studies have in fact found that mean IQs are rising and that very poor outcomes, such as institutionalization, are rare (Schopler 1987); however, community-based supported living situations are still common. As individuals with ASD are diagnosed earlier and provided with state-of-the-art treatments, we expect that the rate of best outcomes, including satisfying careers, independent living, and marriage and family, will continue to increase.

Comorbid Symptoms and Other Associated Features

Autism spectrum disorders can co-occur with a variety of other neurodevelopmental disorders. Best appreciated is the high comorbidity rate of autism and mental retardation. Most studies have found that the majority of individuals with autism (approximately 75%) are intellectually handicapped, with roughly half of the group functioning in the range of mild to moderate mental retardation and half in the severe to profound range. However, recent epidemiologic investigations focusing on preschool children with autism found a decrease (down to 25%–50%) in the percentage of those with mental retardation (Chakrabarti and Fombonne 2001; Honda et al. 1996). This trend is not inconsistent with increasing recognition that autism is a spectrum disorder and with improvements in the detection of mild cases. Rising IQ may also reflect the effect of early intervention.

Another commonly associated symptom is seizures. As discussed in Chapter 5, some children with ASD suffer from seizures, with onset most often occurring during either the preschool or the adolescent years (Volkmar and Nelson 1990). Autism spectrum disorders also seem to co-occur with Tourette syndrome and other tic disorders (Baron-Cohen et al. 1999b; Burd et al. 1986; Marriage et al. 1993; Sverd 1991; Sverd et al. 1993) and ADHD (Ghaziuddin et al. 1992; Jaselskis et al. 1992) at greater than chance levels. As first noted by Kanner, anxiety symptoms are also common (Kim et al. 2000; Muris et al. 1998). Disorders of mood, both depression and mania, are seen (Lainhart and Folstein 1994; Wozniak et al. 1997), particularly in higher-functioning individuals of latency age or beyond. There have been occasional reports of schizophrenia developing in adolescence or young adulthood in individuals diagnosed with ASD in childhood (Petty et al. 1984; Sverd et al. 1993; Volkmar and Cohen 1991), although the frequency of this comorbidity and whether it exceeds chance rates are unclear. As discussed in Chapters 2 and 3, the high rate of comorbidity in ASD complicates differential diagnosis, particularly in the evaluation of children school-age or older, for whom other psychiatric or learning disorders have often been previously identified. Comorbid symptoms can take a great toll on affected individuals and families and significantly reduce functioning, so it is essential to account for them in evaluation and treatment planning. Psychiatrists can be of particular help in this endeavor.

Kanner's first impression of autism as more common in males than females has proven true, with a ratio of 4:1 widely reported across samples (Fombonne 2002). However, his suggestion that it is a disorder of high–socioeconomic status (SES), high-achieving families has proven to be incorrect. It is now accepted that autism occurs across all socioeconomic levels, in all cultures, and in all racial and ethnic groups (Dyches et al. 2001). As further discussed in Chapter 9, research has generally neglected multicultural issues, but epidemiologic studies that have examined such variables suggest that autism prevalence rates do not differ significantly between ethnic and SES groups (Powell et al. 2000; see review in Dyches et al. 2001 and in Chapter 9).

Major Scientific Advances Since Kanner

Autism Is a Spectrum Disorder

As with many conditions, the most severe manifestations are the first recognized. Early diagnostic criteria for infantile autism, as it was originally called, were quite faithful to Kanner's original description. Most affected children displayed severely incapacitating symptoms, impaired intelligence, and poor outcomes. With time, however, it has become recognized that there is a range of potential manifestations, from readily apparent disabilities to subtle differences that are not always handicapping. For many years it was believed that autism was one of the most categorical of disorders (you either had it or you did not), but there is now thought to be a continuum of "autistic propensity" (Rutter 1999). In DSM-IV and DSM-IV-TR, the addition of the Asperger syndrome diagnosis reflected the growing realization that there are individuals with symptoms of autism who are normal in intelligence and do not show marked impairments in structural language. The most recent epidemiologic investigation of autism spectrum disorders suggests that the majority of children with these conditions do *not* have mental retardation (Chakrabarti and Fombonne 2001). Autism can also be found in individuals with severe or profound mental retardation. Such individuals do not always show the strengths exhibited by Kanner's first patients. It can be very complex to sort out the features that are due to general impairment and those that are specific to autism. An understanding of the wide range of manifestations of ASD is extremely important in the evaluation process, and the practical implications of this research are discussed in more detail in Chapter 3.

Autism Spectrum Disorders Are Not Rare

Concerns regarding the apparently increasing prevalence of ASD are expressed frequently by both parents and service providers and have been the focus of much media attention. Early research suggested that autism (strictly limited to children meeting full criteria for the disorder) occurred at the rate of 4 to 6 affected individuals per 10,000 (Lotter 1967; Wing and Gould 1979). An influential study conducted in the mid-1980s broadened diagnostic criteria somewhat and found a rate of 10 per 10,000 in a total population screening of a circumscribed geographic region in Canada (Bryson et al. 1988). In a departure from previous research, new studies have focused on preschool children, utilized standardized diagnostic measures of established reliability and validity, and employed active ascertainment techniques. These surveys have given prevalence estimates of 60–70 per 10,000, or approximately 1 in 150, across the spectrum of autism and 1 in 500 for children with the full syndrome of autistic disorder (Baird et al. 2001; Bertrand et al. 2001; Chakrabarti and Fombonne 2001). One obvious reason for the rise in rates is that more recent research has examined all autism spectrum disorders, whereas early surveys looked at rates of only strictly defined autism. However, in studies that have broken down the rates by specific DSM-IV-TR PDD subtypes, it is clear that the prevalence of classic autism itself is increasing, and thus better detection of high-functioning cases does not alone account for the rise in prevalence. Chakrabarti and Fombonne (2001) reported a rate of 16.8 per 10,000 for DSM-IV autistic disorder, which is 3 to 4 times higher than suggested in the 1960s and 1970s and over 1.5 times higher than thought in the 1980s and 1990s. This same study reported the rates of Asperger syndrome and PDDNOS as 8.4/10,000 and 36.1/10,000, respectively.

Several reasons for this increase have been proposed, from artifactual explanations to newly emerging environmental and biological risk factors. Included in the first category are increased awareness among clinicians, better identification and referral practices, more sensitive diagnostic tools, and broader classification systems. There is no doubt that the ability of clinicians to identify milder and more subtle manifestations of ASD has improved and that the current diagnostic system of DSM-IV-TR is broader in the net it casts than were previous classification systems (Wing 1996). However, the argument that these changes in referral and practice alone can account for the large increase in prevalence is no longer convincing. As discussed in detail later in this and several subsequent chapters, factors may have emerged in the last few decades that put infants and young children at greater risk for developing autism. There is currently a tremendous press to study environmental factors that might contribute to the growing number of cases now being seen. We do not yet have the evidence needed to answer these questions. Nevertheless, it is clear that ASD is a much more common problem than previously thought, as Kanner presciently suggested, and it is likely that clinicians will need to evaluate and treat it on a regular basis in their general practice.

Autism Is a Developmental Disorder

Despite Kanner's original assertion that autism was distinct from schizophrenia, it soon came to be seen as a form of psychosis and called "schizophrenic syndrome of childhood" and "infantile psychosis" (Creak 1961, 1963a, 1963b). However, research by Kolvin (1971) that carefully compared autism with schizophrenia eventually demonstrated clear differences between the conditions in both phenomenology and age of onset. Rutter (1972) argued persuasively that the two were distinct conditions requiring separate diagnostic criteria. It was at this time that autism was conceived as a developmental disorder and the need to take a developmental perspective in evaluation and treatment began to be appreciated.

Autism is unique in the incredible range of developmental levels involved, from toddlers functioning at a 6-month level, to school-age children with precocious reading ability and memory for facts, to adults whose cognitive and linguistic abilities can range from profound impairment to several standard deviations above the mean. This vast landscape requires that those involved with diagnosis be sophisticated developmentalists. Unlike conditions such as mental retardation or learning disorders, where the disability is defined by objective criteria and performance on quantitative measures, the diagnosis of autism requires developmentally informed clinical judgment. Autism is defined by the presence of both positive and negative symptoms. Positive symptoms involve the presence of behaviors that are not typical for the person's age and developmental level and that should not be a prominent part of their behavioral repertoire. Negative symptoms involve the absence or unusually low frequency of behaviors that are expected for a person's age and developmental level. Thus, diagnosis of autism requires significant knowledge of typical social, communication, cognitive, and play development and age-appropriate behavioral profiles from which individuals may deviate. These issues and how they inform both evaluation and intervention are discussed more fully in Chapters 3 and 6.

Autism Is a *Neuro*developmental Disorder With a Biological Basis

Kanner suggested that autistic children were born with "an innate inability to form the usual, biologically provided affective contacts with people" (Kanner 1943, p. 42). Later, however, his thinking came into line with that of his contemporaries trained in the psychoanalytic tradition predominant at the time. It was suggested that autism is the result of inadequate nurturance by emotionally cold, rejecting parents (Bettelheim 1967; Kanner 1943), a theory that prevailed until the late 1960s and did a great deal of harm to many families. Rimland (1964) did a tremendous service to the field when he provided powerful arguments that autism had an organic etiology. Rutter's (1970) finding that approximately 25% of children with autism developed seizures in adolescence also strongly suggested that autism was a neurodevelopmental condition with underlying organic brain dysfunction (Rutter 1999). It is now abundantly clear that autism is a biological disorder and is not caused by parenting deficiencies or other social factors. It is now also apparent that parents, far from being to blame, are integral members of the treatment team and are critical instruments of change. Many of the chapters in this book discuss the evidence for biological etiology in detail. Here, a few central research findings that have been instrumental to moving the field forward are highlighted.

Genetic factors appear to play a strong role in the development of autism (Bailey et al. 1995; International Molecular Genetic Study of Autism Consortium 2001). Evidence comes from four primary sources (Rutter et al. 1990). First, the recurrence risk for autism after the birth of one child with the disorder is 3%–6%, a rate that far exceeds that of the general population (Bailey et al. 1998b). Second, the concordance rate for autism in monozygotic twins is greatly elevated relative to that for dizygotic twins. The most recent twin studies, which used standardized diagnostic measures and total population screening, found a concordance rate for autistic disorder of 60% in monozygotic pairs, compared with only 5% in dizygotic pairs. Monozygotic concordance rates of up to 90% are reported when social and communication abnormalities broader than autistic disorder are included. Twin studies yield a heritability estimate greater than 0.90 (Bailey et al. 1995; Le Couteur et al. 1996). Third, autism occurs in association with a variety of known genetic abnormalities, including fragile X syndrome (Levitas et al. 1983; Watson et al. 1985), tuberous sclerosis (Gillberg et al. 1994; Hunt and Shepherd 1993), and many different chromosomal abnormalities (Gillberg and Wahlstrom 1985; Mariner et al. 1986), as discussed in Chapters 4 and 5. Finally, it appears that something is transmitted in the families of autistic probands that is not present in the families of children with other disorders. Research suggests that what is inherited is not autism itself, but an extended set of familial cognitive and social anomalies that are milder than but qualitatively similar to autism (the so-called broader autism phenotype, or BAP) (Bailey et al. 1998b; Piven et al. 1997). Family members also suffer from higher-than-average rates of anxiety and affective disorders (DeLong 1994; Piven et al. 1991; Smalley et al. 1995) and learning disabilities (Bailey et al. 1998b). BAP has been found in 15%–45% of family members of people with autism in different samples (Bailey et al. 1998b). One important implication of this research is that multiple members of a family may be affected, either with autism itself or with a broader set of difficulties that require clinical attention. These BAP-related symptoms, including slow language development and shyness in younger siblings, and psychiatric difficulties such as anxiety in first-degree adult relatives, must be attended to and handled expertly and sensitively.

With acceptance of the possibility of a genetic etiology and with the genome mapping efforts of the Human Genome Project, advances have been rapid, but the results are so far inconclusive. One reason is that the inheritance pattern appears to be far from simple, with statistical models suggesting that several, perhaps as many as 10, genes are involved in conferring susceptibility (Pickles et al. 1995; Risch et al. 1999). Case reports have demonstrated an association between autism and a wide variety of chromosomal anomalies (see Chapters 4 and 5 for more detail). One review (Gillberg 1998) found autism associated with all but three chromosomes. It is not yet clear which associations are random and which may provide clues about etiology. The one cytogenetic abnormality that has been consistently replicated in a small proportion of children with autism is a duplication of material on chromosome 15 (Cook et al. 1998; Rutter 2000). Molecular genetic studies have found associations with a number of different chromosomes, but the location with the highest log of odds (LOD) score across studies is on chromosome 7 (Barrett et al. 1999; Collaborative Linkage Study of Autism 2001; International Molecular Genetics Study of Autism Consortium 2001; Wassink et al. 2001). Genetic heterogeneity and the spectrum of affectedness make the implications for genetic counseling very complex (Simonoff 1998).

It is likely that autism is not a purely genetic disorder, and that other factors influence its development and severity. There is tremendous phenotypic variability even among monozygotic twins, with one twin displaying severe autism and the other the broader phenotype, for example. Fifty-point IQ differences between monozygotic twins have been reported (Rutter 1999). In recent years, environmental factors have been put forth as either moderating influences or full etiologic agents, including vaccination, heavy metal or pesticide exposure, viral agents, and food products, to name but a few (Bernard et al. 2002; Levy and Hyman 2002; Wakefield et al. 1998; Warren 1998). These issues are explored in detail in Chapter 8.

It is also abundantly clear that autism is an organic brain disorder. Evidence from numerous fields, including neuropathology, neuroimaging, and neuropsychology, point toward both structural and functional brain differences in individuals with autism. This topic is reviewed in Chapters 2 and 5. To highlight some of the more important and salient findings, it has become clear that autism has a specific neuropsychologic phenotype that involves particular deficits in social cognition, executive function, and abstract reasoning (Baron-Cohen et al. 1999a; Happe and Frith 1996; Minshew et al. 1997; Ozonoff et al. 1994). These functional deficits suggest difficulties in particular brain regions, including the limbic system and related medial temporal structures and the frontostriatal system (dorsolateral and orbital prefrontal cortex, anterior cingulate, basal ganglia structures). Structural imaging and neuropathology studies have found defects in the cerebellum, the limbic system, the brain stem, and several cortical regions (Bailey et al. 1998a; Courchesne et al. 1988; Kemper and Bauman 1993; Piven et al. 1990; Rodier 2002). Several studies have confirmed Kanner's original observation of macrocephaly (head circumference greater than the 97th percentile) in approximately 20% of individuals with autism (Fombonne et al. 1999; Lainhart et al. 1997; Piven et al. 1996b; Woodhouse et al. 1996). The increased head volume reflects a larger brain volume, which is not apparent at birth but is present by the late preschool years and is hypothesized to be due to failure of normal pruning mechanisms (Courchesne et al. 2001; Piven et al. 1996b).

Functional imaging techniques that have more recently become available shed light on how the brains of people with autism process information. In a study published in 1999, Baron-Cohen and his colleagues used functional magnetic resonance imaging (fMRI) to examine brain function while people with and without ASD looked at pictures of eyes and made judgments about what emotion the eyes conveyed. They found that typical adults relied heavily on both the amygdala and the frontal lobes to perform this task. Adults with either high-functioning autism or Asperger syndrome used the frontal lobes much less than the normal adults and did not activate the amygdala at all when looking at the pictures of eyes. Instead they used the superior temporal gyrus, which is not typically active during this task in people without ASD (Baron-Cohen et al. 1999a). A study by Schultz et al. (2000) found that people with autism or Asperger syndrome use the inferior temporal gyrus, the part of the brain that normally makes sense of objects, when they look at faces and do not activate typical face-processing structures, such as the fusiform gyrus. These studies suggest that even when people with ASD can figure out what someone's eyes or face conveys, they do so in a different, possibly less efficient manner. The medial temporal area of the brain is being hotly investigated by research teams around the world and may turn out to be one (but probably not the only) region that is abnormal in autism spectrum disorders. More review of the neurobiology literature is provided in Chapter 5.

Autism Can Be Identified Early

The onset of ASD is early in life, always occurring before age 3 (with the very rare exception of some cases of disintegrative disorder). It is not usually recognized until many months or years later (Rogers and DiLalla 1990; Short and Schopler 1988; Volkmar et al. 1985), however. Children with milder forms of the disorder may be identified even later, often after school entry (Howlin and Asgharian 1999). The most common initial symptom recognized by parents is delayed or abnormal speech development (DeMyer 1979). However, several other symptoms, particularly social-communicative ones, appear to predate the language abnormalities that parents report at the time of recognition. Research using detailed retrospective parent interviews and family home videos has found that a number of typical social milestones are markedly delayed or fail to develop. These behaviors, which typically appear in the first and second years of life, include eye contact, social referencing, imitation, orientation to name, and shared attention and affect (Baron-Cohen et al. 1992; Osterling and Dawson 1994; Stone et al. 1999).

One question that now occupies researchers is how early these specific developmental differences can be identified reliably. Several studies have shown that very low levels of these early social behaviors can distinguish children who are later diagnosed with autism from those with other developmental delays as early as 12 to 24 months of age (Baranek 1999; Dahlgren and Gillberg 1989; Lord 1995). One study found these developmental differences evident in home videotapes of first-year birthday parties (Osterling and Dawson 1994). Recent research has pushed the age at which some of these social delays can be documented through retrospective video analysis up to 8 months (Werner et al. 2000). Early differences in sensory and motor behaviors may also be potential markers of autism in the first year of life (Baranek 1999; Teitelbaum et al. 1998).

These results suggest that it should be possible to identify autism far earlier than is current practice. The need for earlier recognition has been spurred by studies demonstrating substantial cortical plasticity during early development (Huttenlocher 1984) and improved outcomes from certain intensive early intervention approaches (Lovaas 1987; Rogers 1998). This highlights the need for clinicians to be aware of the early symptoms and act upon them quickly through evaluation and referral. As discussed in Chapters 3 and 4 and in Filipek et al. (1999), the clinician's responsibilities typically begin when parental questions are directed to a primary care physician or public school teacher. The first set of activities prompted by parental voicing of concerns should involve screening. Screening is generally a relatively brief and inexpensive procedure that assists decision making about resource management. Screening activities involve determination of the probability that the child indeed has some type of disorder or is at risk of developing one. Chapter 3 lists recommended screening procedures and specific screening instruments. A main purpose of screening is to determine whether the child should be referred for the more expensive and time-consuming diagnostic procedures and laboratory evaluations outlined in later chapters of this book.

Assessment and Diagnosis of Autism Can Be Challenging

As the brief review of the biology of autism has suggested, there is no specific biomarker, laboratory test, or behavioral assessment procedure that identifies autism. Diagnosis of autism spectrum disorders is a complex clinical process that is dependent on informed clinical judgment. Development of such clinical competency requires sophisticated advanced clinical training. Unfortunately, there are currently few places in the country where professionals are thoroughly trained in the diagnostic (let alone treatment) process. Diagnostic procedures are not easily learned in 2-day workshops or several sessions in a conference. Clinical judgment requires training, supervision, and feedback from experts, as well as experience with many children of different functioning levels and ages.

Further complicating this situation is that autism is a moving target. Autism is defined by behavioral symptoms. The clinical description and boundaries of the syndrome have changed over the past two decades, as have methods of assessment. As discussed earlier in this chapter, we are increasingly able to recognize autism in early childhood and now appreciate that there is a broad spectrum of affectedness that goes well beyond the "classic" presentation first described by Kanner. The challenges of screening, evaluation, and diagnosis vary throughout the lifespan and at different developmental levels. As recently as 10 years ago, autism was diagnosed through subjective clinical opinion, without a requirement for any particular objective measures of development or behavior. As consensus about the diagnosis has been achieved, a number of standardized interviews and observational measures have been developed; these are reviewed in Chapter 3. Competent clinical evaluation now assumes the use of objective measures; funding and publication *require* it. However, many professionals involved in the assessment of autism lack familiarity with the new tools that are available and knowledge of their psychometric strengths and weaknesses. Thus, even those with strong training need regular review of the rapid developments in the research literature and ongoing access to the changing clinical face of autism.

There Are Many Effective Treatments for Autism

Autism was once thought to be a hopeless diagnosis, with little prospect of improvement, even with treatment. Few interventions had been demonstrated to be efficacious. Diagnosis was sometimes delayed or not made at all because of the paucity of community resources and the apparently dismal prognosis. Now, however, research suggests that children with autism can improve a great deal with certain kinds of interventions. These treatment approaches, discussed in detail in Chapters 6 and 7, include intensive early behavioral and language interventions, psychoactive medication, social skills training, and school-based interventions. Several features shared by most efficacious treatments, regardless of model, philosophy, or type, have been identified: they begin early, are intensive (at least 25 hours a week), are individualized and developmentally appropriate, and are family centered, involving parents at every level (Dawson and Osterling 1997; Rogers 1998). There are few comparative studies that directly contrast different approaches while controlling for central variables (such as number of hours of treatment), so it is difficult to firmly claim superiority for any one intervention for all people with autism. Most research has been done on behavioral approaches, but persons with autism of all ages and all levels of severity have demonstrated positive responses to a variety of different treatments. Intervention needs to begin as early as possible and be relatively intense to be of maximum long-term benefit.

Research over the past six decades has both refined and expanded syndrome delineation and notions about cause. The clinical and etiologic heterogeneity suggests that multiple approaches to management may be necessary, with different treatments used with distinct subgroups of children or targeting different symptoms. In the past decade there has been a movement, reasonable enough in theory, to require that only treatments that are "empirically supported" or "empirically validated" be used, particularly with vulnerable groups such as children. This creates a tension, however, since some interventions with little research support, both existing and newly emerging approaches, often appeal to parents, who desire to leave no stone unturned in helping their children. As discussed in detail in Chapter 8, clinicians have an opportunity to establish a partnership with their patients in observing and quantifying behavioral effects of alternative treatments, both potential benefits and side effects. The clinician must strike a balance between restricting treatments to those with empirical support on the one hand and recommending approaches that are potentially dangerous or that replace those known to be efficacious on the other hand. The goal is to work with patients and families in a way that is simultaneously open-minded, safe, and objective (no small feat). Chapters 6 through 8 discuss in more detail examples of treatments for autism that have promised false hopes or whose risks clearly outweigh their benefits. Rutter (1999) tells the following cautionary tale. In the 1980s, the Nobel laureate Tinbergen claimed that "many cases of autism can be cured and even prevented" through "reparenting" therapy (Tinbergen and Tinbergen 1983), an intervention being refuted on multiple grounds. Tinbergen's scientific reputation certainly gave this statement more credibility than it deserved. Rutter concludes that we need to pay careful attention to the evidence, regardless of the status of the researcher or appeal of the claim. If a treatment sounds too good to be true, it probably is.

Approach to Working With Families

How should the scientific advances reviewed in this chapter and throughout the book inform the way we work with families? To begin with, it is important to remember that old ideas about etiology are still around in different forms. Outdated books remain in many library collections and parents may still access them. It is an almost universal experience for families to have someone—perhaps a well-meaning relative, a member of the public, or even a professional—suggest that their child's struggles are the result of poor discipline, inadequate language stimulation, or other parenting shortfalls. Parents may be told, "He'll talk when you stop talking for him" or be given other forms of advice that subtly or not so subtly make them complicit in their child's problems. Regardless of the specific diagnosis, it is a natural inclination of parents to feel guilt for a child's difficulties. Therefore, it is important to state unequivocally to every family seen in a diagnostic setting that autism is not caused by poor parenting or any other social-environmental variable. This knowledge cannot be assumed. Some explanation of what we currently know about etiology can help put things in perspective. Do not brush aside or otherwise devalue a family's concerns and theories about what caused their child's difficulties. Listen well and respond both compassionately and scientifically.

The former hopelessness associated with the autism label is still felt by many parents. It was not long ago that children with autism were given a terrible prognosis. Tragically, parents are still sometimes told that little can be done for their child and advised to place him or her outside the home (see Chapter 10). Clinicians working with families need to stress the hope inherent in early interventions and emerging treatments. With what we now know about intervention, it is certainly possible to help parents feel hopeful about their child's future.

One of the most powerful therapeutic interventions a clinician can perform is to enable parents to actively participate in their child's treatment and development. All efficacious treatments involve parents in some role (Rogers 1998). There has been tremendous growth in grassroots parent self-help organizations since Kanner's time. As discussed in Chapter 10, parents have helped to create legislation, secure and allocate funds for research, encourage research initiatives, and lobby for better and more accessible treatment resources. Beginning with Rimland (1964), etiologic theories have been proposed by parents, most recently exemplified by the surge in interest in potential environmental causes of autism (see Chapter 8).

Clinicians need to ask parents about their hopes for their child on many occasions because, understandably, these change with time. What is at first a reasonable hope for cure may later turn into hopes of social participation, self-determination, and self-esteem—in other words, into hopes that the child will lead a happy, productive, and meaningful life, at whatever level possible (Ruble and Dalrymple 1996). Important outcomes must always include functionality and generalization. The task of the clinician is to carefully sort through available therapies and help families choose those most likely to result in skills that will be useful in daily living and eventual independence.

In working with families, another central tenet is highlighting and using strengths. The emphasis during the diagnostic process is, not surprisingly, on deficits. Stressing weaknesses is often necessary to ensure that the child is eligible for special services and resources. However, autism is by no means a disorder devoid of strengths. Kanner's initial description of very affected children with the syndrome was rife with examples of talents. He mentioned their precocious reading, prodigious memories, and well-developed visual-spatial skills. To this list we might add the passion and conviction that people with autism display for certain topics, and their desire for order and consequent willingness to follow rules and routines (Ozonoff et al. 2002). Parents will be more accustomed to hearing some of these strengths described as deficits (e.g., echolalia, perseveration, monologues, rigidity, circumscribed interests), yet they are legitimate aptitudes that can far exceed the abilities of typical siblings or peers. Helping parents recognize and use these strengths can set a hopeful and helpful tone for a grief-stricken family.

In closing, the clinician-parent relationship is crucial for enhancing the skills and outcomes of children with autism. Treatment outcome research has for many years made it clear that seemingly "simple" and nonspecific interventions—attention, compassionate care, management of fears, setting of expectations, self-determination, self-awareness—can be extremely powerful. The quality of the patient-professional relationship is a potent factor in outcome. Providing a clear diagnosis, instilling hope for the future, applying effective interventions, and allowing an opportunity for dialogue have all been linked with improvement in the management of chronic physical disease (Bass et al. 1986; Stewart 1995). Make the most of these opportunities as you work with the families who seek you out.

References

American Psychiatric Association: Diagnostic and Statistical Manual of Mental Disorders, 4th Edition. Washington, DC, American Psychiatric Association, 1994

American Psychiatric Association: Diagnostic and Statistical Manual of Mental Disorders, 4th Edition, Text Revision. Washington, DC, American Psychiatric Association, 2000

Amir RE, Van Den Veyver IB, Wan M, et al: Rett syndrome is caused by mutations in X-linked *MECP2*, encoding methyl CpG binding protein 2. Nat Genet 23:185–188, 1999

Asperger H: "Autistic psychopathy" in childhood. Archiv fur Psychiatrie und Nervenkrankheiten 117:76–136, 1944

Bailey A, Le Couteur A, Gottesman I, et al: Autism as a strongly genetic disorder: evidence from a British twin study. Psychol Med 25:63–77, 1995

Bailey A, Luthert P, Dean A, et al: A clinicopathological study of autism. Brain 121:889–905, 1998a

Bailey A, Palferman S, Heavey L, et al: Autism: the phenotype in relatives. J Autism Dev Disord 28:369–392, 1998b

Baird G, Charman T, Santosh PJ: Clinical considerations in the diagnosis of autism spectrum disorders. Indian Pediatr 68:439–449, 2001

Baranek G: Autism during infancy: a retrospective video analysis of sensory-motor and social behaviors at 9–12 months of age. J Autism Dev Disord 29:213–224, 1999

Baron-Cohen S, Allen J, Gillberg C: Can autism be detected at 18 months? The needle, the haystack, and the CHAT. Br J Psychiatry 161:839–843, 1992

Baron-Cohen S, Ring H, Wheelwright S, et al: Social intelligence in the normal and autistic brain: An fMRI study. Eur J Neurosci 11:1891–1898, 1999a

Baron-Cohen S, Scahill VL, Izaguirre J, et al: The prevalence of Gilles de la Tourette syndrome in children and adolescents with autism: a large scale study. Psychol Med 29:1151–1159, 1999b

Barrett S, Beck JC, Bernier R, et al: An autosomal genomic screen for autism: collaborative linkage study of autism. Am J Med Genet 88:609–615, 1999

Bass MJ, Buck C, Turner L, et al: The physician's actions and the outcome of illness in family practice. J Fam Pract 23:43–47, 1986

Bernard S, Enayati A, Rogers H, et al: The role of mercury in the pathogenesis of autism. Mol Psychiatry 7 (suppl):S42–S43, 2002

Bertrand J, Mars A, Boyle C, et al: Prevalence of autism in the United States population: the Brick Township New Jersey investigation. Pediatrics 108:1155–1161, 2001

Bettelheim B: The Empty Fortress. New York, Free Press, 1967

Bryson SE, Clark BS, Smith IM: First report of a Canadian epidemiological study of autistic syndromes. J Child Psychol Psychiatry 29:433–445, 1988

Burd L, Kerbeshian J, Wikenheiser M, et al: Prevalence of Gilles de la Tourette's syndrome in North Dakota adults. Am J Psychiatry 143:787–788, 1986

Chakrabarti S, Fombonne E: Pervasive developmental disorders in preschool children. JAMA 285:3093–3099, 2001

Collaborative Linkage Study of Autism: An autosomal genomic screen for autism. Am J Med Genet 105:609–615, 2001

Cook EH, Courchesne R, Cox NJ, et al: Linkage disequilibrium mapping with 15q11–13 markers in autistic disorder. Am J Hum Genet 62:1077–1083, 1998

Courchesne E, Yeung-Courchesne R, Press GA, et al: Hypoplasia of cerebellar vermal lobules VI and VII in autism. N Engl J Med 318:1349–1354, 1988

Courchesne E, Karns CM, Davis HR, et al: Unusual brain growth patterns in early life in patients with autistic disorder: an MRI study. Neurology 57:245–254, 2001

Creak M: Schizophrenic syndrome in childhood: progress report of a working party. Cerebral Palsy Bulletin 3:501–504, 1961

Creak M: Childhood psychosis: a review of 100 cases. Br J Psychiatry 109:84–89, 1963a

Creak M: Schizophrenia in early childhood. Acta Paedopsychiatrica 30:42–47, 1963b

Dahlgren SO, Gillberg C: Symptoms in the first two years of life: a preliminary population study of infantile autism. Eur Arch Psychiatry Neurol Sci 283:169–174, 1989

Dawson G, Osterling J: Early intervention in autism, in The Effectiveness of Early Intervention. Edited by Guralnick MJ. Baltimore, Paul H. Brookes, 1997, pp 307–326

DeLong R: Children with autistic spectrum disorder and a family history of affective disorder. Dev Med Child Neurol 36:674–687, 1994

DeMyer MK: Parents and Children in Autism. Washington, DC, Victor Winston and Sons, 1979

Dyches TT, Wilder LK, Obiakor FE: Autism: multicultural perspectives, in Educational and Clinical Interventions. Edited by Wahlberg T, Obiakor F, Burkhardt S, et al. Oxford, UK, Elsevier Science Ltd, 2001, pp 151–177

Eisenmajer R, Prior M, Leekam S, et al: A comparison of clinical symptoms in individuals diagnosed with autism and Asperger syndrome. J Am Acad Child Adolesc Psychiatry 35:1523–1531, 1996

Filipek PA, Accardo PJ, Baranek GT, et al: The screening and diagnosis of autistic spectrum disorders. J Autism Dev Disord 29:439–484, 1999

Fombonne E: Epidemiological trends in rates of autism. Mol Psychiatry 7 (suppl 2):S4–S6, 2002

Fombonne E, Roge B, Claverie J, et al: Microcephaly and macrocephaly in autism. J Autism Dev Disord 29:113–119, 1999

Ghaziuddin M, Tsai L, Ghaziuddin N: Comorbidity of autistic disorder in children and adolescents. Eur Child Adolesc Psychiatry 1:209–213, 1992

Gillberg C: Outcome in autism and autistic-like conditions. J Am Acad Child Adolesc Psychiatry 30:375–382, 1991

Gillberg C: Chromosomal disorders and autism. J Autism Dev Disord 28:415–425, 1998

Gillberg C, Wahlstrom J: Chromosome abnormalities in infantile autism and other childhood psychosis: a population study of 66 cases. Dev Med Child Neurol 27:293–304, 1985

Gillberg IC, Gillberg C, Ahlsen G: Autistic behaviour and attention deficits in tuberous sclerosis: a population-based study. Dev Med Child Neurol 36:50–56, 1994

Gonzalez NM, Murray A, Shay J, et al: Autistic children on follow-up: change of diagnosis. Psychopharmacol Bull 29:353–358, 1993

Grandin T: Thinking in Pictures and Other Reports from My Life with Autism. New York, Vintage Books, 1996

Happe F, Frith U: The neuropsychology of autism. Brain 119:1377–1400, 1996

Honda H, Shimizu Y, Misumi K, et al: Cumulative incidence and prevalence of childhood autism in children in Japan. Br J Psychiatry 169:228–235, 1996

Howlin P, Asgharian A: The diagnosis of autism and Asperger syndrome: findings from a survey of 770 families. Dev Med Child Neurol 41:834–839, 1999

Howlin P, Goode S: Outcome in adult life for people with autism and Asperger's syndrome, in Autism and Pervasive Developmental Disorders. Edited by Volkmar FR. New York, Cambridge University Press, 1998

Hunt A, Shepherd C: A prevalence study of autism in tuberous sclerosis. J Autism Dev Disord 23:323–339, 1993

Huttenlocher P: Synapse elimination and plasticity in developing human cerebral cortex. Am J Ment Defic 88:488–496, 1984

International Molecular Genetic Study of Autism Consortium: A genomewide screen for autism: strong evidence for linkage to chromosomes 2q, 7q, and 16p. Am J Hum Genet 69:570–581, 2001

Jaselskis CA, Cook EH, Fletcher KE: Clonidine treatment of hyperactive and impulsive children with autistic disorder. J Clin Psychopharmacol 12:322–327, 1992

Kanner L: Autistic disturbances of affective content. Nervous Child 2:217–250, 1943

Kemper TL, Bauman ML: The contribution of neuropathologic studies to the understanding of autism. Neurol Clin 11:175–187, 1993

Kerr A: Rett syndrome: recent progress and implications for research and clinical practice (annotation). J Child Psychol Psychiatry 43:277–287, 2002

Kim JA, Szatmari P, Bryson SE, et al: The prevalence of anxiety and mood problems among children with autism and Asperger syndrome. Autism 4:117–132, 2000

Klin A, Volkmar FR, Sparrow SS, et al: Validity and neuropsychological characterization of Asperger syndrome: convergence with nonverbal learning disabilities syndrome. J Child Psychol Psychiatry 36:1127–1140, 1995

Kolvin I: Psychosis in childhood: a comparative study, in Infantile Autism: Concepts, Characteristics, and Treatment. Edited by Rutter M. Edinburgh, Churchill Livingstone, 1971, pp 7–26

Kurita H: Infantile autism with speech loss before the age of thirty months. J Am Acad Child Psychiatry 24:191–196, 1985

Lainhart JE, Folstein SE: Affective disorders in people with autism: a review of published cases. J Autism Dev Disord 24:587–601, 1994

Lainhart JE, Piven J, Wzorek M, et al: Macrocephaly in children and adults with autism. J Am Acad Child Adolesc Psychiatry 36:282–290, 1997

Lainhart JE, Ozonoff S, Coon H, et al: Autism, regression, and the broader autism phenotype. Am J Med Genet 113:231–237, 2002

Le Couteur A, Bailey AJ, Goode S, et al: A broader phenotype of autism: the clinical spectrum in twins. J Child Psychol Psychiatry 37:785–801, 1996

Levitas A, Hagerman RJ, Braden M, et al: Autism and the fragile X syndrome. J Dev Behav Pediatr 4:151–158, 1983

Levy SE, Hyman SL: Alternative/complementary approaches to treatment of children with autistic spectrum disorders. Infants and Young Child 14:33–42, 2002

Lord C: Follow-up of two-year-olds referred for possible autism. J Child Psychol Psychiatry 36:1365–1382, 1995

Lotter V: Epidemiology of autistic conditions in young children, II: some characteristics of parents and their children. Soc Psychiatry 1:163–173, 1967

Lotter V: Factors related to outcome in autistic children. J Autism Child Schizophr 4:263–277, 1974

Lovaas OI: Behavioral treatment and normal educational and intellectual functioning in young autistic children. J Consult Clin Psychol 55:3–9, 1987

Manjiviona J, Prior M: Comparison of Asperger syndrome and high-functioning autistic children on a test of motor impairment. J Autism Dev Disord 25:23–39, 1995

Mariner R, Jackson AW, Levitas A, et al: Autism, mental retardation, and chromosomal abnormalities. J Autism Dev Disord 16:425–440, 1986

Marriage K, Miles T, Stokes D, et al: Clinical and research implications of the co-occurrence of Asperger and Tourette syndromes. Aust N Z J Psychiatry 27:666–672, 1993

McEachin JJ, Smith T, Lovaas OI: Long-term outcome for children with autism who received early intensive behavioral treatment. Am J Ment Retard 97:359–372, 1993

Miller JN, Ozonoff S: Did Asperger's cases have Asperger disorder? J Child Psychol Psychiatry 38:247–251, 1997

Minshew NJ, Goldstein G, Siegel DJ: Neuropsychologic functioning in autism: profile of a complex information processing disorder. Int Neuropsychol Soc 3:303–316, 1997

Muris P, Steerneman P, Merckelbach H, et al: Comordid anxiety symptoms in children with pervasive developmental disorders. J Anxiety Disord 12:387–393, 1998

Osterling J, Dawson G: Early recognition of children with autism: a study of first birthday home video tapes. J Autism Dev Disord 24:247–259, 1994

Ozonoff S, Griffith EM: Neuropsychological function and the external validity of Asperger syndrome, in Asperger Syndrome. Edited by Klin A, Volkmar F, Sparrow SS. New York, Guilford, 2000, pp 72–96

Ozonoff S, Strayer DL, McMahon WM, et al: Executive function abilities in autism and Tourette syndrome: an information processing approach. J Child Psychol Psychiatry 35:1015–1032, 1994

Ozonoff S, South M, Miller JN: DSM-IV-defined Asperger syndrome: cognitive, behavioral, and early history differentiation from high-functioning autism. Autism 4:29–46, 2000

Ozonoff S, Dawson G, McPartland J: A Parent's Guide to Asperger Syndrome and High-Functioning Autism: How to Meet the Challenges and Help Your Child Thrive. New York, Guilford, 2002

Petty LK, Ornitz EM, Michelman JD, et al: Autistic children who become schizophrenic. Archives of General Psychology 41:129–135, 1984

Pickles A, Bolton PF, MacDonald H, et al: Latent-class analysis of recurrence risks for complex phenotypes with selection and measurement error: a twin and family history study of autism. Am J Hum Genet 57:717–726, 1995

Piven J, Berthier ML, Starkstein SE, et al: Magnetic resonance imaging evidence for a defect of cerebral cortical development in autism. Am J Psychiatry 147:734–739, 1990

Piven J, Chase GA, Landa R, et al: Psychiatric disorders in the parents of autistic individuals. J Am Acad Child Adolesc Psychiatry 30:471–478, 1991

Piven J, Harper J, Palmer P, et al: Course of behavioral change in autism: a retrospective study of high-IQ adolescents and adults. J Am Acad Child Adolesc Psychiatry 35:523–529, 1996a

Piven J, Arndt S, Bailey J, et al: Regional brain enlargement in autism: a magnetic resonance imaging study. J Am Acad Child Adolesc Psychiatry 35:530–536, 1996b

Piven J, Palmer P, Jacobi D, et al: Broader autism phenotype: evidence from a family history study of multiple incidence families. Am J Psychiatry 154:185–190, 1997

Powell JE, Edwards A, Edwards M, et al: Changes in the incidence of childhood autism and other autistic spectrum disorders in preschool children from two areas of the West Midlands, UK. Dev Med Child Neurol 42:624–628, 2000

Rimland ER: Infantile Autism: The Syndrome and Its Implications for a Neural Theory of Behavior. New York, Appleton-Century-Crofts, 1964

Risch N, Spiker D, Lotspeich L, et al: A genomic screen of autism: evidence for a multilocus etiology. Am J Hum Genet 65:493–507, 1999

Rodier PM: Converging evidence for brain stem injury. Dev Psychopathol 14:537–557, 2002

Rogers SJ: Empirically supported comprehensive treatments for young children with autism. J Clin Child Psychol 27:167–178, 1998

Rogers SJ, DiLalla DL: Age of symptom onset in young children with pervasive developmental disorders. J Am Acad Child Adolesc Psychiatry 29:863–872, 1990

Ruble LA, Dalrymple NJ: An alternative view of outcome in autism. Focus on Autism and Other Developmental Disabilities 11:3–14, 1996

Rumsey JM, Rapoport JL, Sceery WR: Autistic children as adults: psychiatric, social, and behavioral outcomes. J Am Acad Child Adolesc Psychiatry 24:465–473, 1985

Rutter M: Autistic children: infancy to adulthood. Semin Psychiatry 2:435–450, 1970

Rutter M: Childhood schizophrenia reconsidered. Autism Child Schizophr 2:315–337, 1972

Rutter M: Autistic children growing up. Dev Med Child Neurol 26:122–129, 1984

Rutter M: Autism: two-way interplay between research and clinical work. J Child Psychol Psychiatry 40:169–188, 1999

Rutter M: Genetic studies of autism: from the 1970s into the millennium. J Abnorm Child Psychol 728:3–14, 2000

Rutter M, MacDonald H, Le Couteur A, et al: Genetic factors in child psychiatric disorders: II. empirical findings. J Child Psychol Psychiatry 31:39–83, 1990

Schopler E: Specific and nonspecific factors in the effectiveness of a treatment system. Am Psychol 42:376–383, 1987

Schultz RT, Gauthier I, Klin A, et al: Abnormal ventral temporal cortical activity during face discrimination among individuals with autism and Asperger syndrome. Arch Gen Psychiatry 57:331–340, 2000

Short AB, Schopler E: Factors relating to age of onset in autism. J Autism Dev Disord 18:207–216, 1988

Simonoff E: Genetic counseling in autism and pervasive developmental disorders. J Autism Dev Disord 28:447–456, 1998

Smalley SL, McCracken J, Tanguay P: Autism, affective disorders, and social phobia. Am J Med Genet 60:19–26, 1995

Stewart MA: Effective physician-patient communication and health outcomes: a review. Can Med Assoc J 152:1423–1433, 1995

Stone WL, Lee EB, Ashford L, et al: Can autism be diagnosed accurately in children under 2 years? J Child Psychol Psychiatry 40:219–226, 1999

Sverd J: Tourette syndrome and autistic disorder: a significant relationship. Am J Med Genet 39:173–179, 1991

Sverd J, Montero G, Gurevich N: Cases for an association between Tourette syndrome, autistic disorder, and schizophrenia-like disorder. J Autism Dev Disord 23:407–413, 1993

Szatmari P, Tuff L, Finlayson AJ, et al: Asperger's syndrome and autism: neurocognitive aspects. J Am Acad Child Adolesc Psychiatry 29:130–136, 1990

Szatmari P, Archer L, Fisman S, et al: Asperger's syndrome and autism: differences in behavior, cognition, and adaptive functioning. J Am Acad Child Adolesc Psychiatry 34:1662–1671, 1995

Szatmari P, Bryson SE, Streiner DL, et al: Two-year outcome of preschool children with autism or Asperger syndrome. Am J Psychiatry 157:1980–1987, 2000

Teitelbaum P, Teitelbaum O, Nye J, et al: Movement analysis in infancy may be useful for early diagnosis of autism. Proc Natl Acad Sci U S A 95:13982–13987, 1998

Tinbergen N, Tinbergen EA: Autistic Children: New Hope for a Cure. Boston, MA, George Allen and Unwin, 1983

Tuchman RF, Rapin I: Regression in pervasive developmental disorders: seizures and epileptiform electroencephalogram correlates. Pediatrics 99:560–566, 1997

Volkmar FR, Cohen DJ: Comorbid association of autism and schizophrenia. Am J Psychiatry 148:1705–1707, 1991

Volkmar FR, Nelson DS: Seizure disorders in autism. J Am Acad Child Adolesc Psychiatry 29:127–129, 1990

Volkmar FR, Rutter M: Childhood disintegrative disorder: results of the DSM-IV autism field trial. J Am Acad Child Adolesc Psychiatry 34:1092–1095, 1995

Volkmar FR, Stier DM, Cohen DJ: Age of recognition of pervasive developmental disorder. Am J Psychiatry 142:1450–1452, 1985

Volkmar FR, Klin A, Siegel B, et al: Field trial for autistic disorder in DSM-IV. Am J Psychiatry 151:1361–1367, 1994

Wakefield AJ, Murch SH, Anthony A, et al: Ileal-lymphoid-nodular hyperplasia, non-specific colitis, and pervasive developmental disorder in children. Lancet 351:637–641, 1998

Warren RP: An immunologic theory for the development of some cases of autism. CNS Spectrum 3:71–79, 1998

Wassink TH, Piven J, Vieland VJ, et al: Evidence supporting *WNT2* as an autism susceptibility gene. Am J Med Genet 105:406–413, 2001

Watson MS, Leckman JF, Annex B, et al: fragile X syndrome in a survey of 75 autistic males. N Engl J Med 310:462, 1985

Werner E, Dawson G, Osterling J, et al: Recognition of autism spectrum disorders before one year of age: a retrospective study based on home videotapes. J Autism Dev Disord 30:157–162, 2000

Werner B, Munson JA: Regression in autism: a description and validation of the phenomenon using parent report and home videotapes. Paper presented at the biannual meeting of the Society for Research in Child Development, Minneapolis, MN, 2001

Willey LH: Pretending to Be Normal: Living With Asperger's Syndrome. London, Jessica Kingsley, 1999

Wing L: Autistic spectrum disorders: no evidence for or against an increase of prevalence. Br Med J 312:327–328, 1996

Wing L, Gould J: Severe impairments of social interaction and associated abnormalities in children: epidemiology and classification. J Autism Dev Disord 9:11–29, 1979

Woodhouse W, Bailey A, Rutter M, et al: Head circumferences in autism and other pervasive developmental disorders. J Child Psychol Psychiatry 37:665–671, 1996

Wozniak J, Biederman J, Faraone SV, et al: Mania in children with pervasive developmental disorder revisited. J Am Acad Child Adolesc Psychiatry 36:1552–1559, 1997

Part II

Interdisciplinary Approaches to Assessment

Chapter 2

Contributions of the Psychiatrist

Robert L. Hendren, D.O.

Introduction

The psychiatrist may be involved in the evaluation and treatment of children with autism spectrum disorders (ASD) as the primary provider, as a member of a treatment team, or as a consultant. Each role requires a different level of involvement. If the psychiatrist is the primary provider, he or she needs to gather the thorough medical and neurologic history described in Chapters 4 and 5 of this book. This chapter describes the contributions of the psychiatrist as a unique member of the assessment and treatment team or as a consultant to providers from other specialties. These contributions fall into three areas: 1) clarifying the diagnosis when multiple symptoms are present, 2) providing treatment recommendations in complicated pharmacotherapy (covered more completely in Chapter 7), and 3) working with families and other providers to unravel medical issues and optimize engagement in effective treatment programs.

Clarifying the Diagnosis

Once a medical evaluation has ruled out alternative or contributing etiologies for the presenting symptoms (as described in Chapters 4 and 5), the

next challenge in determining the diagnosis is to be certain that the presenting symptoms are actually representative of ASD and not another major
mental illness (Tanguay 2000). Historically, children with "classic autism"
were relatively easy to distinguish from children with other mental disorders. Now, as we have become increasingly better at recognizing higher-
functioning and milder forms of autism (Chakrabarti and Fombonne 2001),
symptom presentation is less "classic." Symptoms appear to be more continuous than categorical, and we find an overlap with other mental disorders (Frazier et al. 2002; Lainhart 1999; Szatmari et al. 2000, 2002). The
task of the psychiatrist is to determine whether certain symptoms are part
of a disorder other than ASD or represent one that is comorbid with or sub-
sumed under the ASD diagnosis. An example of the former is that ASD,
prodromal schizophrenia, and early-onset bipolar disorder have certain
similarities, and it is important to examine all the evidence to determine
which is the most accurate diagnosis or diagnoses. An example of the latter
is that obsessive-compulsive symptoms or attention deficits are often sub-
sumed under ASD and may warrant an additional diagnosis. Identifying
these comorbidities may suggest alternative treatment approaches, including psychopharmacologic methods (Gillberg and Billstedt 2000).

Research has demonstrated that ASD can also be associated with symptoms of hyperactivity, impulsivity, anxiety, cognitive disorganization, affective instability, aggression, and distractibility (Volkmar et al. 1999).
Potential comorbid diagnoses include attention-deficit/hyperactivity disorder (ADHD), oppositional defiant disorder, obsessive-compulsive disorder and other anxiety disorders, tics and Tourette syndrome, affective
disorders, and even psychotic disorders (Tsai 1996). It is often unclear
whether these additional symptoms are distinct from or part of the ASD.
In a study of 35 patients with ASD, 65% presented with symptoms of an
additional psychiatric disorder at the time of the initial evaluation or during the 2-year follow-up (Ghaziuddin et al. 1998). The most common diagnosis in the children in the sample was ADHD, and depression was the
most common diagnosis in the adolescents and adults. In the next section,
symptoms that suggest potential comorbidity with ASD are reviewed.

Symptom Presentation

Many factors influence the presentation of psychiatric disorders in individuals with ASD and complicate their diagnosis. The decrement in functioning
associated with ASD means that the baseline is already lower than average
and that a change in behavior has to be relatively marked to be identifiable.
Autism, by itself, causes a variety of psychosocial deficits and maladaptive

behaviors, and their presence may mask other psychiatric symptoms or make them difficult to identify. Cognitive limitations may mean that the range and quality of symptoms differ. For example, anxiety may be manifest as obsessive talking about a topic or the insistence on sameness, rather than as rumination or somatic complaints. Individuals with ASD may not demonstrate certain symptoms, such as the feelings of guilt often seen in depression or the grandiosity and inflation of self-esteem typical of mania. The diminished ability to think abstractly, communicate effectively, and be aware of and describe internal states also means that interview and self-report measures are often of less use. People with autism may lack either the self-insight to recognize symptoms or the motivation and social relatedness needed to report them (Howlin 1997; Perry et al. 2001). Thus, the assessment of comorbid psychiatric illness can be quite tricky (implications of this issue for evaluation are addressed in Chapter 3). Table 2–1 contains some tips for identifying such problems. It is of tremendous importance to identify major changes in behavior from the typical baseline, usually through careful interview of parents and caregivers. Comorbidity should also be carefully investigated in the presence of severe or worsening symptoms that are not responding to traditional methods of treatment (Lainhart 1999).

Table 2–1.   When to consider comorbidity in ASD

1. When signs of problems outside the autism spectrum are apparent

Hyperactivity, distractible inattention

Sad or irritable mood, decreased pleasure in activities, increased withdrawal, vegetative signs

Increased anxiety

Affective instability

Cognitive disorganization

2. When there is an abrupt change in behavior from "baseline"

First rule out a medical problem (seizures, migraine, medication side effect)

3. When there is a severe and incapacitating problem behavior

Aggression

Self-injury

Agitation

Sleep disturbance

4. When there is a worsening of symptoms already present

Decreased communication

Increased hand flapping or motor stereotypies

Decreased adaptive behavior and daily living skills

5. When patient does not respond as expected to treatment

Inattention

Impairments in attention are common in youngsters with ASD, but they may take various forms and it is important to evaluate the nature of the "inattention." For example, the inattention seen in ADHD is a distractible inattention, with deterioration in attention and vigilance over time. In contrast, children with ASD are more likely to have difficulty shifting attention. Caretakers may refer to this as inattention, but it is qualitatively different from the distractible inattention of ADHD. Children with ASD may also appear to be inattentive due to a lack of arousal, but again this is not the classic attentional dysfunction of ADHD. However, when the child with ASD also meets the criteria for ADHD (e.g., distractible inattention, hyperactivity, impulsivity) and the symptoms require treatment, the additional diagnosis of ADHD should be made.

Oppositional Behavior

Individuals with ASD may show signs of oppositional defiant disorder, including negativistic, defiant, and disobedient behavior toward authority figures. This behavior may at times be secondary to the strong preoccupations and rigidity associated with ASD. For example, some children so strongly prefer their own activities that their resistance to the suggestions of others is interpreted as defiance or oppositionality. Clinically, it is not uncommon for such negativism to be associated with Asperger syndrome and high-functioning autism. Rarely, antisocial behavior (possibly consistent with conduct disorder) has been reported, but in many instances it appears that the antisocial acts reflect social naivete or a lack of understanding of social norms. For example, there have been reports of individuals with ASD stealing because they did not understand the necessity of paying, and having unreciprocated sexual behavior interpreted as assault (Ghaziuddin et al. 1991; Kohn et al. 1998).

Tics

Symptoms ranging from chronic motor and vocal tics to full-blown Tourette syndrome are commonly reported in people with ASD (Stern and Robertson 1997). One small study found a prevalence rate for Tourette syndrome of 8.1% in children with ASD who also had a strong family history of tics (Baron-Cohen et al. 1999). At times, parents may describe impulsive or stereotypic behaviors of their children as being similar to the involuntary motor tics of Tourette syndrome, but the differential diagnosis can usually be clarified by further history taking and careful observation of the behaviors in question. Simple motor tics are involuntary, nonrhythmic, sudden, and of rapid onset/offset, whereas the stereotypies of autism tend to be voluntary, rhythmic, and of longer duration. The differentiation of complex motor tics from ASD-type repetitive behaviors is more challenging, but, in general, the latter are more intentional, are more driven, and may serve soothing, self-regulating, discharge, or self-stimulatory functions (American Psychiatric Association 2000).

Anxiety

Symptoms of anxiety are common in ASD, and children may meet criteria for obsessive-compulsive disorder, avoidant disorder, separation anxiety disorder, phobia, and generalized anxiety disorder (Tsai 1996). A study that involved interviewing parents of 44 children with ASD using the Diagnostic Interview Schedule for Children found that 84.1% met full criteria for at least one anxiety disorder (Muris et al. 1998). Another study found that children with high-functioning autism demonstrated significantly more anxiety symptoms than children with language impairment and typical children, with the highest scores on measures of separation anxiety and obsessive-compulsive disorder (Gillott et al. 2001). Anxiety may increase stereotyped behaviors, such as echolalia, hand flapping, and repetitive questioning. It has been suggested that these behaviors serve a calming function for individuals with ASD when they are anxious (Howlin 1997), but there is little in the way of empirical data to support this view at this time.

Affective Symptoms

Many authors have described affective disorders in both individuals with ASD (for a review, see Lainhart and Folstein 1994) and their relatives (Bolton et al. 1998; DeLong 1994; DeLong and Dwyer 1988; Smalley et al. 1995). Children with ASD are reported to have an increased risk of developing a mood disorder, particularly those with average intellectual abilities, and symptoms often worsen with puberty (Ghaziuddin and Tsai 1991; Gillberg 1984). One survey of parents reported that 16.9% of their children and adolescents had elevated scores on the depression subscale of the Child Behavior Checklist (Kim et al. 2000). Youths with ASD who are found to be depressed are reported to present with accentuated symptoms of autism, including more stereotypies and preoccupations, and greater social withdrawal, hyperactivity, and agitation (Lainhart 1999).

Although less often described than major depression, symptoms of bipolar disorder have also been reported in children and adolescents with ASD (Frazier et al. 2002; Steingard and Biederman 1987; Wozniak et al. 1997). Suggestive symptoms include irritability, affective instability, and

tantrums. Children displaying these symptoms are more frequently referred to psychiatrists for evaluation, and these symptoms tend to impair
their functioning more significantly than do their core autism deficits. Estimates in the literature of the incidence of comorbid bipolar disorder and
ASD range from 5% to 21% (Lainhart 1999). Tantum reported that approximately 10% of adult patients with Asperger syndrome presented with
mania (Tantum 1991). Studying a sample of children with ASD referred
for medication, Wozniak et al. (1997) reported that 21% met the criteria
for bipolar disorder. Another study found a symptom cluster of irritability,
moodiness, attention difficulties, poor frustration tolerance, and explosive
behavior with anger outbursts in 29 of 40 children with ASD (Chilakamarri
et al. 2001). A lifetime diagnosis of bipolar disorder was identified in 3 of
the 40 children (7.5%), and subthreshold bipolar disorder was evident in
an additional 2 of the 40 (5%). DeLong (1994) described a group of 40 children with symptoms of both ASD and bipolar disorder. He argued that
their mood instability, severe temper outbursts, and marked irritability
caused more impairment for these children and created far more management problems for their families and schools than children with typical
ASD and urged that this group be a focus of more in-depth study.

Psychosis

It is increasingly appreciated that the prodrome of schizophrenia can be
recognized in childhood (Erlenmeyer-Kimling et al. 2000; Weinberger
1987). It often presents as social withdrawal, lack of motivation, affective
flattening, and poverty of speech; all of these symptoms can be confused
with ASD. Symptoms and course clarify the differential diagnosis in most
cases, but there does appear to be some overlap such that some individuals
with ASD also display signs of schizophrenia (Goldstein et al. 2002). When
marked deterioration in functioning appears in adolescence in an individual with ASD, accompanied by positive symptoms such as hallucinations
and delusions, the diagnosis of schizophrenia spectrum disorder should be
made. Transient psychosis can also be present in ASD.

Mixed Symptoms

At times, children with ASD present with multiple symptoms of other disorders, particularly affective instability and cognitive disorganization, causing confusion about what is the primary diagnosis. Research groups have
created two new categories to explain these complexities, but as yet neither
is validated or widely used. Researchers at Yale University identified a
group of children who had some features in common with ASD, particularly

a limited capacity for relating, but who also demonstrated basic defects in affect modulation and stability of thinking (Dahl et al. 1986; Towbin et al. 1993). These children demonstrated "peculiar fears, chronic anxiety, frequent incidents of intense anger and extreme behavioral reactions" distinguishing them from children with ASD (Towbin 1997, p. 135). They also exhibited recurrent episodes of disorganized thought and perceptual distortions, although these were not of the severity or pervasiveness seen in psychotic disorders. These researchers coined the term *multiple complex developmental disorder* (MCDD) to describe this group of children. Although they proposed a new diagnostic category, they felt that MCDD was part of the autism spectrum, sharing both serious limitations in reciprocal social interaction and onset in infancy with ASD (Towbin 1997). It was noted that the affective instability, behavioral dysregulation, and disorganized thinking associated with MCDD were often precipitated by changes in routine or structure, as in ASD. It was recommended that, until the external validity of MCDD was clarified, children falling in this category should be classified under the "wider umbrella of PDDNOS [pervasive developmental disorder not otherwise specified]" (Cohen et al. 1986; Towbin 1997, p. 135).

A separate research group, this one at the National Institute of Mental Health, identified children similar to those described as having MCDD. In a study of early-onset schizophrenia, they encountered a number of children who did not fit in the schizophrenia category or in any other DSM-IV diagnosis (Kumra et al. 1998). They displayed affective instability with nearly daily outbursts of tantrums, poor social skills in spite of eagerness to relate to peers, poor ability to distinguish fantasy from reality, and attention deficit symptoms. Some had symptoms of ASD but did not meet the full criteria. This research group used the term *multidimensionally impaired disorder* (MDI) to describe these children.

Symptoms similar to the MDI and MCDD categories have also been identified in a study of 8- to 12-year-old children with psychotic spectrum disorder (Hendren et al. 1995). These children exhibited negative symptoms consistent with schizotypal disorder but not of sufficient severity to meet the diagnosis of schizophrenia. Some of these symptoms were similar to the symptoms of ASD, such as poor social relationships, odd and peculiar thinking, and communication deficits and deviances. Unlike children with "uncomplicated" ASD, they also demonstrated impaired reality testing and affective instability.

This group of children with mixed symptoms of ASD, affective instability, and cognitive disorganization needs further characterization and study before any new categories are used in routine diagnosis. For now, it is useful in clinical practice to know that others are seeing this pattern of symptoms and considering if treatment should be directed at affective instability and/or cognitive disorganization.

Psychiatric Symptoms and the Broader Autism Phenotype

Psychiatric symptoms should also be considered in evaluating family members of children with ASD (Piven and Palmer 1999; Piven et al. 1991). Motor tics, obsessive-compulsive disorder, and affective disorders are significantly more common in family members of a child with ASD compared with family members of a child with Down syndrome (Bolton et al. 1998). Social phobia has been reported in 20% of family members with ASD and affective disorders in 37% of first-degree relatives (Smalley et al. 1995).

Neurodevelopmental Signs

The presence of neurodevelopmental signs suggests neurologic vulnerability or dysfunction and may help in clarifying the diagnosis, although no single sign or cluster of signs is diagnostic of any DSM category. As discussed in more detail in Chapters 4 and 5, neurodevelopmental abnormalities are occasionally present in individuals with ASD and may be helpful in distinguishing them from children with other psychiatric disorders. Although not documented in published studies, our clinical experience suggests that children with ASD generally have neurodevelopmental signs greater in number and severity than children with bipolar disorder or ADHD, but fewer than children with early-onset schizophrenia. Research has demonstrated physical anomalies including macrocephaly, low-seated ears, and high-steepled palate (Green et al. 1994); neurologic soft signs such as difficulties with right-left discrimination or rapid alternating movements (Pine et al. 1997); and poor coordination and integration difficulties. Phenotypically abnormal children are 10 times more likely to be diagnosed with a known genetic syndrome (Miles et al. 2000), as discussed in Chapter 4, indicating the need for a thorough genetic evaluation. Rapin (1996) provides a nice summary of the neurologic examinations, common findings, and their implications for assessment.

Contribution of Neuroimaging

Recent advances in neuroimaging technology have enhanced the potential for studying neurodevelopmental psychiatric disorders at the brain mechanisms level. Magnetic resonance imaging (MRI), magnetic resonance spectroscopy (MRS), and functional MRI (fMRI) can provide reliable and precise quantitative measures of brain regions, structures, tissue types and composition, site-specific function, and functional pathways. These technologies are relatively safe and noninvasive. Structural brain abnormalities identified by neuroimaging technology hold promise for serving as biological markers (*biomarkers*) for psychopathology in childhood. Recently, Pantelis et al. (2003) reported the ability to predict which at-risk family members would develop schizophrenia from volumetric MRI measurements. Identification of similar biomarkers predictive of autism would be of assistance in understanding the natural history of the pathology and the potential effect of therapeutic manipulations (Bristol-Power and Spinella 1999), in addition to being potentially helpful in diagnosis. Using pharmacologic probes with MRI may elucidate brain regions and functions involved in neurodevelopmental disorders and help to identify potential responders (Buchsbaum et al. 2001; Casey et al. 2000). However, to date, neuroimaging has demonstrated its value primarily as a research tool and not as a diagnostic or treatment-matching tool (Hendren et al. 2000).

Evidence for brain abnormalities that can explain the heterogeneity of ASD has proven elusive, and many believe that biomarkers specific to the DSM category of autism will not be found (Ciesielski et al. 1997; Deb and Thompson 1998). Methodologic inconsistencies make it difficult to validate and compare results across studies. Despite these complexities, neuroimaging research in ASD has increased in recent years. Neuroimaging studies of subjects with autism provide inconsistent results (see Chapter 5), but the most replicated findings suggest increased total brain volume (Cody et al. 2002; Courchesne 1997; Filipek et al. 1992; Piven et al. 1995, 1996) and changes in cerebellar and temporal lobe structures (Cody et al. 2002; Sparks et al. 2002). Decreased function in the temporal lobe is consistently reported on fMRI (Abell et al. 1999; Howard et al. 2000; Schultz et al. 2000; Sweeten et al. 2002). Proton MRS in children with ASD also demonstrates findings that may be unique to ASD (Filippi et al. 2002; Fitzgerald et al. 2000) and are worth researching further. Someday these differences may help to better identify children early in the developmental trajectory of their disorder and suggest effective treatment interventions.

Other Evaluation Procedures

When the diagnosis is in question, other specialty evaluations can be very helpful in determining the most productive focus for intervention. The structured and semistructured interviews described in Chapter 3 can provide a systematic review of symptomatology and course of the disorder. The neuropsychologic testing suggested in Chapter 3 can be useful in determining specific areas of impairment. Speech and language evaluations can identify the nature of the impairment associated with communication difficulties and suggest specific interventions. Other specialty evaluations are described in this book and are valuable especially when symptoms other than those of ASD are present, when the diagnosis is in question, or when a patient is not responding to interventions.

Psychopharmacology

There have been few controlled clinical trials of psychopharmacologic agents in the treatment of children with ASD. In current clinical practice, the medications believed to provide the greatest benefit in reducing core and associated autistic symptomatology are selective serotonin reuptake inhibitors (SSRIs) and atypical antipsychotics (Buitelaar and Willemsen-Swinkels 2000; Posey and McDougle 2000; Scahill and Koenig 1999; Volkmar 2001). Within these two classes of medications, however, only the atypical antipsychotic agent risperidone has been proven efficacious in a controlled clinical trial in children with autism (Research Units on Pediatric Psychopharmacology Autism Network 2002). Current pharmacotherapy for children with ASD often includes extended treatment with a single agent or a combination of agents, but there are few data on the long-term safety and efficacy of such interventions. Here we provide some suggestions for the psychiatrist engaged in pharmacologic management of ASD, but the reader is referred to Chapter 7 for a review of the empirical literature and a more complete discussion of practical guidelines for selecting and combining agents.

In the assessment for pharmacologic intervention, symptoms should be carefully characterized over time. Those of particular relevance to psychopharmacologic treatment include inattention and distractibility; impulsivity; affect expression and regulation; anxiety; aggression; thought disorganization; and language, cognitive, and social skills. Once the family and physician have agreed to use a pharmacologic intervention to treat the child's disorder, the target symptoms should be reviewed and the medication options to treat these symptoms described. The prioritized problem list should be matched with appropriate interventions based on evidence from the scientific literature regarding the potential of the medication to benefit the target symptoms and its side effects. For instance, distractible inattention is more highly associated with a good response to stimulant medication, whereas difficulty shifting attention is more likely to respond to an SSRI. The experience of the child or family members with other medication treatments, ease of administration, and length of time for treatment response should also be considered in the selection of agents. Medication management provides the opportunity to develop a relationship with the child and the family. Asking about medication benefits and side effects in the context of school and home life provides the family an opportunity to talk about how the disorder and the medication are affecting their lives. We turn to this aspect of the psychiatrist's role in the final section of this chapter.

Working With the Family

The psychiatrist can play an important role for the family in helping them process the implications of the diagnosis and their feelings associated with it, consider treatment alternatives, manage difficult behavior, and remain engaged in treatment.

The Initial Meeting

Several models exist for the initial meeting with the family. Some prefer the child guidance model of first meeting with the parents without the child, discussing the concerns they have, and later seeing the child alone. Another model is to meet with the parents and the child together to see how the family defines the problem with the child present, watch the child play, and observe the parent–child interaction. Unless the child is very active and impulsive, I prefer the latter model, as it helps me feel what it is like to be in the family and to see the child in a more "natural" setting. One can get a sense of the child's inner world, see the nature of the child's attention and impulse control, and observe how the child regulates his or her mood.

Medical Aspects of ASD

Children with ASD may have a number of medically complex associated conditions. The referring physician may have little expertise in neurodevelopmental disorders. Given the training and expertise of child psychiatrists in this area, it is crucial that they work with primary care doctors to ensure that medical aspects of ASD receive appropriate attention. These issues are thoroughly discussed in later chapters of this book (particularly Chapters 4, 5, and 8) and are not reiterated here. The important point is that one role of the psychiatrist is to examine and address medical issues associated with autism.

Processing the Diagnosis and Considering Treatment Alternatives

The meaning of an ASD diagnosis to the child and family should be considered. Denial and confusion about the illness may not be expressed directly.

Each parent may process the information differently. Parents need assistance in finding resources and becoming effective advocates. Pointing them to the parent information and advocacy groups described in the Appendix of this book can make a huge difference in how they and their children cope with ASD.

The treatment plan should be multimodal, targeting all impairing symptoms and including psychosocial, psychoeducational, and other allied health interventions, as well as consideration of medication. Treatment alternatives should be described and the advantages and disadvantages of each discussed. Families should be informed of additional interventions such as speech and language therapy, occupational therapy, and behavioral interventions and given referrals to regional providers. In considering medications with families, education efforts should include

- Why medications are being suggested
- Changes they are hoped to achieve and how quickly
- Common and rare potential side effects and when they might emerge
- Activities, foods, drinks, and other medications that are contraindicated or require caution
- Recommended parental response to potential side effects
- Duration of treatment

Compliance With Treatment

Noncompliance with medication treatment can be the result of multiple factors in children and adolescents and occurs more frequently than physicians recognize. A recent study found that only 38% of adolescent psychiatric patients were compliant with medication treatment 14 months after inpatient hospitalization (Lloyd et al. 1998) despite a relatively low level (23%) of side effects. Potential reasons for noncompliance include resistance to taking medication in either the child, the parent, or both; incomplete or poorly understood directions for taking the medication; and poor organization of medication administration. It is crucial that these reasons be evaluated and that the psychiatrist help the family overcome the barriers to using helpful medications. Behavioral interventions with the child and family may be useful in obtaining medication compliance.

Therapeutic Alliance

The initial assessment begins to establish the therapeutic alliance between the physician and the family. A working partnership with the parents and the youngster is essential for comprehensive treatment and compliance.

The physician should be a collaborator with the child and family to empower them to effect improvements in their lives. Active participation and collaboration from parents and the child to identify target symptoms and select the medication improves the therapeutic alliance. Respect for the child's autonomy and control over his or her mind and body also improves the treatment alliance.

Conclusion

The psychiatrist member of the evaluation and treatment team for a child with ASD can

- Help identify alternative psychiatric diagnoses and comorbid diagnoses that may be the focus of successful treatment
- Examine and address medical issues of autism
- Suggest and implement pharmacologic strategies when initial efforts have not been successful
- Suggest psychological interventions that may help control behavior and lead to more successful socialization
- Work in concert with other professionals and take active responsibility for encouraging the team process

Psychiatrists are often particularly experienced in working with complex family situations and interdisciplinary teams and can help coordinate successful treatments. In the near future, research on neurodevelopmental processes, using neuroimaging and molecular genetics, will enable psychiatrists and other health care professionals to better diagnose children's disorders early in their trajectory, leading to earlier intervention and effective treatment matching.

References

Abell F, Krams M, Ashburner J, et al: The neuroanatomy of autism: a voxel-based whole brain analysis of structural scans. Neuroreport 10:1647–1651, 1999

American Psychiatric Association: Diagnostic and Statistical Manual of Mental Disorders, 4th Edition, Text Revision. Washington, DC, American Psychiatric Association, 2000

Baron-Cohen S, Mortimore C, Moriarty J, et al: The prevalence of Gilles de la Tourette's syndrome in children and adolescents with autism. J Child Psychol Psychiatry 40:213–218, 1999

Bolton PF, Pickles A, Murphy M, et al: Autism, affective and other psychiatric disorders: patterns of familial aggregation. Psychol Med 28:385–395, 1998

Bristol-Power M, Spinella G: Research on screening and diagnosis in autism: a work in progress. J Autism Dev Disord 29:435–438, 1999

Buchsbaum M, Hollander E, Haznedar M, et al: Effect of fluoxetine on regional cerebral metabolism in autistic spectrum disorders: a pilot study. Int J Neuropsychopharmacol 4:119–125, 2001

Buitelaar J, Willemsen-Swinkels S: Medication treatment in subjects with autistic spectrum disorders. Eur Child Adolesc Psychiatry 9 (suppl 1):I85–I97, 2000

Casey B, Giedd J, Thomas K: Structural and functional brain development and its relation to cognitive development. Biol Psychiatry 54:241–257, 2000

Chakrabarti S, Fombonne E: Pervasive developmental disorders in preschool children. JAMA 285:3093–3099, 2001

Chilakamarri J, Patzer D, Scahill L, et al: Prevalence of bipolar disorders in pervasive developmental disorder population. Paper presented at the annual meeting of the American Academy of Child and Adolescent Psychiatry, Honolulu, HI, 2001

Ciesielski K, Harris R, Hart B, et al: Cerebellar hypoplasia and frontal lobe cognitive deficits in disorders of early childhood. Neuropsychologia 35:643–655, 1997

Cody H, Pelphrey K, Piven J: Structural and functional magnetic resonance imaging of autism. Int J Dev Neurosci 20:421–438, 2002

Cohen DJ, Paul R, Volkmar FR: Issues in the classification of pervasive developmental disorders: toward DSM-IV. J Am Acad Child Adolesc Psychiatry 25:213–229, 1986

Courchesne E: Brainstem, cerebellar and limbic neuroanatomical abnormalities in autism. Curr Opin Neurobiol 7:269–278, 1997

Dahl EK, Cohen DJ, Provence S: Clinical and multivariate approaches to the nosology of pervasive developmental disorders. J Am Acad Child Adolesc Psychiatry 25:170–180, 1986

Deb S, Thompson B: Neuroimaging in autism. Br J Psychiatry 173:299–302, 1998

DeLong GR, Dwyer JT: Correlation of family history with specific autistic subgroups: Asperger's syndrome and bipolar affective disease. J Autism Dev Disord 18:593–600, 1988

DeLong R: Children with autistic spectrum disorder and a family history of affective disorder. Dev Med Child Neurol 36:674–688, 1994

Erlenmeyer-Kimling L, Rock D, Roberts SA, et al: Attention, memory and motor skills as childhood predictors of schizophrenia-related psychosis: the New York High-Risk Project. Am J Psychiatry 157:1416–1422, 2000

Filipek P, Richelme C, Kennedy D: Morphometric analysis of the brain in developmental language disorders and autism (abstract). Ann Neurol 32:475, 1992

Filippi C, Ulug A, Deck M, et al: Developmental delay in children: assessment with proton MR spectroscopy. Am J Neuroradiol 23:882–888, 2002

Fitzgerald K, Moore G, Paulson L, et al: Proton spectroscopic imaging of the thalamus in treatment-naive pediatric obsessive-compulsive disorder. Biol Psychiatry 47:174–182, 2000

Frazier J, Doyle R, Chiu S, et al: Treating a child with Asperger's disorder and co-morbid bipolar disorder. Am J Psychiatry 159:13–21, 2002

Ghaziuddin M, Tsai L: Depression in autistic disorder. Br J Psychiatry 159:721–723, 1991

Ghaziuddin M, Tsai L, Ghaziuddin N: Brief report: violence in Asperger syndrome, a critique. J Autism Dev Disord 21:349–354, 1991

Ghaziuddin M, Weidmer-Mikhail E, Ghaziuddin N: Comorbidity of Asperger syndrome: a preliminary report. J Intellect Disabil Res 42:279–283, 1998

Gillberg C: Autistic children growing up: problems during puberty and adolescence. Dev Med Child Neurol 26:122–129, 1984

Gillberg C, Billstedt E: Autism and Asperger syndrome: coexistence with other clinical disorder. Acta Neurol Scand 102:321–330, 2000

Gillott A, Furniss F, Walter A: Anxiety in high-functioning children with autism. Autism 5:277–286, 2001

Goldstein G, Minshew NJ, Allan DN, et al: High-functioning autism and schizophrenia: a comparison of an early and late onset neurodevelopmental disorder. Arch Clin Neuropsychol 17:461–475, 2002

Green M, Satz P, Christenson C: Minor physical anomalies in schizophrenia patients. Schizophr Bull 20:433–440, 1994

Hendren R, Hodde-Vargas J, Yeo R, et al: Neuropsychophysiological study of children at risk for schizophrenia: a preliminary report. J Am Acad Child Adolesc Psychiatry 34:1284–1291, 1995

Hendren R, DeBacker I, Pandina G: Review of neuroimaging studies of child and adolescent psychiatric disorders from the past 10 years. J Am Acad Child Adolesc Psychiatry 39:815–828, 2000

Howard M, Cowell P, Boucher J, et al: Convergent neuroanatomical and behavioral evidence of an amygdala hypothesis of autism. Neuroreport 11:2931–2935, 2000

Howlin P: Autism: Preparing for Adulthood. London, Routledge, 1997

Kim JA, Szatmari P, Bryson SE, et al: The prevalence of anxiety and mood problems among children with autism and Asperger syndrome. Autism 4:117–132, 2000

Kohn Y, Fahum T, Ratzoni G, et al: Aggression and sexual offense in Asperger's syndrome. Isr J Psychiatry Relat Sci 35:293–299, 1998

Kumra S, Jacobsen L, Lenane M, et al: Multidimensionally impaired disorder: is it a variant of very early onset schizophrenia? J Am Acad Child Adolesc Psychiatry 37:91–99, 1998

Lainhart J: Psychiatric problems in individuals with autism, their parents and siblings. Int Rev Psychiatry 11:278–298, 1999

Lainhart JE, Folstein SE: Affective disorders in people with autism: a review of published cases. J Autism Dev Disord 24:587–601, 1994

Lloyd A, Horan W, Borgaro S, et al: Predictors of medication compliance after hospital discharge in adolescent psychiatric patients. J Child Adolesc Psychopharmacol 8:133–141, 1998

Miles J, Hadden L, Takahashi T, et al: Head circumference is an independent clinical finding associated with autism. Am J Med Genet 95:339–350, 2000

Muris P, Steerneman P, Merckelbach H, et al: Comorbid anxiety symptoms in children with pervasive developmental disorders. J Anxiety Disord 12:387–393, 1998

Pantelis C, Velakoulis D, McGorry PD, et al: Neuroanatomical abnormalities before and after onset of psychosis: a cross-sectional and longitudinal MRI comparison. Lancet 361:281–288, 2003

Perry D, Marston G, Hinder S, et al: The phenomenology of depressive illness in people with learning disability and autism. Autism 5:265–275, 2001

Pine D, Wasserman G, Fried J, et al: Neurological soft signs: one-year stability and relationship to psychiatric symptoms in boys. J Am Acad Child Adolesc Psychiatry 36:1579–1586, 1997

Piven J, Palmer P: Psychiatric disorder and the broad autism phenotype: evidence from a family study of multiple-incidence autism families. Am J Psychiatry 156:557–563, 1999

Piven J, Chase G, Landa R, et al: Psychiatric disorders in the parents of autistic individuals. J Am Acad Child Adolesc Psychiatry 30:471–478, 1991

Piven J, Arndt S, Bailey J, et al: An MRI study of brain size in autism. Am J Psychiatry 152:1145–1149, 1995

Piven J, Arndt S, Bailey J, et al: Regional brain enlargement in autism: a magnetic resonance imaging study. J Am Acad Child Adolesc Psychiatry 35:530–536, 1996

Posey D, McDougle C: The pharmacotherapy of target symptoms associated with autistic disorder and other pervasive developmental disorders. Harv Rev Psychiatry 8:45–63, 2000

Rapin I: Neurological examination, in Preschool Children With Inadequate Communication. Edited by Rapin I. London, Mac Keith Press, 1996

Research Units on Pediatric Psychopharmacology Autism Network: Risperidone in children with autism and serious behavioral problems. N Engl J Med 347:314–321, 2002

Scahill L, Koenig K: Pharmacotherapy in children and adolescents with pervasive developmental disorders. J Child Adolesc Psychiatr Nurs 12:41–43, 1999

Schultz RT, Gauthier I, Klin A, et al: Abnormal ventral temporal cortical activity during face discrimination among individuals with autism and Asperger syndrome. Arch Gen Psychiatry 57:331–340, 2000

Smalley SL, McCracken J, Tanguay P: Autism, affective disorders, and social phobia. Am J Med Genet 60:19–26, 1995

Sparks B, Friedman S, Shaw D, et al: Brain structural abnormalities in young children with autism spectrum disorder. Neurology 59:184–192, 2002

Steingard R, Biederman J: Lithium responsive manic-like symptoms in two individuals with autism and mental retardation. J Am Acad Child Adolesc Psychiatry 26:932–935, 1987

Stern JS, Robertson MM: Tics associated with autistic and pervasive developmental disorders. Neurol Clin 15:345–355, 1997

Sweeten T, Posey D, Shekhar A, et al: The amygdala and related structures in the pathophysiology of autism. Pharmacol Biochem Behav 71:449–455, 2002

Szatmari P, Bryson SE, Streiner DL, et al: Two-year outcome of preschool children with autism or Asperger's syndrome. Am J Psychiatry 157:1980–1987, 2000

Szatmari P, Merette C, Bryson S, et al: Quantifying dimensions in autism: a factor-analytic study. J Am Acad Child Adolesc Psychiatry 41:467–474, 2002

Tanguay PE: Pervasive developmental disorders: a 10-year review. J Am Acad Child Adolesc Psychiatry 39:1079–1095, 2000

Tantum D: Asperger syndrome in adulthood, in Autism and Asperger Syndrome. Edited by Frith U. Cambridge, UK, Cambridge University Press, 1991, pp 147–183

Towbin K: Pervasive developmental disorder not otherwise specified, in Handbook of Autism and Pervasive Developmental Disorders, 2nd Edition. Edited by Cohen D, Volkmar F. New York, Wiley, 1997, pp 123–147

Towbin KE, Dykens ED, Pearson GS, et al: Conceptualizing "borderline syndrome of childhood" and "childhood schizophrenia" as developmental disorders. J Am Acad Child Adolesc Psychiatry 32:775–782, 1993

Tsai L: Comorbid psychiatric disorders of autistic disorder. J Autism Dev Disord 26:159–163, 1996

Volkmar F: Pharmacological interventions in autism: theoretical and practical issues. J Clin Child Psychol 30:80–87, 2001

Volkmar F, Cook E, Pomeroy J, et al: Summary of the practice parameters for the assessment and treatment of children, adolescents, and adults with autism and other pervasive developmental disorders. J Am Acad Child Adolesc Psychiatry 38:1611–1615, 1999

Weinberger DR: Implications of normal brain development for the pathogenesis of schizophrenia. Arch Gen Psychiatry 44:660–669, 1987

Wozniak J, Biederman J, Faraone SV, et al: Mania in children with pervasive developmental disorder revisited. J Am Acad Child Adolesc Psychiatry 36:1552–1559, 1997

Chapter 3

Contributions of Psychology

Beth L. Goodlin-Jones, Ph.D.
Marjorie Solomon, Ph.D.

Introduction

Psychologists can play an important role in many aspects of caring for children with autism spectrum disorders (ASD). Psychologists, working in partnership with physicians, speech and language pathologists, and occupational therapists, can lead or contribute to multidisciplinary diagnostic teams in clinical settings. Psychologists are skilled in diagnostic practices and assessment of cognitive and behavioral function. After the evaluation is complete, they often play important roles in treatment and case management, making referrals to community resources, setting up interventions in schools and homes, and providing various therapies for both children and families.

This chapter focuses on the psychologist's role in the evaluation process, and Chapter 6 summarizes treatments that psychologists (and other professionals) may provide. This chapter provides a synopsis of important issues in the assessment of ASD, highlighting many of the tools and measures used by psychologists and outlining best practices in the psychological evaluation of individuals with ASD. The chapter begins with an overview of the assessment process. It then describes measures used to diagnose autism, evaluate intellectual and adaptive function, and identify neuropsychologic strengths and weaknesses. The chapter ends with a discussion of ways that psychologists can assist in the evaluation of comorbid psychiatric illness.

Important Considerations in the Assessment Process

The psychological evaluation of a child includes assessment of

- Level of intellectual ability
- Problem-solving and learning style
- Neuropsychologic strengths and weaknesses (e.g., memory skills, communication, executive functions)
- Adaptive functioning
- Family systems and needs
- Social, communication, and behavioral problems

Specific practice parameters for the assessment of ASD recently have been published by the American Academy of Neurology (Filipek et al. 2000), the American Academy of Child and Adolescent Psychiatry (Volkmar et al. 1999), and a consensus panel with representation from multiple professional societies (Filipek et al. 1999). These practice parameters describe two levels of screening/evaluation. Level 1 screening involves routine developmental surveillance by all providers of services for young children. Level 2 evaluation involves a comprehensive diagnostic assessment by experienced clinicians for children who fail the initial screening (Filipek et al. 1999, 2000; Volkmar et al. 1999). These publications are significant milestones in the field of autism and are written for both the physician and psychologist as clinician. The components of these diagnostic steps that involve psychologists will be described later.

The first step of the assessment process is to review with parents the child's neonatal and early developmental history. The critical aspects of this history taking are described in Chapter 4. After this review, the psychologist begins to evaluate the child's behavioral capacities and social interactions. Specific diagnostic measures for ASD are obtained with the parent by means of an interview or questionnaire format. An assessment of the child's cognitive ability, learning style, and adaptive behavior skills typically follows. Evaluation of language ability may be conducted by the psychologist or by a speech-language pathologist. Occasionally, a neuropsychologic battery may be employed for determining specific strengths and weaknesses. Psychiatric status may be assessed when indicated, since psychiatric comorbidities often play a significant role in the effectiveness of intervention and in the child's adaptation to daily challenges. Finally, defining the social network of the child—family, school, and community characteristics that might interact with symptoms—should be included in the assessment.

There are several important considerations that should inform the assessment process. First, an interactionist-developmental perspective that explores both delays and deviance in the child should be maintained in the evaluation. Autism is a lifelong disorder, defined at all stages by the individual's interactive difficulties. It initially is diagnosed in early childhood and continues to be apparent throughout a person's life. It is characterized by unevennesses in development that vary over the lifespan of the individual. Studying a child within an interactionist-developmental framework provides a benchmark for understanding the severity or quality of delays or deviance. Delays in one developmental aspect can significantly affect the achievement of later developmental milestones, such as when early levels of joint attention predict later language acquisition (Mundy et al. 1990) and play abilities (Charman 1997). Autism symptoms frequently peak in severity between the ages of 4 and 5 years. Children who have very poor eye contact and make few social initiations at this age may have quite different social symptoms when they become teenagers. They may be relatively interested in social engagement by this later stage and may have acquired some more advanced social skills. Their social difficulties may then be manifest as awkwardness or inappropriateness rather than the lack of interest seen in young childhood. There are also characteristic patterns of delays in ASD that differ across domain and developmental level. For example, a child with autism may have meaningful expressive language, a large vocabulary, and adequate syntactic abilities, but not be able to participate in a conversation or even adequately answer questions. A final consideration is that experiences affect outcome. This is what makes determining a prognosis from early symptoms so difficult. Understanding symptom presentation requires an understanding of the child's social experiences to date.

A second important consideration is that the evaluation of a child with ASD must include information from multiple sources and environmental contexts. Measures of parent report, teacher report, child observation across settings, cognitive and adaptive behavior assessments, and clinical judgments all should be employed to provide a balanced and comprehensive picture (Filipek et al. 1999). This is vital because children with ASD may exhibit different symptoms depending on the characteristics of the environment. For example, high-functioning ASD children may present as charming, precocious, and highly intelligent when provided with one-on-one attention and conversational scaffolding from a well-meaning adult professional. The same child may appear much more symptomatic with peers on a playground or in a distracting classroom situation where individual adult attention is unavailable. Conversely, children with severe learning and behavioral deficits may seem much more competent in a known environment, such as the classroom, than in an evaluation room without familiar, well-practiced routines.

Third, it is recommended that assessments of ASD include participation of professionals from different disciplines, including psychology, psychiatry, pediatrics, neurology, speech and language therapy, and occupational therapy whenever possible. Each specialty has a unique perspective that focuses on different symptoms. Multidisciplinary assessment may generate a richer selection of potential treatment options. For example, to manage distractibility in a child, a psychiatrist may recommend stimulant medication, a psychologist may recommend cognitive-behavioral techniques to encourage the development of metacognition, and an occupational therapist may suggest environmental modifications designed to enhance attention and decrease distractions.

Finally, the psychologist may act as the evaluation and treatment coordinator. In this role, the psychologist communicates with parents and referring professionals before the evaluation to understand the referral questions, organizes appropriate team members, plans the components of the assessment, and establishes contact with the service providers in the community who will implement the recommendations from the evaluation. This type of coordination is critical to the successful outcome of an evaluation. Without this direct gathering and conveyance of pertinent information, the results of the evaluation are less likely to answer the referral questions and influence the child's progress. Direct contact with the professionals implementing the recommendations provides important assistance to parents as they integrate technical information derived from evaluations to improve the health and education of their child.

Autism Diagnostic Measurement

Several diagnostic measures, both labor-intensive "gold standards" and brief screening instruments, are reviewed in this section. All professional practice parameters state the necessity of both observing the child and interviewing the parents about early development and specific symptoms of autism (Filipek et al. 1999, 2000; Volkmar et al. 1999), ideally using the types of standardized instruments reviewed here. In the relatively brief observation of the child done in most clinic settings the range of difficulties experienced by the child will likely not be evident, so parent report is required. Parents, however, do not have the professional expertise and experience to recognize all difficulties or interpret them, so observation and testing by informed practitioners in a controlled setting is also necessary. The information gained from these sources can then be integrated into a DSM-IV-TR (American Psychiatric Association 2000) diagnosis. Next we describe both parent report and observational tools for the diagnostic assessment of children with autism.

It is important to understand the impact of relatively new instruments for the assessment of ASD. Clinical impression, oral traditions, and clinical observations have dominated the assessment process of ASD until recently (Klinger and Renner 2000). In the past, use of standard criteria and recognition of symptoms differed across clinical settings. The particular details and emphasis of each tradition were not explicitly documented, and the interpretation of DSM-III-R (American Psychiatric Association 1987) and DSM-IV varied between university clinics, private practice settings, and research projects. The publication of two standardized assessment tools, the parent-interview Autism Diagnostic Interview–Revised (ADI-R; Lord et al. 1994) and the performance-based Autism Diagnostic Observation Schedule–Generic (ADOS-G; Lord et al. 2000), have eliminated many of these disparities and are currently considered the "gold standards" for diagnosis of ASD. Use of these and other tools described here has advanced scientific progress and improved the accuracy and reliability of diagnostic assessment (Filipek et al. 1999).

An additional significant and highly beneficial development in the evaluation of autism is the availability of instruments to assist in earlier recognition and identification of children with ASD. Consensus regarding the importance of early intervention for children with ASD is universal (Filipek et al. 1999, 2000; Volkmar et al. 1999). With this recognition has come the development of standardized screening instruments for infants and toddlers that assist in early identification, including the Screening Tool for Autism in Two-Year-Olds (STAT; Stone et al. 2000), the Pervasive Developmental Disorders Screening Test (PDDST; Siegel 1998), the Checklist for Autism in Toddlers (CHAT; Baron-Cohen et al. 1992, 1996), and the Modified Checklist for Autism in Toddlers (M-CHAT; Robins et al. 2001), each of which is described here. Research that retrospectively analyzes home videos suggests that impairments in social-communicative behaviors are present and measurable by 12 months of age (Baranek 1999; Osterling and Dawson 1994) and possibly as young as 8 to 10 months (Werner et al. 2000). In the future, it is possible that video-coding systems will become available to screen very young children, who can then be referred for diagnostic evaluations (Rogers 2001).

Autism Diagnostic Interview–Revised

The ADI-R (Lord et al. 1994) is a comprehensive parent interview that probes for symptoms of autism. It is administered by a trained clinician using a semistructured interview format. It is closely linked to the diagnostic criteria set forth in DSM-IV-TR and ICD-10 (World Health Organization 1993), and it has an algorithm and cutoff scores for the diagnosis of autistic disorder. There are no thresholds yet established for other autism spectrum disorders, such as Asperger syndrome or pervasive developmental disorder not otherwise specified (PDDNOS). The "research" or "long" version of the ADI-R requires approximately 3 hours to administer and score. A "short edition" of the ADI-R, which includes only the items on the diagnostic algorithm, may be used for clinical assessment and takes less time, approximately 90 to 120 minutes (Lord et al. 1994). The use of the ADI-R for research purposes requires attending a 3-day training seminar with a certified trainer and completion of reliability testing with the developers of the instrument. Training to use the ADI-R as a clinical tool is also available; it is helpful, but not required for routine use by practitioners who do not participate in research protocols. Training information is included in the Appendix at the end of this book.

The long (research) form of the ADI-R elicits information from the parent on over 100 questions regarding the child's current behavior and developmental history. The significant developmental time point on the ADI-R is age 4 to 5 years for most behaviors; research suggests that symptoms are often at their peak at this age, making it the most sensitive time period for identification. The items that empirically distinguish children with autism from those with other developmental delays are summed into three algorithm scores measuring social difficulties, communication deficits, and repetitive behaviors. Excellent psychometric properties are reported (Lord et al. 1997).

The ADI-R is an extremely helpful tool, but it does have some limitations. It is not sensitive to differences among children with mental ages below 20 months or IQ below 20 (Cox et al. 1999; Lord 1995) and is not advised for use with such children. It is not designed to assess change through repeated administrations and is best suited to confirm the initial clinical diagnosis of autism (Arnold et al. 2000). It is also less helpful for individuals who do not have an informant familiar with the child's early development available to interview. Research has demonstrated that the diagnostic judgment based on current behavior is similar to that based on historical data (Boelte and Poustka 2000; Lord et al. 1997). However, the current behavior of individuals who have improved substantially may not be judged as autistic by the ADI-R algorithm and would be missed if the historical information was not present (Boelte and Poustka 2000). This may also be the case for other diagnostic measures, and thus it is critical to have information about behavior during the preschool years available when possible.

Social Communication Questionnaire

The Social Communication Questionnaire (SCQ, formerly known as the Autism Screening Questionnaire or ASQ; Berument et al. 1999) is a parent report questionnaire based on the ADI-R. It contains the same questions included on the ADI-R algorithm, presented in a briefer, yes/no parent report format. It is thus an efficient way to obtain diagnostic information, but may be less sensitive than a detailed interview with the parent. There are two versions available—one for current behavior and one for lifetime behavior. The lifetime version is helpful for screening and diagnostic purposes, and the current version is more appropriate for assessment of change over time in an individual. A cutoff score of 15 differentiates ASD from other diagnoses for children age 4 and older, and a cutoff of 22 distinguishes children with autistic disorder from those with other autism spectrum disorders (e.g., PDDNOS or Asperger syndrome).

Autism Diagnostic Observation Schedule–Generic

The Autism Diagnostic Observation Schedule–Generic (ADOS-G; DiLavore et al. 1995; Lord et al. 2000) is a semistructured interactive assessment conducted with a child, teenager, or adult during an evaluation for ASD. There are four different modules, graded according to language and developmental level. Most diagnostic observation instruments are hampered by the short time period of assessment. One cannot always be sure that a behavior is deficient after only an hour of observation, but this is often all the time a professional has with a patient. The ADOS-G minimizes this problem by including multiple opportunities or "presses" for social interaction and communication. For example, a number of different activities and situations are set up that would, in a typical child, elicit eye contact or a question. Once several chances to display these typical social behaviors are missed, a clinician can be reasonably certain that the behavior in question is difficult for the child being assessed. For children with younger mental and chronological ages, items from modules 1 and 2 of the ADOS-G assess social interest, joint attention, communicative behaviors, symbolic play, and atypical behaviors (e.g., excessive sensory interest, hand mannerisms). For older and more capable individuals, modules 3 and 4 of the ADOS-G focus on conversational reciprocity, empathy, insight into social relationships, and special interests. The ADOS-G takes approximately 30–45 minutes to administer and provides two empirically defined cutoff scores, one for autistic disorder and the other for broader autism spectrum disorders (e.g., PDDNOS or Asperger syndrome). As with the ADI-R, use of the ADOS-G for research purposes requires attending a training workshop and establishing reliability with a certified trainer. There are shorter clinical trainings for clinicians not involved in research that are, like those for the ADI-R, very helpful but not required for routine clinical use of the instrument.

Diagnostic Interview of Social and Communication Disorders

A newly published instrument, the Diagnostic Interview of Social and Communication Disorders (DISCO; Wing et al. 2002), is an alternative to the ADI-R that takes a more dimensional approach to diagnosis. The DISCO is designed to cover a range of developmental domains (e.g., motor, language, self-care, imitation, communication) as well as behaviors with autistic features. The ADI-R was designed as a diagnostic instrument, whereas the DISCO is designed to compile developmental history on a wider range of typical and atypical behaviors. Its use for clinical research presently is expanding (Wing et al. 2002).

Childhood Autism Rating Scale

The Childhood Autism Rating Scale (CARS; Schopler et al. 1988) is a 15-item structured observation instrument that is appropriate for children over 24 months of age. Items focus on the three core features of autism and are scored on a 7-point scale (from typical to severely deviant). The items are summed into one score and compared to a scale that distinguishes typical behavior from mild to moderate/severe autistic behavior. Although it is sometimes used as a parent report instrument (e.g., questionnaire or interview), it was developed as a tool to rate behavior observed during developmental evaluation. The CARS requires approximately 30 minutes to administer.

Screening Tool for Autism in 2-Year-Olds

The STAT is an interactive measure for children between ages 24 and 35 months (Stone et al. 2000). Similar in purpose and scope to the ADOS module 1 but briefer to administer, the STAT requires a 20-minute play session in which several different activities are presented to the child. The child's symbolic play, reciprocal social behavior, joint attention, motor imitation, and communication are assessed. The STAT provides mean scores that differentiate autism from other developmental delays in 2-year-olds.

Pervasive Developmental Disorders Screening Test

The PDDST (Siegel 1998) is a parent questionnaire for children up to 36 months of age. There are three stages of the PDDST: stage 1 is designed for use in the primary care clinic, stage 2 is for more specialized developmental disorders clinics, and stage 3 is for specialty ASD clinics. Items cover positive symptoms, negative symptoms, general development, and regression. The PDDST provides cutoff scores and an algorithm to differentiate autism from general developmental delay, but it has not yet been published or peer reviewed. Information about how to obtain the PDDST is included in the Appendix.

Checklist for Autism in Toddlers

The CHAT is a screening instrument developed for use in primary care settings (Baron-Cohen et al. 1992, 1996, 2000). There are two sections; the first section is an interview including nine questions for the parent, and the second section contains five items to be administered to the child. The CHAT requires little training to administer. It was designed for use at well-child pediatric visits. The original study was done at the 18-month visit, but a recent paper showed that the CHAT continued to distinguish those at risk from autism from those with other developmental delays at age 2 (Scambler et al. 2001). It was developed to identify children who meet full criteria for autism and does not appear to be sensitive to the broader spectrum of ASD (Baron-Cohen et al. 1996). The high false-negative rate of the CHAT makes it most appropriate for initial screening purposes, and it should not be used for diagnosis. Another version of the CHAT, called the Q-CHAT (Q for *quantitative*), currently is under development to increase the CHAT's sensitivity and specificity for screening purposes (Charman 2002).

Another modification of the CHAT, the M-CHAT, expands the number of items to 23 for the parent to complete and eliminates the portion administered to the child (Robins et al. 2001). It is a simple screening test designed to be given to all parents during the 24-month well-child pediatric visit. There are 6 critical items on the M-CHAT, and any child who fails 2 or more receives a follow-up phone call and possible referral for an evaluation. The sensitivity (0.87) and specificity (0.99) of the M-CHAT were quite impressive in a large screening study involving 1,293 toddlers. The tool identified 58 children at risk of autism, all of whom were found to have developmental disorders upon further evaluation and 39 of whom had autism.

Asperger Syndrome Screening Tools

Several parent report measures that provide information about the Asperger syndrome diagnosis have been developed recently. The Autism Spectrum Screening Questionnaire (ASSQ; Ehlers et al. 1999) is a 27-item checklist standardized for completion by lay informants. It assesses symptoms of both Asperger syndrome and high-functioning autism and does not purport to provide a differential diagnosis between the two. The ASSQ has high internal consistency and good validity (Ehlers and Gillberg 1993). The Gilliam Asperger Disorder Scale (GADS; Gilliam 2001) is based on DSM-IV criteria for Asperger syndrome. It was standardized on a multicultural sample of 371 subjects. The GADS has subscales for social interaction, restricted patterns of behavior, cognitive patterns, pragmatic skills, and early development. It also provides an overall quotient. There are no published psychometric studies of the GADS. The Asperger Syndrome Diagnostic Scale (ASDS; Myles et al. 2001) is appropriate for children and adolescents age 5 through 18. Items are based on DSM-IV (American Psychiatric Association 1994) and ICD-10 criteria, as well as the research literature on Asperger syndrome. It has five subscales—language, social behavior, maladaptive behavior, cognitive characteristics, and sensorimotor behaviors—as well as an overall quotient. There are no published studies of the ASDS's psychometric qualities.

Unfortunately, none of the tools currently available provides an adequate differential diagnosis between Asperger syndrome and other high-functioning autism spectrum disorders (e.g., high-functioning autism or PDDNOS). Most were not standardized on well-characterized groups of subjects with confirmed diagnoses of Asperger syndrome, and none can reliably rule out other ASD diagnoses. Although all three scales are based on DSM-IV characteristics, all include other symptoms that are not part of the diagnostic criteria and are controversial aspects of the phenotype (e.g., clumsiness). Thus, these measures may have some utility for broadly identifying any high-functioning autism spectrum disorder but should not be used for differential diagnosis of Asperger syndrome and high-functioning autism.

Intellectual Assessment

A second important domain assessed by the psychologist is intellectual function. Intellectual assessment helps frame the interpretation of many observations about the child. Level of intellectual functioning is associated with severity of symptoms, ability to acquire skills, level of adaptive functioning, and outcome (Filipek et al. 1999). Major goals of intellectual assessment include generating a profile of the child's cognitive strengths and weaknesses, facilitating educational planning, suggesting prognosis, and determining eligibility for certain IQ-related services.

Intellectual assessment may have been completed prior to the clinic visit. For example, schools are required to conduct cognitive and academic test batteries as part of their determination of eligibility for special education. It is important to ask parents for the results of any previous cognitive assessments. If testing was completed within the past year or two, the report appears congruent with the child's presentation, there are no concerns about its validity or reliability, and there have been no significant medical events or changes in health status, then there is typically no reason to repeat it.

There are numerous published intellectual test batteries available for use in evaluating a child with ASD. The child with suspected ASD often presents an assessment challenge due to social difficulties, unusual use of language, frequent off-task behaviors, high distractibility, and variable motivation (Ozonoff et al. 2002a). Motivation can have a tremendous influence on test results, and assessment procedures that incorporate motivational variables can result in very different test scores (Koegel et al. 1997). It is the psychologist's responsibility to 1) enhance motivation as much as possible without altering the standard administration of the instrument and 2) consider the motivational element when interpreting scores. Furthermore, a child's level of anxiety may impede his or her ability to attend and respond to performance-based measures. Obviously, the testing environment and the particular test battery used must minimize any difficulties for the child while ensuring that the validity of the battery is maintained. More frequent reinforcement breaks may be needed, and testing may need to be conducted over multiple, shorter sessions. When experienced psychologists evaluate young children with autism, few should be "untestable." Untestability reflects primarily a lack of availability of appropriate test instruments.

Intelligence Tests for Children With Spoken Language

The Wechsler Intelligence Scales are the most widely used intellectual tests for people with ASD who have relatively good verbal language. There are three different age-graded Wechsler tests (see Table 3–1), as well as an abbreviated form that is suitable for a broad age range from childhood to adulthood. The Wechsler scales assess both verbal and nonverbal intelligence, yielding a verbal and a performance IQ score, as well as a full-scale IQ measure that is a composite of the two. Additional "factor scores" can be derived, representing freedom from distractibility, perceptual organization, verbal comprehension, and processing speed. The Wechsler tests rely heavily on language skills, have many timed items, and are lengthy (taking an hour or more to administer), so they are not usually appropriate for younger or more compromised children with ASD.

Individuals with ASD frequently exhibit uneven subtest score profiles on Wechsler tests (Lincoln et al. 1995; Ozonoff 1995), complicating the interpretation of test results. Performance IQ (PIQ) may be higher than verbal IQ (VIQ) (Lincoln et al. 1995), which is generally interpreted to mean that visuospatial skills are stronger than verbal abilities. However, the verbal-performance discrepancy is severity dependent, and the majority of individuals with ASD do not show a significant split (>12 points) (Siegel et al. 1996). When present, a PIQ > VIQ pattern can have important implications for how the child learns best and what activities may be most and least enjoyable. For example, we have worked with a 10-year-old boy with high-functioning autism (VIQ = 60, PIQ = 118) who was extremely interested in Disney characters and videos (both very visual in nature) and was very good at drawing. Interestingly, he was also surprisingly adept at interpreting facial expressions and social situations in video clips, possibly due to his very good visual skills. This boy learned best when visual cues were used to supplement verbal instruction. He benefited from social skills training that incorporated video modeling, a visual approach described in Chapter 6. This boy was handsome and well coordinated, and appeared to others to be typically developing, leading many to assume that he understood far more language than he actually did. This was frustrating for him, and he frequently withdrew from social situations or became irritable and uncooperative when the verbal content of interactions was too high.

Children with Asperger syndrome may exhibit the opposite intellectual test profile, with VIQ significantly higher than PIQ (Klin et al. 1995), but this is by no means universal and has not been replicated in

Table 3–1. Wechsler Intelligence Scales

Wechsler Preschool and Primary Scale of Intelligence–Revised (WPPSI-R; Wechsler 1989) for ages 3 to 7 years

Wechsler Intelligence Scale for Children–Third Edition (WISC-III; Wechsler 1991) for ages 6 to 16 years

Wechsler Adult Intelligence Scale–Third Edition (WAIS-III; Wechsler 1997) for ages 16 and up

Wechsler Abbreviated Scale of Intelligence (WASI; Wechsler 1999) for ages 6 to 89 years

all studies (see Ozonoff and Griffith 2000 for a review). Thus, intellectual test profiles should *never* be used for diagnostic confirmation or differential diagnosis of ASD subtypes (e.g., Asperger syndrome versus high-functioning autism). However, when a $VIQ > PIQ$ profile is evident, the child may benefit from verbal instruction (e.g., verbal explanations rather than visual supports) and may excel in subjects that require good verbal processing, such as foreign language classes. At the extreme, some children with ASD may exhibit the so-called nonverbal learning disability (NLD) profile (Myklebust 1975; Rourke 1995). Children with NLD have difficulties in tactile perception, psychomotor coordination, mathematic reasoning, visual-spatial organization, and nonverbal problem solving. They have well-developed rote verbal skills, as well as strong verbal memory and auditory linguistic capabilities. Some children with Asperger syndrome and high-functioning autism display an NLD profile. They may require additional interventions, such as occupational therapy and math tutoring. This is an academic diagnosis that does not take the place of the primary ASD diagnosis, which is a more complete description of the full range of the child's behavioral and developmental limitations.

The Stanford-Binet Intelligence Test–Fourth Edition (SB-IV; Thorndike et al. 1986) provides multiple IQ scores that measure verbal reasoning, abstract/visual reasoning, quantitative reasoning, and memory, as well as an overall composite. A newly revised fifth edition (Roid 2003) is now available. The fifth edition provides a wider variety of items requiring nonverbal responses, so it is better suited for children with communication disorders or limited English skills. Relative to the instruments discussed in the next section, however, it still makes significant demands on language and may not be appropriate for children with ASD who have significant limitations in using and understanding language.

Intellectual Assessment for Children With the Most Severe Communication Difficulties

There are special concerns about the validity of testing younger, lower-functioning, and nonverbal children, and care must be taken in choosing an appropriate test instrument. It is important that the test chosen 1) is appropriate for both the chronological *and* mental age of the child, 2) provides a full range (in the lower direction) of standard scores, and 3) measures verbal and nonverbal skills separately (Filipek et al. 1999). In this section we review several other intellectual tests available for children with more severe communication difficulties.

The Kaufman Assessment Battery for Children (K-ABC; Kaufman and Kaufman 1983) is very useful, with its wide age range (2 through 12 years) and reduced (but not absent) demands on verbal abilities. The K-ABC measures both sequential and simultaneous processing abilities, which can be useful in identifying a child's strengths and learning style. The Sequential Processing Scale includes problems that require arrangement of stimuli in sequential or serial order (e.g., hand movements, memory for number or word order), and the Simultaneous Processing Scale measures holistic or gestalt abilities (e.g., face recognition, figural closure). The K-ABC provides an overall General Cognitive Index that is similar (although not identical) to an IQ score. It also provides achievement (e.g., academic) tests that may be completed if that information is also needed. A nonverbal IQ score may be calculated separately, and appropriate norms are provided for interpretation; however, the K-ABC does require that the child understand some spoken language, and this may limit its usefulness for some children with ASD.

The Leiter International Performance Scales–Revised (Roid and Miller 1997), a purely nonverbal intelligence test, is a reasonable choice for assessing a child who has limited language ability or is nonverbal. The age range (2 to 21 years) is wide. Two batteries are available: the Visualization and Reasoning scale measures general nonverbal intelligence, and the Attention and Memory scales measure discrete neuropsychologic abilities. Tasks can be administered with no language; instructions and demonstrations are nonverbal (e.g., pantomime). There is no time limit on any item, which is useful for children who do not understand the demands of a timed administration. The Leiter instrument is not appropriate for children with mental age less than 2 years and who cannot perform visual matching tasks reliably. It does not provide any measure of verbal intellectual abilities.

The Differential Ability Scales (DAS; Elliott 1990) is a battery of cognitive and achievement (academic) tests that is growing in popularity given the very wide chronological and mental age range for which it is useful (2½ through 17 years). Both verbal and nonverbal intelligence are assessed.

Tasks vary in developmental range, beginning with those appropriate for preschoolers and continuing all the way up to items appropriate for typically developing adolescents. It is thus a very useful test for repeat administrations, to track progress, and for research projects, in which the developmental range of participants may vary considerably.

For younger children (below 5) or those with skills that fall below the entry levels of the tests just described, there are a few additional choices for assessment of intellectual functioning. Well-known instruments include the Bayley Scales of Infant Development–II (for ages 1 to 42 months; Bayley 1993) and the Mullen Scales of Early Learning (MSEL) (for ages 1 to 60 months; Mullen 1995). For children suspected of having ASD, the MSEL is often chosen over the Bayley because of its wider age range and five distinct scales (gross motor, visual reception, fine motor, receptive language, expressive language) that allow separate assessment of verbal and nonverbal abilities. The MSEL provides an age-normed T-score for each scale and an overall Early Learning Composite. The Bayley has a longer research tradition than the MSEL, but is difficult to administer and score (with a recommendation of 50 administrations with supervision prior to independent use). Additionally, it yields less-detailed information, with one score, the Performance Developmental Index (PDI), averaging infant memory, problem solving, communication, and mathematical abilities. The Motor Developmental Index (MDI) evaluates body control, muscle coordination, postural imitation, and praxis. These instruments provide both standard scores and developmental age equivalents. Thus, they can be used to evaluate children who are older than the test norms but whose developmental skills are not high enough for administration of more age-appropriate instruments.

Language Assessment

Although the participation of a speech-language pathologist on the team is very important in the evaluation of a child with ASD, the psychologist may need to administer a screening test to obtain an estimate of verbal expressive and receptive abilities. Expressive language level is a good predictor of long-term outcome, so it is an especially important characteristic to measure in terms of future prognosis (Stone and Yoder 2001). If a verbal child with ASD has already completed the verbal scales of an intelligence test, however, the tests described in this section may not provide further informative data, and a comprehensive evaluation by a speech-language pathologist will be more appropriate.

The Peabody Picture Vocabulary Test–Third Edition (PPVT-III; Dunn and Dunn 1997) provides a brief estimate of receptive language ability. Its administration requires that the child point to or touch a picture that matches a single word said aloud by the examiner. A parallel instrument for assessing expressive language is the Expressive One-Word Picture Vocabulary Test (Brownell 2000). These instruments may overestimate a child's language ability since there is no requirement for sentence production or comprehension or for single words to be used or understood in context. Other tests that evaluate expressive and receptive skills together and provide broader measures of language ability (e.g., formulating and comprehending sentences, following directions) include the Clinical Evaluation of Language Fundamentals–Third Edition (CELF-III; Semel et al. 1995) and the Preschool Language Scales–Third Edition (PLS-3; Zimmerman et al. 1991).

Children with ASD are typically limited in the use of language in a social context, even when receptive and expressive abilities are within normal limits (Wetherby and Prizant 1992). Pragmatic communication includes body language, turn taking, and understanding intention and interest of others. The structured tests just mentioned do not assess pragmatic communication, but there are other measures available to examine this important domain, including the Communication and Symbolic Behavior Scales (CSBS; Wetherby and Prizant 1993) and the Test of Language Competence (TLC; Wiig and Secord 1989). The TLC examines the ability to understand and interpret inferences and figurative expressions and to produce conversational sentences—all skills that research has shown are impaired in ASD (Ozonoff and Miller 1996).

Adaptive Behavior Assessment

The assessment of children's adaptive functioning examines their ability to take care of themselves and function independently in their day-to-day settings, including school and home. When measuring intelligence, it is also necessary to measure adaptive behavior. A diagnosis of mental retardation cannot be made unless functioning is compromised across both standardized tests of intelligence and real-life measures of adaptive function. Measuring adaptive behavior is also important for setting appropriate goals in treatment planning.

The most widely used measure of adaptive behavior is the Vineland Adaptive Behavior Scales (Sparrow et al. 1984). The domains of functioning include communication, daily living skills, socialization, and, for children under 5, motor skills. The Vineland is completed during an interview with a parent or teacher and is appropriate for children up to age 17 and mentally retarded adults (separate norms are provided for each population). Standard scores are summed across the domains to provide an overall Adaptive Behavior Composite. The Vineland provides sufficient detail for planning interventions. This instrument is currently undergoing restandardization and will include supplemental norms for children with ASD (S. Sparrow, personal communication, October 2002).

The Adaptive Behavior Assessment System (ABAS; Harrison and Oakland 2000) examines 10 different aspects of daily functioning. Two versions exist, one for report by either parents/caregivers or teachers on children ages 5 to 21, and the other for persons over 18 years of age who are able to understand the written questions and report on themselves. The ABAS provides four domain scores and an overall Adaptive Behavior Composite, similar to the Vineland. The Scales of Independent Behavior–Revised (SIB-R; Bruininks et al. 1996) is another useful instrument for measuring adaptive behavior. On all measures of adaptive behavior, the most common areas of deficit for children with ASD are socialization and communication.

Psychological Assessment of Individuals Without Receptive or Expressive Language

Some of the most difficult assessment challenges involve children and adults with autism who do not use or understand speech. Although there are some intellectual tests developed to assess cognition without the use of speech (cited previously), these instruments may require a level of comprehension that is beyond the ability of some persons with autism. Additionally, the testing situation requires a level of attention to another person and cooperation with adult requests that a young child with autism may not have experienced before. Poor test response may reflect age and lack of experience, rather than lack of the abilities that the task measures.

Intellectual assessment of very young children is usually a part of the initial diagnostic evaluation. While research has consistently documented that IQ at age 5 correlates with adult outcomes, we have no such information about test scores at age 2 or 3. In our experience, developmental quotients of very young children with autism, especially those who had normal early motor development (suggesting less neurodevelopmental dysfunction), are generally not predictive of response to treatment and potential for growth. That is, many children who do poorly on tests will still improve significantly with intervention.

For preverbal preschoolers, the MSEL, described earlier, provides a useful tool for assessment of developmental skills. However, the child may need to learn the test-taking format in order to give his or her best performance.

Pre-teaching of certain test-taking skills can dramatically improve motivation to attend to the adult and complete tasks, resulting in better test performance. The first lesson involves teaching children to sit in a chair at a table with an adult for 5 to 10 minutes at a stretch. Next, it is helpful to prepare children for the give-and-take of the testing situation. They can be taught to accept and trade toys and reinforcers and become familiar with the pattern of adult demonstration, child performance, adult removal of items, and reward. Once there is good cooperation in this kind of task, the child is ready for the actual test items. This preparation can be done in short bursts within the evaluation format, but it also may require several short sessions prior to testing. The value of preparing the child in this way comes in knowing that the test scores are valid indicators of current ability, rather than an index of the child's lack of experience with the test-taking format.

For older children and adults who have very severe cognitive delays, the usual purpose of the assessment is for planning educational or other intervention approaches. The psychologist needs to look broadly at functional skills, examining cognition, behavior, communication style, and recreational, community, domestic, and vocational skills. This provides a comprehensive look at a person's current abilities and needs for supports. In this kind of evaluation, the goal is to determine what supports the person needs for meaningful, enjoyable, inclusive activities and to identify the barriers that prevent the person from participation in all of life's basic activities. For this kind of assessment, a standardized tool may not be necessary; using real-life tasks and objects may allow a person to demonstrate more skills than a standardized test can. Using developmental knowledge of cognition, psychologists can probe understanding of the spatial and causal attributes of objects, relationships among objects, and object characteristics such as color, shape, number, category, and functional use. Tasks from standardized tools may also be helpful in eliciting samples of a person's behavior for programming purposes. The Adolescent and Adult Psychoeducational Profile (AAPEP; Mesibov et al. 1988) is an especially helpful tool that measures independent living, vocational, leisure, and functional communication skills. Adaptive behavior scales (reviewed earlier) are also helpful in assessing the ability of individuals with autism who have minimal language and severe cognitive limitations.

Neuropsychologic Assessment

The neuropsychology of ASD has been studied extensively. As a group, persons with ASD exhibit spared rote, mechanical, and visual-spatial processes and deficient higher-order conceptual processes, such as abstract reasoning (Minshew et al. 1997). They often perform acceptably on simple language, memory, and perspective-taking tasks but show deficits when tasks become more complex. Persons with ASD also have deficits in executive functions, particularly higher-order skills such as planning and shifting cognitive set (Ozonoff et al. 1991).

Data from neuropsychologic testing may be able to provide greater clarity about the individual's profile of strengths and weaknesses, an important foundation for treatment and educational planning (Ozonoff et al. 2002a). However, neuropsychologic testing is costly and time consuming. The decision to carry out neuropsychologic assessment and the choice of tests should be done thoughtfully, emphasizing domains with relevance for educational and treatment plans (Klin and Shepard 1994; Ozonoff et al. 2002a). Neuropsychologic assessment is not usually useful (or even possible) with nonverbal or mentally retarded children with ASD. It *may* be warranted for higher-functioning individuals when there are unexplained discrepancies or weaknesses in school performance, behavioral difficulties that appear to stem from undiagnosed learning disorders, and suspected organic problems. Although there are typical neuropsychologic profiles associated with ASD, they should never be used for diagnostic clarification or differential diagnosis. Two children referred for neuropsychologic assessment at the M.I.N.D. Institute Clinic illustrate the potential utility of this type of evaluation. The first child was a 10-year-old girl experiencing school failure and behavioral outbursts at school despite intellectual testing results in the low average range. The neuropsychologic assessment clarified that she had deceptively low receptive language ability and very poor attention, leading to frustration and anxiety when she was given instructions that she could not follow. In the second example, another child experiencing school underachievement, this time with superior intelligence, was found to have serious problems shifting cognitive set, inhibiting impulses, organizing, and planning. Several of the neuropsychologic domains that can provide helpful information are outlined next.

Attention

Attention is a multidimensional construct that encompasses several components, including focusing, sustaining, and shifting operations (Mirsky et al. 1991, 1999). Children with ASD do not usually have problems with sustained attention (Garretson et al. 1990). However, they do have problems with focusing attention, although their pattern is different than children with attention-deficit/hyperactivity disorder (ADHD). Those with ASD tend to "miss the forest for the trees" or overfocus attention on extraneous details while missing meaning (Fein et al. 1990); this difficulty has also been called impaired central coherence (Happe and Frith 1996). Children with ASD are more distracted by internal phenomena (e.g., special interests) than those with ADHD, whose attention is more typically diverted by external stimuli in the environment. Some children with ASD do exhibit classic ADHD symptoms of distractibility and hyperactivity (Ghaziuddin et al. 1992). For these children, a traditional ADHD workup is indicated and stimulant medications may be appropriate (see Chapter 7). Chapter 2 provides an overview of the important issues in the comorbid diagnosis of ADHD and ASD. Here we discuss particular test instruments that may be helpful in the evaluation.

Assessment of attention and activity level should examine the child's behavior across multiple contexts, including both school and home. Some of the most frequently used parent and teacher report questionnaires are the Conners Rating Scales (Conners 1996), the Achenbach Child Behavior Checklist (CBCL; Achenbach 1991), and the Behavior Assessment System for Children (BASC; Reynolds and Kamphaus 1998). It is also useful to obtain performance data about behaviors of interest. Continuous performance tests (CPTs) are administered by computer and measure sustained attention, vigilance, and response inhibition. Most CPTs measure performance under several different conditions, some requiring responses to one particular stimulus only (e.g., the letter X), others to combination stimuli (e.g., A-X), and still others to duplicate stimuli (e.g., X-X). The primary variables of interest are the accuracy and time taken to identify targets and the number of omission and commission errors.

Many different continuous performance tests are available; one of the most commonly used versions is published by Gordon (1983). The Integrated Visual Auditory Performance Test (IVA; Sandford and Turner 2000) is a unique CPT in that it measures impulsivity and inattention in both auditory and visual modalities. It is appropriate for ages 5 to 90 years. However, it is relatively lengthy and is not appropriate for younger and more severely impaired children. The Conners' Kiddie Continuous Performance Test (K-CPT; Conners 2001) is designed to screen for attention disorders in 4- and 5-year-old children. It is much shorter than the CPTs intended for older children (7.5 minutes vs. typical 13–15 minutes), and common objects, rather than letters and numbers, are presented as targets and distracters.

The Test of Everyday Attention for Children (TEA-Ch; Manly et al. 2001) is a comprehensive battery of tests of attention that may be more ecologically valid than CPTs. It includes nine subtests that are designed to be more interesting and relevant to real life than a CPT. For example, one of the subtests revolves around an imaginary scenario of a vacation trip to a large city, and others involve identification of spaceship targets and specific tones reminiscent of video games. The TEA-Ch has two parallel versions, allowing readministration without concern about practice effects. This can be helpful in measuring treatment outcome, for example, in medication trials. It is appropriate for clients age 6 to 16.

Executive Functions

One of the most consistently replicated cognitive deficits in individuals with ASD is executive dysfunction (Hughes et al. 1994; Ozonoff and Jensen 1999; Russell 1997). The executive function domain includes the many skills required to prepare for and execute complex behavior, including planning, inhibition, organization, self-monitoring, mental representation of tasks and goals, and cognitive flexibility and set shifting.

The Wisconsin Card Sorting Test (WCST; Heaton et al. 1993) is often considered the "gold standard" of executive function tests. It measures cognitive flexibility and set shifting. Subjects are asked to sort cards based on an undisclosed sorting rule (by either shape, color, or number). They are given feedback about whether they are sorting correctly or incorrectly. Once the individual has correctly completed 10 sorts, the rule is changed without any warning or comment, and the individual is expected to shift to a new sorting set. The most relevant score is the number of perseverative responses, defined as the number of sorts that use an old sorting rule despite feedback that it is incorrect. Norms are available for ages 6½ to 89. The WCST takes approximately 20 minutes to complete and can be challenging and frustrating for some children. It is available in both an examiner-administered and a computer version. Persons with ASD often perform better on the computer version of the test (Ozonoff 1995). If this executive function test is being given to document deficits for the purposes of treatment eligibility, it may therefore be best to use the examiner administration format. If, however, the examiner wants to evaluate achievement under supportive conditions, to see how well the child is potentially capable of performing, then the computer administration format may be preferable (Ozonoff et al., in press).

The Delis-Kaplan Executive Function System (D-KEFS; Delis et al. 2001) provides a battery of tests that assess cognitive flexibility, concept formation, planning, impulse control, and inhibition in children and adults. The D-KEFS was standardized on a sample of over 1,700 children and adults age 8 to 89. Most of its nine subtests are adaptations of traditional research measures of executive function that have been refined to examine skills more precisely, with fewer confounding variables. Subtests include Trail Making, Verbal

Fluency, Design Fluency, Color-Word Interference (similar to a Stroop test), Sorting (similar to the WCST), Twenty Questions, Tower (similar to the Towers of Hanoi or London), Word Context, and Proverbs.

The Behavioral Rating Inventory of Executive Function (BRIEF; Gioia et al. 2000) is a parent- or teacher-rated pen-and-pencil inventory that has 86 questions and takes about 10 minutes to complete. Clinical scales measure inhibition, cognitive flexibility, organization, planning, metacognition, emotional control, and initiation. Specific items tap everyday behaviors indicative of executive dysfunction that may not be captured by performance measures, such as organization of the school locker or home closet, monitoring of homework for mistakes, or trouble initiating leisure activities. Thus, this measure may have more ecological validity than other executive function tests. It can be especially useful to document the impact of executive function deficits on the child's "real-world" function and to plan treatment and educational accommodations. Correlational analyses with other behavior rating scales and executive function tests provide evidence of both convergent and divergent validity. The BRIEF is appropriate for children age 5 to 18.

Another executive deficit seen in ASD is difficulty with problem solving. Real-life problem solving can be assessed using the Test of Problem Solving (TOPS; Bowers et al. 1994). The TOPS consists of 14 stimulus pictures and accompanying questions that are designed to provide information about a subject's critical thinking and reasoning abilities. Responses are penalized for misinterpreting questions; providing vague, inadequate, perseverative, irrelevant, concrete, or tangential responses; failing to provide context; and inability to generate appropriate solutions. The TOPS-Elementary was designed for children ages 6–11, and the Adolescent Test of Problem Solving (Bowers et al. 1991) is intended for students in grades 7 through 12. The TOPS has shown high levels of test-retest and internal consistency reliability for all age levels. Age norms and percentile ranks are available for these measures.

Academic Functioning

It is crucial to assess academic ability, even in younger children, for the purposes of educational decision making. It is an area of strength that often goes unrecognized. Many children with ASD have precocious reading skills and can decode words at a higher level than others of the same age and functional ability. Reading and other academic strengths can be used to compensate for weaknesses, as when a written schedule is provided to facilitate transitions or written directions are supplied to improve compliance. The good memory of children with ASD may mean that spelling lists and multiplication tables are learned more easily. Conversely, specific areas of weakness also exist, with the most consistently demonstrated one being reading comprehension. This academic profile is quite different from the problem patterns most teachers and school psychologists are trained to detect (e.g., the poor decoding but good comprehension of dyslexia). Thus, it is important that appropriate test batteries that highlight both academic strengths and weaknesses be included in the comprehensive evaluation, the learning patterns they suggest be interpreted in the feedback to parents and the written report, and appropriate educational recommendations be made. For young children, the Bracken Test of Basic Concepts (Bracken 1998), the Young Children's Achievement Test (YCAT; Hresko 2000), and the Psychoeducational Profile (PEP; Schopler et al. 1990) are useful instruments that highlight both the strengths and the challenges typical of ASD. For older children and those who are verbal, the most often used academic tests are the Woodcock-Johnson Test of Achievement (Woodcock et al. 2001) and the Wechsler Individual Achievement Test (WIAT; Wechsler 1992).

Tests Useful for Psychiatric Evaluation

Over the course of development, children with ASD may develop new symptoms and behaviors that disrupt their daily functioning. Behavioral changes can include problems with sleep, appetite, mood, activity level, anger management, and aggression. The psychologist can play a role in the assessment of the child or teen with ASD for psychiatric problems through their knowledge of specific test instruments. In this chapter, we elaborate on the previous chapter's discussion of comorbidity, focusing here on standardized, normed, objective measurements of behavior that can assist in the psychiatric evaluation and differential diagnosis process.

Recent studies have used semistructured interviews to assist in the diagnosis of psychiatric symptoms, such as the Schedule for Affective Disorders and Schizophrenia for School Aged Children–Present Version (K-SADS-IVR; Ambrosini 2000) and the Diagnostic Interview Schedule for Children (DISC; Shaffer et al. 1996). Lainhart, Folstein, and colleagues have developed a K-SADS interview that has been modified to be sensitive to the manifestations of psychiatric illness in individuals with developmental disabilities. It is called the Schedule of Affective Disorders and Schizophrenia for Developmentally Delayed Children and Adolescents (K-SADS-DD-PL; J.E. Lainhart, personal communication, December 2002). Most semistructured interviews, as well as the questionnaires to be described later, require the child to self-report (sometimes, but not always, in addition to parent report). Thus, they are best used with children with average intellectual abilities and those who can read. However, the limited self-insight of ASD makes the validity of such measures questionable, and results, particularly reports of "no problems," should be interpreted with caution. A new trend in assessment is the development of pictorial interviews for child self-report of psychiatric symptoms; instruments such as the Dominic-Revised (Valla et al. 2000) may prove helpful for evaluation of children with ASD.

The Children's Depression Inventory (CDI; Kovacs 1992) is a self-report questionnaire that measures different aspects of child mood, interpersonal problems, feelings of effectiveness, physical symptoms, and self-esteem. It is suitable for children ages 7–17. The child is instructed to select the statement from each group that best describes him or her for the past 2 weeks. The CDI has exhibited acceptable levels of internal consistency, test-retest reliability, and discriminant validity. Other self-report inventories include the Revised Children's Manifest Anxiety Scale (RCMAS; Reynolds and Richmond 1998), the Multidimensional Anxiety Scale for Children (MASC; March et al. 1997), and the Screen for Child Anxiety-Related Emotional Disorders (SCARED; Birmaher et al. 1997).

The Behavioral Assessment System for Children (BASC; Kamphaus et al. 1999) scales include parent report, teacher report, and self-report questionnaires for children age 8–18. There are scales for internalizing, externalizing, and adaptive behaviors. Subscales assess school, clinical, and personal adjustment. The self-report form also measures "sense of inadequacy" and "sense of atypicality," which in our experience are helpful for understanding the struggles of children with Asperger syndrome and high-functioning autism who are able to validly report on their internal states. These subscales may also prove helpful for measuring treatment effects (Ozonoff et al. 2002b). Importantly, each form provides caution indices to inform the clinician of overly positive or negative responses and to provide a measure of the consistency of the respondent's profile. This set of scales may require follow-up of critical items through a clinical interview with the child.

Conclusion

Psychologists can play several helpful roles on interdisciplinary team evaluations of children suspected of ASD. They can

- Help other team members take a developmental perspective in understanding the child
- Select the measures that are most appropriate to the referral question, the child's particular characteristics and developmental level, and the

desired outcome of the testing (e.g., service eligibility, treatment planning, etc.)

- Measure, in an objective and standardized fashion, core autistic symptoms, comorbid psychiatric symptoms, intelligence, adaptive behavior, academic ability, and neuropsychological function
- Translate test results into practical intervention applications (e.g., interpret neuropsychologic test results as particular learning styles and map onto educational accommodations)
- Assist in making community referrals and setting up interventions
- Measure outcomes of therapy (e.g., benefits and side effects of pharmacotherapy)
- Provide psychological treatments (see Chapter 6) and long-term follow-up
- Engage in research

References

Achenbach TM: Child Behavior Checklist (CBCL). Burlington, VT, ASEBA, 1991

Ambrosini P: The historical development and present status of the Schedule for Affective Disorders and Schizophrenia for School-Age Children (K-SADS). J Am Acad Child Adolesc Psychiatry 39:49–58, 2000

American Psychiatric Association: Diagnostic and Statistical Manual of Mental Disorders, 3rd Edition, Revised. Washington, DC, American Psychiatric Association, 1987

American Psychiatric Association: Diagnostic and Statistical Manual of Mental Disorders, 4th Edition. Washington, DC, American Psychiatric Association, 1994

American Psychiatric Association: Diagnostic and Statistical Mannual of Mental Disorders, 4th Edition, Text Revision. Washington, DC, American Psychiatric Association, 2000

Arnold LE, Aman MG, Martin A, et al: Assessment in multisite randomized clinical trials of patients with autistic disorder: the Autism RUPP Network. J Autism Dev Disord 30:99–111, 2000

Bailey A, Phillips W, Rutter M: Autism: towards an integration of clinical, genetic, neuropsychological, and neurobiological perspectives. J Child Psychol Psychiatry 37:89–126, 1996

Baranek GT: Autism during infancy: a retrospective video analysis of sensory-motor and social behaviors at 9–12 months of age. J Autism Dev Disord 29:213–224, 1999

Baron-Cohen S, Allen J, Gillberg C: Can autism be detected at 18 months? The needle, the haystack, and the CHAT. Br J Psychiatry 161:839–843, 1992

Baron-Cohen S, Cox A, Baird G, et al: Psychological markers in the detection of autism in infancy in a large population. Br J Psychiatry 168:158–163, 1996

Baron-Cohen S, Wheelwright S, Cox A, et al: The early identification of autism: the Checklist for Autism in Toddlers (CHAT). J R Soc Med 93:521–525, 2000

Bayley N: The Bayley Scales of Infant Development, 2nd Edition. San Antonio, TX, Psychological Corporation, 1993

Berument SK, Rutter M, Lord C, et al: Autism screening questionnaire: diagnostic validity. Br J Psychiatry 175:444–451, 1999

Birmaher B, Khetarpal S, Brent D, et al: The screen for child anxiety-related disorders (SCARED): scale construction and psychometric characteristics. J Am Acad Chil Adolesc Psychiatry 36:545–553, 1997

Boelte S, Poustka F: Diagnosis of autism: the connection between current and historical information. Autism 4:382–390, 2000

Bowers L, Barrett M, Huisingh R, et al: Adolescent Test of Problem Solving. East Moline, IL, LinguiSystems, 1991

Bowers L, Huisingh R, Barrett M, et al: Elementary Test of Problem Solving Revised. East Moline, IL, LinguiSystems, 1994

Bracken BA: The Bracken Basic Concept Scale–Revised. San Antonio, TX, Psychological Corporation, 1998

Brownell R: Expressive One-Word Picture Vocabulary Test. Novato, CA, Academic Therapy Publications, 2000

Bruininks RH, Woodcock RW, Weatherman RE, et al: Scales of Independent Behavior–Revised (SIB-R). Chicago, IL, Riverside, 1996

Charman T: The relationship between joint attention and play in autism. Dev Psychopathol 9:1–16, 1997

Charman T: Progress in screening and surveillance for autism spectrum disorders. Paper presented at the annual meeting of the International Meeting for Autism Research, Orlando, FL, 2002

Conners CK: Conners' Rating Scales Revised (CRS-R). San Antonio, TX, Psychological Corporation, 1996

Conners CK: Conners' Continuous Performance Test for Windows, Kiddies Version (K-CPT). North Tonawanda, NY, MHS, 2001

Cox A, Klein K, Charman T, et al: Autism spectrum disorders at 20 and 42 months of age: stability of clinical and ADI-R diagnosis. J Child Psychol Psychiatry 40:719–732, 1999

Delis DC, Kaplan E, Kramer JH: Delis-Kaplan Executive Function System. San Antonio, TX, Psychological Corporation, 2001

DiLavore PC, Lord C, Rutter M: Pre-linguistic autism diagnostic observation schedule. J Autism Dev Disord 25:355–379, 1995

Dunn LM, Dunn LM: The Peabody Picture Vocabulary Test, 3rd Edition (PPVT-III). Circle Pines, MN, American Guidance Service, 1997

Ehlers S, Gillberg C: The epidemiology of Asperger syndrome: a total population study. J Child Psychol Psychiatry 34:1327–1350, 1993

Ehlers S, Gillberg C, Wing L: A screening questionnaire for Asperger syndrome and other high-functioning autism spectrum disorders in school age children. J Autism Dev Disord 29:129–141, 1999

Elliott C: Differential Abilities Scale. San Antonio, TX, Psychological Corporation, 1990

Fein D, Lucci D, Waterhouse L: Brief report: fragmented drawings in autistic children. J Autism Dev Disord 20:263–269, 1990

Filipek PA, Accardo PJ, Baranek GT, et al: The screening and diagnosis of autistic spectrum disorders. J Autism Dev Disord 29:439–484, 1999

Filipek PA, Accardo PJ, Ashwal S, et al: Practice parameter: screening and diagnosis of autism. Neurology 55:468–479, 2000

Garretson HB, Fein D, Waterhouse L: Sustained attention in children with autism. J Autism Dev Disord 20:101–114, 1990

Ghaziuddin M, Tsai L, Ghaziuddin N: Comorbidity of autistic disorder in children and adolescents. Eur Child Adolesc Psychiatry 1:209–213, 1992

Gilliam JE: Gilliam Asperger Disorder Scale. Austin, TX, Pro-Ed, 2001

Gioia GA, Isquith PK, Guy SC, et al: Behavior Rating Inventory of Executive Function. Odessa, FL, Psychological Assessment Resources, 2000

Gordon M: The Gordon Diagnostic System. DeWitt, NY, Gordon Systems, 1983

Happe F, Frith U: The neuropsychology of autism. Brain 119:1377–1400, 1996

Harrison P, Oakland T: Adaptive Behavior Assessment System. San Antonio, TX, Psychological Corporation, 2000

Heaton RK, Chelune GJ, Talley JL, et al: Wisconsin Card Sorting Test Manual: Revised and Expanded. Odessa, FL, Psychological Assessment Resources, 1993

Hresko WP, Peak PK, Herron SR, et al: Young Children's Achievement Test. Austin, TX, Pro-Ed, 2000

Hughes C, Russell J, Robbins TW: Evidence for executive dysfunction in autism. Neuropsychologia 32:477–492, 1994

Kamphaus RW, Reynolds CR, Hatcher NM: Treatment planning and evaluation with the BASC: the Behavior Assessment System for Children, in The Use of Psychological Testing for Treatment Planning and Outcomes Assessment, 2nd Edition. Edited by Maruish ME. Hillsdale, NJ, Erlbaum, 1999, pp 563–597

Kaufman AS, Kaufman NL: K-ABC: Kaufman Assessment Battery for Children. Circle Pines, MN, American Guidance Service, 1983

Klin A, Shepard BA: Psychological assessment of autistic children. Child Adolesc Psychiatr Clin N Am 3:53–70, 1994

Klin A, Volkmar FR, Sparrow SS, et al: Validity and neuropsychological characterization of Asperger syndrome: convergence with nonverbal learning disabilities syndrome. J Child Psychol Psychiatry 30:1127–1140, 1995

Klinger LG, Renner P: Performance-based measures in autism: implications for diagnosis, early detection, and identification of cognitive profiles. J Clin Child Psychol 29:479–492, 2000

Koegel LK, Koegel RL, Smith A: Variables related to differences in standardized test outcomes for children with autism. J Autism Dev Disord 27:233–243, 1997

Kovacs M: The Children's Depression Inventory. North Tonawanda, NY, Multi-Health Systems, 1982

Lincoln AJ, Allen MH, Kilman A: The assessment and interpretation of intellectual abilities in people with autism, in Learning and Cognition in Autism. Edited by Schopler E, Mesibov GB. New York, Plenum, 1995, pp 89–117

Lord C: Follow-up of two-year-olds referred for possible autism. J Child Psychol Psychiatry 36:1365–1382, 1995

Lord C, Rutter M, LeCouteur AM: Autism Diagnostic Interview–Revised: a revised version of a diagnostic interview with possible pervasive developmental disorders. J Autism Dev Disord 24:659–685, 1994

Lord C, Pickles A, McLennan J, et al: Diagnosing autism: analyses of data from the Autism Diagnostic Interview. J Autism Dev Disord 27:501–517, 1997

Lord C, Risi S, Lambrecht L, et al: The Autism Diagnostic Observation Schedule–Generic: a standard measure of social and communication deficits associated with the spectrum of autism. J Autism Dev Disord 30:205–223, 2000

Manly T, Anderson V, Nimmo-Smith I, et al: The differential assessment of children's attention: the Test of Everyday Attention for Children (TEA-Ch), normative sample and ADHD performance. J Child Psychol Psychiatry 42:1065–1081, 2001

March JS, Parker JD, Sullivan K, et al: The multidimensional anxiety scale for children (MASC): factor structure, reliability, and validity. J Am Acad Child Adolesc Psychiatry 36:554–565, 1997

Mesibov G, Schopler E, Schaffer B, et al: Adolescent and Adult Psychoeducational Profile. Austin, TX, Pro-Ed, 1988

Minshew NJ, Goldstein G, Siegel DJ: Neuropsychologic functioning in autism: profile of a complex information processing disorder. J Int Neuropsychol Soc 3:303–316, 1997

Mirsky AF, Anthony BJ, Duncan CC, et al: Analysis of the elements of attention: a neuropsychological approach. Neuropsychol Rev 2:109–145, 1991

Mirsky AF, Pascualvaca DM, Duncan CC, et al: A model of attention and its relation to ADHD. Ment Retard Dev Disabil Res Rev 5:169–176, 1999

Mullen EM: Mullen Scales of Early Learning, AGS Edition. Circle Pines, MN, American Guidance Service, 1995

Mundy P, Sigman M, Kasari C: A longitudinal study of joint attention and language development in autistic children. J Autism Dev Disord 20:115–128, 1990

Myklebust HR (ed): Progress in Learning Disabilities: III. New York, Grune & Stratton, 1975

Myles BS, Bock SJ, Simpson RL: Asperger Syndrome Diagnostic Scale. Austin, TX, Pro-Ed, 2001

Osterling J, Dawson G: Early recognition of children with autism: a study of first birthday home videotapes. J Aut Dev Disord 24:247–259, 1994

Ozonoff S: Reliability and validity of the Wisconsin Card Sorting Test in studies of autism. Neuropsychology 9:491–500, 1995

Ozonoff S, Griffith EM: Neuropsychological function and the external validity of Asperger syndrome, in Asperger Syndrome. Edited by Klin A, Volkmar F, Sparrow SS. New York, Guilford, 2000, pp 72–96

Ozonoff S, Jensen J: Specific executive function profiles in three neurodevelopmental disorders. J Autism Dev Disord 29:171–177, 1999

Ozonoff S, Miller JN: An exploration of right-hemisphere contributions to the pragmatic impairments of autism. Brain Lang 52:411–434, 1996

Ozonoff S, Pennington BF, Rogers SJ: Executive function deficits in high-functioning autistic individuals: relationship to theory of mind. J Child Psychol Psychiatry 32:1081–1105, 1991

Ozonoff S, South M, Miller J: DSM-IV-defined Asperger syndrome: cognitive, behavioral and early history differentiation from high-functioning autism. Autism 4:29–46, 2000

Ozonoff S, Dawson G, McPartland J: A Parent's Guide to Asperger Syndrome and High-Functioning Autism: How to Meet the Challenges and Help Your Child Thrive. New York, Guilford, 2002a

Ozonoff S, Provencal S, Solomon M: The effectiveness of social skills training programs for autism spectrum disorders. Paper presented at the annual meeting of the American Academy of Child and Adolescent Psychiatry, San Francisco, CA, 2002b

Ozonoff S, South M, Provencal S: Executive functions, in Handbook of Autism and Pervasive Developmental Disorders, 3rd Edition. Edited by Volkmar FR, Klin A, Paul R. New York, Wiley (in press)

Reynolds CR, Kamphaus RW: BASC: Behavior Assessment System for Children. Circle Pines, MN, American Guidance Service, 1998

Reynolds CR, Richmond BO: Revised Children's Manifest Anxiety Scale. Los Angeles, CA, Western Psychological Services, 1998

Robins DL, Fein D, Barton M, et al: The modified checklist for autism in toddlers: an initial study investigating the early detection of autism and pervasive developmental disorders. J Autism Dev Disord 31:131–144, 2001

Rogers SJ: Diagnosis of autism before the age of 3, in International Review of Research in Mental Retardation: Autism, Vol 23. Edited by Glidden LM. Los Angeles, CA, Academic Press, 2001, pp 1–31

Roid GH: Stanford-Binet Intelligence Scales, 5th Edition. Chicago, IL, Riverside, 2003

Roid G, Miller L: Leiter International Test of Intelligence–Revised. Chicago, IL, Stoelting, 1997

Rourke BP (ed): Syndrome of Nonverbal Learning Disabilities: Neurodevelopmental Manifestations. New York, Guilford, 1995

Russell J (ed): Autism as an Executive Disorder. New York, Oxford University Press, 1997

Sandford JA, Turner A: Integrated Visual and Auditory Continuous Performance Test. Richmond, VA, BrainTrain, 2000

Scambler D, Rogers SJ, Wehner EA: Can the Checklist for Autism in Toddlers differentiate young children with autism from those with developmental delays? J Am Acad Child Adolesc Psychiatry 40:1457–1463, 2001

Schopler E, Reichler R, Renner B: The Childhood Autism Rating Scale (CARS). Los Angeles, CA, Western Psychological Services, 1988

Schopler E, Reichler RJ, Bashford A, et al: Psychoeducational Profile–Revised (PEP-R). Austin, TX, Pro-Ed, 1990

Semel E, Wing EH, Secord WA: Clinical Evaluation of Language Fundamentals–3 Examiner's Manual. San Antonio, TX, Psychological Corporation, 1995

Shaffer D, Fisher P, Dulcan M, et al: The NIMH Diagnostic Interview Schedule for Children (DISC-2): description, acceptability, prevalences, and performance in the MECA study. J Am Acad Child Adolesc Psychiatry 35:865–877, 1996

Siegel B: Early screening and diagnosis in autism spectrum disorder: the pervasive developmental disorders screening test. Paper presented at the NIH State of the Science in Autism: Screening and Diagnosis Working Conference, Rockville, MD, June 1998

Siegel DJ, Minshew NJ, Goldstein G: Wechsler IQ profiles in diagnosis of high-functioning autism. J Autism Dev Disord 26:389–406, 1996

Sparrow S, Balla D, Cicchetti D: Vineland Adaptive Behavior Scales. Circle Pines, MN, American Guidance Service, 1984

Stone WL, Yoder PJ: Predicting spoken language level in children with autism spectrum disorders. Autism 5:341–361, 2001

Stone WL, Coonrod EE, Ousley OY: Screening tool for autism in two-year-olds (STAT): development and preliminary data. J Autism Dev Disord 30:607–612, 2000

Thorndike RL, Hagen EP, Sattler JM: The Stanford-Binet Intelligence Scales, 4th Edition. Chicago, IL, Riverside, 1986

Valla JP, Bergeron L, Smolla N: The Dominic-R: a pictorial interview for 6- to 11-year-old children. J Am Acad Child Adolesc Psychiatry 39:85–93, 2000

Volkmar FR, Pomeroy JCE, Realmuto G, et al: Practice parameters for the assessment and treatment of children, adolescents, and adults with autism and other pervasive developmental disorders. J Am Acad Child Adolesc Psychiatry 38 (suppl 12):32S–54S, 1999

Wechsler D: Wechsler Preschool and Primary Scale of Intelligence, Revised. San Antonio, TX, Psychological Corporation, 1989

Wechsler D: Wechsler Intelligence Scale for Children, 3rd Edition. San Antonio, TX, Psychological Corporation, 1991

Wechsler D: Wechsler Individual Achievement Test. San Antonio, TX, Psychological Corporation, 1992

Wechsler D: Wechsler Adult Intelligence Scale, 3rd Edition. San Antonio, TX, Psychological Corporation, 1997

Wechsler D: Wechsler Abbreviated Scale of Intelligence. San Antonio, TX, Psychological Corporation, 1999

Werner E, Dawson G, Osterling J, et al: Brief report: recognition of autism spectrum disorder before one year of age: a retrospective study based on home videotapes. J Autism Dev Disord 30:157–162, 2000

Wetherby AM, Prizant BM: Profiling young children's communicative competence, in Causes and Effects in Communication and Language Intervention. Edited by Warren SF, Reichle JE. Baltimore, MD, Paul H. Brookes, 1992, pp 217–253

Wetherby AM, Prizant BM: Communication and Symbolic Behavior scales (CSBS)–Normed Edition. Chicago, IL, Applied Symbolix, 1993

Wiig E, Secord W: Test of Language Competence–Expanded Edition. San Antonio, TX, Psychological Corporation, 1989

Wing L, Leekam SR, Libby SJ, et al: The diagnostic interview for social and communication disorders: background, inter-rater reliability and clinical use. J Child Psychol Psychiatry 43:307–325, 2002

Woodcock RW, McGrew KS, Mather N: Woodcock-Johnson III Tests of Achievement. Chicago, IL, Riverside, 2001

World Health Organization: The International Statistical Classification of Diseases and Related Health Problems, 10th Revision. Geneva, Switzerland, World Health Organization, 1993

Zimmerman IL, Steiner VG, Pond RE: Preschool Language Scale–3: Manual. San Antonio, TX, Psychological Corporation, 1991

Chapter 4

Contributions of Pediatrics

Robin L. Hansen, M.D.
Randi J. Hagerman, M.D.

Introduction

Pediatric health care providers play an essential role in the early identification, diagnostic evaluation, and long-term care of children with autism spectrum disorders (ASD). Because most of the etiologies of ASD are unknown and likely to be multifactorial, developing consistent medical assessment guidelines for clinicians that reflect the current state of knowledge is important. We need to identify associated disorders that are treatable or that have important genetic or prognostic implications. It is important to reassure families that a considered, comprehensive search for etiology based on current research has been completed. Widespread clinical use of comprehensive assessment guidelines that are empirically supported by peer-reviewed research can provide a larger data set of well-defined populations of children with ASD for etiologic research. Our efforts to define clinical subgroups or phenotypes will eventually help us understand the common pathophysiologies that lead to autism so that better treatment and, hopefully, prevention methodologies can be developed.

The focus of this chapter is on medical evaluation and diagnostic testing practices presently available to the clinician that are supported by empirical data. The pediatric evaluation is optimally carried out as part of a team evaluation; the contributions of other team members are elaborated in other chapters in this book. Pediatricians can also play an important role in medical treatment approaches, including pharmacologic interventions and alternative therapies, which are covered in subsequent chapters.

Associated Medical Conditions

The relationship of autism spectrum disorders to known medical conditions is the focus of much current research. Autism has been associated with a variety of genetic syndromes, chromosome anomalies, and other medical disorders. It is important to distinguish between associated medical conditions that may be causally related to autistic symptoms and those that coexist because of shared underlying biological conditions. Methodologic problems in previous studies investigating associated medical conditions make it difficult to address causal relationships. These problems include inconsistent or unclear criteria for ASD diagnosis, small sample sizes, ascertainment bias, multiple reports of single case studies, and nonblinded conditions. It is also important to determine whether the association is greater than that expected to appear in the general population or to occur by chance.

The association of medical conditions in children with ASD varies across studies, generally from 5% to 30%, although some studies have identified associated medical conditions in as many as 50% (Dykens and Volkmar 1997). Obvious contributors to this variation are the comprehensiveness of the evaluation; the technological advances available at the time of the study, such as high-resolution cytogenetic and molecular studies; and the sample evaluated. Steffenburg (1991) found associated medical conditions in 18% of children with autism who did not have severe mental retardation, and in 43% of children with autism and severe to profound mental retardation. Similarly, Scott (1994) found associated medical conditions in 50% of children with autism and severe to profound mental retardation. Rutter et al. (1994) suggest that the association of medical conditions is approximately 10%–11% across the autism spectrum, with 8% of those conditions having a plausible causal relationship to autism and the other 3% being unrelated co-occurring conditions. Gillberg (1996) reviewed seven population-based studies that met specific methodologic requirements, including: systematic information collected about associated medical disorders, defined diagnostic criteria for autism, specific age cohorts from a geographically defined population, initial screening for cases made within a population of children broader than only those with autism, and final diagnosis made by a research team. Two studies were from the United States, two from Sweden, and one each from the United Kingdom, France, and Canada. The average rate of associated medical disorders was 24.4%, and the rate was highest in samples that included a larger proportion of individuals with mental retardation.

Physical Anomalies

Previous studies examining physical anomalies in children with autism have described an increased incidence of low-set ears, adherent ear lobes, furrowed tongue, hypertelorism, 2-3 toe syndactyly, shortened fifth finger (Walker 1977), posteriorly rotated ears, small feet, and large hands (Rodier et al. 1997). Thus far, no clear set of anomalies seem to separate affected children into meaningful subgroups. Lauritsen et al. (2002) found congenital anomalies in 5.3% of their sample with autism, in a retrospective review of two population-based Danish registers. They found mainly anomalies of the eyes (coloboma, eyelid anomalies, glaucoma, micropthalmus), ears (cochlear disease, hearing impairment), central nervous system (spina bifida, encephalocele, neurofibromatosis, cerebral atrophy), heart (patent ductus arteriosus [PDA]), extremities (polydactyly, pelvic girdle anomaly), and urinary system (accessory kidney, medullary sponge kidney).

In a study important to the understanding of etiologies for ASD, Miles and Hillman (2000) examined 94 consecutive children referred for clinical evaluation who met DSM-IV (American Psychiatric Association 1994) and Childhood Autism Rating Scale (CARS) diagnostic criteria for autistic disorder. Each of these subjects underwent a comprehensive etiologic examination that included clinical morphology, blood and urine studies, brain magnetic resonance imaging (MRI), electroencephalogram (EEG), and review of historical, medical, and family data. Of these 94 children, 6 were found to have genetic syndromes thought to be associated with autism (tuberous sclerosis, Soto's syndrome, ring chromosome 8, del 8q22, der 15). Fifty-one of the remaining 88 (58%) were phenotypically normal, defined in this study as having three or fewer minor anomalies or abnormal measurements, and three or fewer descriptive traits that occur in a sizable proportion of the population and have a continuous range of variability (e.g., flat feet). Twenty-two percent (19/88) were classified as phenotypically abnormal (defined as six or more minor anomalies, measurement abnormalities, or descriptive traits). The remaining 20% (18/88) were classified as phenotypically equivocal, with four or five minor anomalies or descriptive traits. These data suggest a significant disruption in early embryogenesis in over one-fifth of the sample. The male:female ratio was significantly higher in the phenotypically normal group (7.5:1) than in either the abnormal (1.7:1) or the equivocal group (3.5:1). Fifty-five of the 94 participants consented to brain MRI scans. The phenotypic status judged on the basis of the physical examination directly correlated with the presence of structural malformations of the brain. Fourteen percent of the phenotypically normal subjects had abnormal structure, as opposed to 29% of the phenotypically abnormal individuals and 27% of the equivocal group. On the basis of the differing neurobiology, symptom presentation, and male:female ratios, Miles and Hillman (2000) postulated the existence of multiple different etiologic subgroups, with phenotypically abnormal children having distinct etiologies for their autism compared with those with normal phenotypic exams. This study supports the idea that many cases of autism involve disruptions in early fetal development, a point also made by Bauman and Kemper's brain autopsy studies (1988).

Neural Growth Factors

Nelson et al. (2001) found that concentrations of two neuropeptides (vasoactive intestinal peptide [VIP] and calcitonin gene–related peptide [CGRP]) and two neurotrophins (brain-derived neurotrophin factor [BDNF] and neurotrophin 4/5 [NT4/5]) were significantly elevated in blood samples of newborn children later diagnosed with autism and/or mental retardation, compared with children with cerebral palsy or normal control subjects. This provides additional support for the conjecture that alterations in brain development are present during prenatal development in at least some children with autism. There were no differences in neuropeptide concentrations of substance P or pituitary adenylate cyclase–activating polypeptide or in neurotrophin nerve growth factor or neurotrophin 3. Similar elevations in VIP, CGRP, BDNF, and NT4/5 were found in subgroups of the autistic spectrum, both those with and without mental retardation and those with and without a history of regression. No analyte distinguished children with autism from children with mental retardation alone. Whether these growth factors are part of a causal pathway to autism or mental retardation is unclear, as is the nature of the primary defect(s), and this is an area of active current research at the M.I.N.D. Institute and elsewhere.

Genetic Disorders

Chromosomal abnormalities are seen in up to 9% of patients with autistic disorder or ASD (Wassink et al. 2001) and have been found on virtually every chromosome (Gillberg 1998). Many of these abnormalities do not exceed chance levels and are unlikely to be etiologically meaningful. There are, however, several known genetic disorders that are thought to be causally related to autism. Those discussed in this chapter include 15q duplications, fragile X syndrome (FXS), and tuberous sclerosis (TS) complex. Chapter 5 provides discussion of other genetic syndromes that appear to have strong nonrandom associations with ASD.

Deletions and Duplications at 15q11–13

The 15q11–13 region holds great interest for researchers and clinicians concerned with neurodevelopmental disorders, particularly ASD. Studies have shown that approximately 1%–4% of individuals with autism have abnormality in this region of chromosome 15 (Cook et al. 1997; Thomas et al. in press), making it one of the most common known etiologies for the syndrome. This region is a hot spot for deletions and duplications because large genomic duplications that date back at least 20 million years (Christian et al. 1999) led to homologous unequal recombination events that mediate the frequent rearrangements. This region is also imprinted, so methylation typically occurs here on the chromosome 15 inherited from the mother, but not on the chromosome inherited from the father. Three types of anomalies in the 15q11–13 region have been found to be associated with autism. The first two, deletions that lead to the distinct phenotypes of Prader-Willi and Angelman syndromes, are occasionally associated with autism. The third abnormality in this region involves duplication of genetic material and is frequently associated with ASD. We discuss the two deletion syndromes first, although they are less commonly and clearly associated with autism than the duplication syndrome.

When the 15q11–13 region is missing from the father's chromosome, the child presents with Prader-Willi syndrome (PWS), characterized by severe hypotonia and failure to thrive for the first year or two of life. Then a shift up in appetite and severe hyperphagia develop between 2 and 4 years of age, with a lack of satiation leading to obesity (Cassidy and Morris 2002; Hagerman 1999a). The physical phenotype includes short stature, round face, almond-shaped eyes, short fingers and toes, and hypogonadism secondary to hypothalamic dysfunction. The behavioral phenotype includes voracious eating, insatiable appetite, skin picking, hoarding of food and other objects of interest, tantrums, stubborn and manipulative behavior, and obsessive-compulsive symptoms (Cassidy and Morris 2002). Language and motor milestones are usually delayed, and cognitive abilities range from normal IQ in 5%, borderline IQ in 27%, mild mental retardation in 34%, moderate mental retardation in 27%, and profound mental retardation in 6% (Curfs and Fryns 1992).

Approximately 1 individual in 10,000 has PWS. In 75% of cases, there is a paternally derived deletion at 15q11–13. Most of the rest have maternal uniparental disomy, meaning that they have inherited two copies of their mother's chromosome 15 and they have no copies of their father's chromosome 15. Most individuals with PWS do not have autism, but a few cases have been reported; all have maternal uniparental disomy (Cassidy and Morris 2002; Schroer et al. 1998). It is presumed, therefore, that autism may be related to overexpression of a gene in this region.

When the maternal region of 15q11–13 is missing, through either a deletion (75% of cases), uniparental disomy of the paternal chromosome 15 (2%–5% of cases), or an imprinting defect (2%–5% of cases), then a different phenotype occurs: Angelman syndrome. This phenotype has been found to be related to the *UBE3A* gene, which codes for the E6AP-3A ubiquitin protein ligase that is important for protein degradation in neurons. The ubiquitin-mediated proteolytic pathway plays a major role in regulation of protein turnover. This gene is differentially imprinted in different maternal tissues, and it is inactive in certain regions of the brain but active in blood. Twenty percent to 25% of cases of Angelman syndrome have a mutation in the *UBE3A* gene. In addition, the 5′ end of *UBE3A* was recently reported to be in linkage disequilibrium in 94 siblings of families with idiopathic autism (Nurmi et al. 2001). Perhaps this locus is important as an additive effect with other genes associated with autism.

Angelman syndrome occurs in approximately 1 individual in 15,000. The phenotype typically involves seizures, hyperactivity, microcephaly, no speech, wide mouth, and a movement disorder with ataxia and tremulous or stiff limb movements that reminded Dr. Angelman of a puppet on a string. Generally, these individuals are happy, with frequent and prolonged bouts of laughter, so the term *happy puppet syndrome* was used in the past to describe them (Hagerman 1999a). Because of the lack of speech, presence of repetitive movements such as hand flapping, and social deficits, autism has been diagnosed frequently in Angelman syndrome (Schroer et al. 1998; Steffenburg et al. 1996). However, given the severe mental retardation that characterizes Angelman syndrome, differential diagnosis of autism is a challenge. Abnormalities on EEG, treatment of seizures, and other details of Angelman syndrome are described in Chapter 5.

The phenotypes of Angelman syndrome and PWS are relatively easy to detect, but duplications in the region of 15q11–13 are often not obvious clinically. Individuals who have an interstitial duplication in this region that is maternally inherited may present with an autism spectrum disorder (Browne et al. 1997; Cook et al. 1997; Mao and Jalal 2000; Schroer et al. 1998; Thomas et al., in press). They therefore have three copies of 15q11–

13 (Cook et al. 1997). Others have found this genotype in 2%–4% of patients with autism of unknown etiology (Cook et al. 1997). Their phenotype usually includes down-slanting eyes, epicanthal folds, broad nasal bridge, hypotonia, hyperextensible finger joints, and minor partial syndactyly, cryptorchidism, and a large head circumference in a smaller number (Thomas et al., in press). They typically have mild mental retardation or borderline IQ, and hyperactivity is common (Bolton et al. 2001; Thomas et al., in press).

Although several studies indicate that almost all patients with this duplication are on the autism spectrum, a careful study by Bolton et al. (2001) suggests otherwise. They studied 21 individuals with 15q duplications from six families and unaffected controls from the same families, using the Autism Diagnostic Observation Scale (ADOS), Autism Diagnostic Interview–Revised (ADI-R), clinical assessment, and cognitive and adaptive measures. Of the 17 patients with maternal inheritance of the duplication, ASD was documented in 4, although milder social or language deficits were common in the others. Epilepsy was seen in 2 patients, and motor clumsiness was also common. Eleven had mild mental retardation, 3 had borderline IQ, and 3 had normal IQ. Many of these patients did not have dysmorphic features, although hypotonia, joint laxity, down-slanting palpebral fissures, and thick or pouting lips were seen in several (Bolton et al. 2001).

More severely affected patients may have an additional extra chunk of chromosomal material, which is usually chromosome 15 material that is inverted and duplicated from this region. This material is termed a *supernumerary inverted duplicated marker chromosome 15*, so overall the patient has four copies of this region, typically causing autism and moderate to severe mental retardation (Gillberg 1998; Mignon et al. 1996). It is almost always maternally inherited, perhaps because spermatozoa bearing this marker have lower fertilizing capacity (Mignon et al. 1996). Cantú et al. (1990) first reported this marker after screening 67 individuals who were institutionalized with severe autism. They detected one female with this marker chromosome. Many of these individuals also have seizures that are difficult to control and which may be partially responsible for severe regression and loss of milestones. The duplicated region also includes three GABA (gamma-aminobutyric acid) receptor subunit genes (*GABRB3*, *GABRA5*, *GABRG3*). Since GABA is an inhibitory neurotransmitter that may be important for suppressing seizures, dysfunction of the receptors of GABA or perhaps dysfunction of *UBE3A* may add to the seizure problem in these patients.

In summary, the 15q11–13 region appears to show an association with autism, particularly duplication of maternally inherited material. Any

abnormalities in this region should be looked for with high-resolution cytogenetic studies, in addition to fluorescent in situ hybridization (FISH)
analysis and methylation studies, as described later.

Fragile X Syndrome

FXS is the most common inherited cause of mental retardation and represents 30% of X-linked causes of mental retardation. Approximately 2%–
8% of boys with autism have FXS (Bailey et al. 1993; Brown et al. 1986;
Gillberg 1993; Li et al. 1993; Wassink et al. 2001). Therefore, children
who present with either mental retardation or autism of unknown etiology
should undergo DNA testing for the fragile X mental retardation 1 gene
(*FMR1*). This recommendation has been made by the American Society of
Human Genetics, the American Academy of Pediatrics, the American
Academy of Neurology (Filipek et al. 2000), the California Department of
Developmental Services (2002), and numerous research publications
(Blomquist et al. 1985; Brown et al. 1986; Li et al. 1993; Hagerman 2002b;
Hagerman et al. 1994).

FXS is a trinucleotide-repeat disorder. Individuals affected with the full
syndrome have over 200 CGG repeats. A smaller expansion or "premutation" (55 to 200 repeats) is seen in carriers, who are usually unaffected.
Male premutation carriers will pass only the premutation to all of their offspring because only the premutation is present in sperm. Female premutation carriers are at high risk to pass on a full mutation to their offspring.
If a mother has greater than 90 repeats, almost 100% of the time that the
mutated X is passed on, it will expand to a full mutation. The full mutation
is usually completely methylated, which significantly decreases transcrip-
tion (the making of messenger RNA [mRNA]) and leads to reduced trans-
lation (the making of the FMR1 protein [FMRP] from *FMR1* mRNA). It
is the deficiency of FMRP that causes FXS.

The *FMR1* gene was sequenced in 1991 (Verkerk et al. 1991), which subsequently allowed for development of an accurate *FMR1* DNA diagnostic
test, less expensive than the laborious cytogenetic techniques previously
used to look for a fragile site at Xq27.3. The cytogenetic test had been used
to diagnose fragile X for more than a decade before 1991. The cytogenetic
technique does not identify carriers of the premutation (55 to 200 CGG repeats) or high-functioning individuals (IQ>70), who are often lacking methylation. The polymerase chain reaction (PCR) technique is used in DNA
studies to identify the exact number of CGG repeats in those with the premutation, and the Southern blot is used to identify the full mutation.

Almost all children with FXS display some symptoms that are associated with autism; the most common are hand flapping, hand biting, poor

eye contact, tactile defensiveness, perseverative speech, and social deficits. Unlike children with classic autism, most children with FXS are interested in social interactions, although sensory hyperarousal and anxiety may interfere with optimal socialization. The number who meet criteria for autism varies across studies, from 15% to 33% depending on the criteria and the evaluation tools used (Bailey et al. 1998; Hagerman et al. 1986; Reiss and Freund 1990; Rogers et al. 2001; Turk and Graham 1997). A study by Rogers et al. (2001) found the highest rate (33%) in preschoolers with FXS, utilizing autism research diagnostic tools (ADI-R and ADOS-G, described in Chapter 3). In this study, the children who had both FXS and autism had a lower IQ than those with FXS alone or those with autism alone, a result that has also been found by Bailey et al. (2001a, 2001b). This suggests that children with FXS and autism may have had an additional hit, either genetic or environmental, that contributes to the development of autism.

In addition to ASD, there are several other aspects of the behavioral phenotype of FXS important for evaluation, differential diagnosis, and treatment recommendations. Young children with FXS often present with hypotonia in infancy. The majority have reflux, leading to frequent emesis and feeding problems in the first few months of life. A poor suck and irritability are common. Sleeping problems, with difficulty settling down at bedtime and frequent wakefulness in the middle of the night, are seen in over 50%, and this leads to parent exhaustion and frustration. Hyperactivity, impulsivity, a short attention span, and tantrums are common. Sensory hyperarousal and sensory integration dysfunction are seen in the majority of patients, with many intolerant of light touch, certain textures of clothes, large crowds, alarms, or loud noises, for example. The physiologic basis of these symptoms appears to be enhanced sympathetic responsivity to all modalities of sensory input and decreased vagal tone (Belser and Sudhalter 2001; Miller et al. 1999; Roberts et al. 2001). These difficulties can be improved by medications described in Chapter 7 and by occupational therapy (Hagerman 2002a; Scharfenaker et al. 2002).

We have reported autism in a subgroup of children with the premutation, suggesting that even the premutation can cause significant central nervous system (CNS) dysfunction, particularly if the level of FMRP is lower than normal (Goodlin-Jones et al. 2002; Hagerman 2002b). These children are less likely than those with the full mutation to show typical physical features of FXS, such as prominent ears. Thirty percent of those with the full mutation do not have obvious physical features, and at least 25% do not have a family history of mental retardation (Hagerman 2002b). Therefore, all individuals with either autism or mental retardation of unknown etiology should have *FMR1* DNA testing, as recommended by the American Society of Human Genetics and the American Academy of Pediatrics. Once the diagnosis of FXS is made in a proband, genetic counseling is essential for the extended family (Gane and Cronister 2002); a variety of treatments, including medication (Hagerman 1996) and educational interventions, can be helpful for these children (Braden 2002; Hills-Epstein et al. 2002; Scharfenaker et al. 2002).

Tuberous Sclerosis Complex

Approximately 2%–4% of individuals with autism have TS, making it another common identifiable cause of autism. The overall prevalence of TS in the general population is approximately 1 per 10,000 (O'Callaghan 1999). Bourneville, a French physician, first described TS in 1880 in a 3-year-old girl who had had seizures since infancy as well as learning problems (Bourneville 1880). When she died from seizures, he described the cortical anomalies as resembling the cut surface of potatoes—hence the French name *sclerose tubereuse.* Subsequently, Vogt (1908) described the association between cortical tubers and facial angiomas, which led to a clinical diagnosis that could be made before death. Other skin manifestations of TS include hypomelanotic macules or ash leaf patches, shagreen patches, ungual fibromas, café au lait spots, and soft fibromas (de Vries and Bolton 2000). TS can affect many other organs, including the kidneys with cysts and angiolipomas, the heart with rhabdomyomata, the lungs with lymphangiomyomatosis, the retina with hamartomas and visual field defects, and the lens with cataracts (Roach et al. 1998). In the CNS, subependymal nodules (SENs) are usually present. In 5%–10% of cases they can develop into subependymal giant cell astrocytomas (SEGAs), which lead to clinical deterioration including vomiting, headaches, and papilledema.

Two different gene mutations can cause TS. The *TSC1* gene is located at 9q34 and it produces a protein called hamartin, which is a tumor suppressor gene. The *TSC2* gene is on 16p13.3 and it produces tuberin, which works together with hamartin, perhaps as a chaperone. An abnormal copy of one of these genes is inherited from the parent in an autosomal dominant fashion, or it can be a spontaneous mutation. It is hypothesized that a second hit must take place at some point in cell division before phenotypic features occur. When the second normal allele is eliminated, the absence of either hamartin or tuberin leads to dysregulation of the cell cycle and cell proliferation. These cells then migrate to other cortical areas in a disorganized fashion that causes cortical tubers. The tubers are abnormal neurons and glial cells with demyelination. They often calcify when the central portion degenerates, and the MRI is the best way to demonstrate them. SENs occur when there is a lack of migration from the periventricular zone. When they calcify, they are stone hard and they typically occur in the walls of the lateral and third ventricles (de Vries and Bolton 2000). Seizures occur in about 84% of those with TS, and they usually start before 5 years of age (Gomez 1999). Many different seizure types occur, including infantile spasms. See Chapter 5 for more information regarding seizures.

Cognitive deficits and emotional/behavioral problems are common in TS. They occur because of the abnormal brain structure, including the tubers, the SENs, and the migration abnormalities that can also lead to more subtle deficits such as heterotopias and white matter changes. The seizures may also lead to further brain damage. The prevalence of mental retardation in TS varies from 38% to 80%, with the lower figure obtained from secondarily ascertained cases as families are further evaluated (de Vries and Bolton 2000). Even in those with normal intellectual abilities, learning disabilities are common, including attentional difficulties and spatial working memory deficits. Behavioral problems include hyperactivity, aggressive outbursts, self-injury, and sleep difficulties. High levels of anxiety and social deficits (e.g., extreme shyness) have been reported in those without mental retardation or learning disabilities (Asano et al. 2001; Smalley et al. 1994). These authors hypothesize that even mild forms of this genetic disorder lead to migrational abnormalities and changes in brain architecture that can produce behavioral and emotional issues.

Autism or autistic features are common findings in those affected by TS, although the rates vary in different studies. Between 24% and 61% of individuals with TS have been reported to have autism, and 43%–86% are said to have some form of ASD (Gillberg et al. 1994; Hunt and Shepherd 1993). Location of the tubers in the temporal lobes was found to be associated with the presence of ASD (Bolton and Griffiths 1997). The presence of mental retardation and seizures was also found to be associated with autism, but they are not necessary or sufficient for the development of autism (de Vries and Bolton 2000). Recent work by Asano et al. (2001) utilizing PET scanning in TS patients, both with and without autism, found glucose hypermetabolism in the deep cerebellar nuclei and increased serotonin (5-HT) uptake in the caudate to be associated with impaired social interactions, communication deficits, and stereotypic behavior. In addition, a history of infantile spasms and glucose hypometabolism in the lateral temporal gyri were both associated with communication deficits. It appears that the combination of these problems creates the symptom complex seen in autism. Elucidating why some individuals with a single disorder have autism and others do not, and relating this to the same process in other disorders, will help us understand the commonalities in brain dysfunction that lead to autism.

The diagnosis of TS is a clinical diagnosis that is dependent on finding the physical manifestations. TS can present in infancy with infantile spasms or developmental delay. The white patches can be seen from birth onward by using a Wood's light, whereas the shagreen patches and angiofibromas may not develop until adolescence. The tubers are best seen on MRI. DNA diagnostic studies for the *TSC1* and *TSC2* mutations are not clinically utilized at this time, but are likely to become part of the routine medical evaluation in the near future. Some preliminary genotype-phenotype correlations suggest that the *TSC1* gene mutation produces a milder phenotype than the *TSC2* mutation (de Vries and Bolton 2000).

Evaluation

In this section, the clinical implications of this literature review are discussed, particularly those related to evaluation. Treatment implications are the focus of other chapters, especially Chapters 7 and 8. The core of the pediatrician's evaluation of the child with suspected ASD is in a detailed medical history and physical examination. The components of the medical evaluation are summarized in Table 4–1.

Medical History

While pre- and perinatal risk factors have contributed little to the etiologic understanding of ASD, they represent additive brain trauma that is important to understand (Nelson 1991; Rodier 1996). Therefore, details regarding maternal infections, bleeding during gestation, prematurity, multiple births, respiratory problems at the time of birth, course in a neonatal intensive care unit, any CNS bleeding episode, and results of prenatal or neonatal ultrasounds or MRIs are important to collect. Inconsistent findings across studies are likely due to differences in comparison populations, case definitions, and controls for potential confounding variables. Croen et al. (2002) investigated the association between selected infant and maternal characteristics and autism risk in a total population of 3.5 million live births in California over 6 successive years, using multivariate analysis. Increased risks were found for males, multiple births, and children born to African-American mothers. Risk increased as maternal age and education increased. Despite increasing prevalence over the 6 years studied, there were no changes in the patterns of risk. Several prior studies have found similar risks (Bolton and Griffiths 1997; Lord et al. 1991; Nel-

Table 4–1. Components of the medical evaluation

History

    Pregnancy and birth history

    Prenatal exposures to drugs, alcohol, or other neurotoxins

    Review of systems

    Allergy and immune history

    Immunization history and reactions

    Family history

Examination

    Vision and hearing

    Growth parameters and head circumference

    Skin examination

    Dysmorphology examination

    Neurologic examination

Laboratory studies

    FMR1 DNA studies for fragile X

    FISH studies for 15q duplications or deletions

    Selective ordering of tests for *MECP2* and other mutations, dependent on
        clinical phenotype

    Complete blood count with differential

Note.   FISH = fluorescent in situ hybridization.

son 1991; Piven et al. 1993). Intrauterine infections such as rubella, cytomegalovirus, herpes, and HIV have also been associated with ASD,
although they likely represent additive brain trauma to a vulnerable child
(Dykens and Volkmar 1997) rather than a distinct etiology of ASD.

It is essential to ask about exposure during gestation to any potential
neurotoxins that increase risk for abnormal brain development, including
drugs or alcohol, in a nonjudgmental fashion. Prenatal alcohol exposure
has been linked to fetal alcohol syndrome (FAS), the most common preventable cause of mental retardation, as well as alcohol-related neurodevelopmental disabilities (ARNDs) which, combined, are found in nearly
1 per 100 live births (Hagerman 1999b). FAS has been diagnosed in children with autism (Elia et al. 1991), but because FAS/ARND is so common,
the association may be due to chance rather than being a causal association.
Exposures to thalidomide and valproate early in pregnancy have been reported to be associated with autism in humans and social deficits in knockout mice (Rodier et al. 1996). The timing of exposure, at the time of closure
of the neural tube, appears critical and results in a selective loss of neurons
derived from the basal plate of the rhombencephalon. Several etiologic

studies are under way to look further at environmental factors, both prenatal and postnatal, such as maternal hormonal variations, diet, immunologic alterations, and unrecognized exposure to neurotoxins, which may interact with genetic susceptibility to increase the risk of autism. More on this aspect of the evaluation process is included in Chapter 8.

Other parts of the pediatric evaluation include careful assessment and documentation of developmental and behavioral status. A careful history of language development, the age at recognition of language delays, and any history of regression in language and social interactions are important to collect. Some parents are initially concerned about hearing deficits, given the lack of response to speech that is typical in young children with autism. Atypical play behaviors, lack of interest in siblings or peers, and repetitive behaviors emerge as somewhat later concerns. More information on assessment procedures that may be useful in the workup is included in Chapter 3.

A complete medical history and review of systems is important, with an emphasis on symptoms relevant to medical conditions known to be related to autism or to proposed etiologies. The review of systems and past medical history must include vision or hearing problems, including otitis media and placement of polyethylene tubes; unusual or frequently recurring infections suggesting immune dysfunction; thyroid problems, presence of arthritis, or rashes suggestive of autoimmune disorders; an allergy history to foods or environmental triggers; gastrointestinal symptoms such as diarrhea, constipation, bloating, cyclic vomiting, and presence of abdominal pain; and weight or growth problems. The presence of major congenital anomalies such as cardiac or renal abnormalities should be documented, even if not currently medically significant. Chapter 8 contains more detail about assessment and treatment for some of these symptoms. Careful attention must be paid to seizures or seizurelike episodes (eye blinking, staring, abrupt swings in behavior, facial jerking or extremity twitching, etc.). The decision to order an EEG is based on the medical history, so the clinician should ask enough questions to clarify whether an EEG should be done. See Chapter 5 for more detail.

Attention should also focus on the immunization history, especially possible reactions that may have occurred after each dose, such as high fevers, seizures, persistent and prolonged episodes of unsoothable crying, vascular collapse or shock, or any event that required medical attention. A careful history of regression in language or motor behavior around the time of immunization is essential. This topic is covered in more detail in Chapter 8.

The family history is also essential to obtain because of the possibility of the broader autism phenotype, including language deficits, social problems, obsessive-compulsive behavior, learning disabilities, or mental retardation. These findings may suggest increased genetic loading or a specific genetic etiology. Families should be asked specifically about a history of epilepsy, mental retardation, TS, FXS, chromosomal abnormalities, schizophrenia, anxiety, depression, bipolar disorder, and other genetic conditions. In addition, a family history of immunologic diseases such as lupus, Crohn's disease, ulcerative colitis, and thyroid disease should be obtained. Positive family history for any of these may be important in determining etiologic testing in the child being evaluated for ASD. Positive findings may also suggest that further evaluation of identified family members is indicated, particularly those exhibiting the broader autism phenotype.

Examination

The medical examination should include hearing and visual screening. If either is abnormal, then referral for audiometric testing and an ophthalmologic examination is indicated. Vital signs and growth parameters, including height, weight, and head circumference, should be obtained to document abnormalities in growth that may suggest associated medical conditions (e.g., short stature, low weight, and microcephaly in FAS, obesity in PWS).

Research demonstrates that although brain size is usually normal at birth, by 2–4 years the head circumference has shifted upward to a mean at the 67th percentile, with 14%–37% of children with autism above the 97th percentile (Lainhart et al. 1997; Minshew et al. 1997). Neuroimaging studies by Courchesne (2002) showed an anterior to posterior gradient, with frontal lobes being the most abnormally enlarged (dorsolateral and medial prefrontal cortex) and occipital lobes showing the smallest effects. Interestingly, the time of accelerated brain growth appears to coincide with onset of clinical symptoms (Kemper and Bauman 2002). The presence of microcephaly is unusual in autism and suggests a complex etiology that needs further investigation. Thus, it is important to measure and monitor head circumference regardless of the child's age. Isolated macrocephaly without other abnormalities on physical or neurologic examination does not indicate the need for neuroimaging. See Chapter 5 for further discussion of macrocephaly in ASD.

The skin examination should include a careful look for the neurocutaneous features of neurofibromatosis, tuberous sclerosis or hypomelanosis of Ito, such as café au lait spots, hypopigmented macules or swirls (best seen with Wood's lamp), shagreen patches, or angiofibromas. Features of elastic skin or hyperextensible joints are seen in FXS, Williams syndrome, or other connective tissue disorders.

Major and minor congenital anomalies are important to search for and document during the exam. All dysmorphic features such as ear anomalies, epicanthal folds, hypertelorism, mid-face hypoplasia, and dental anomalies must be documented. Coarse facies and enlargement of liver or spleen suggest mucopolysaccharidosis or storage diseases that are rare but require further diagnostic testing, as noted subsequently. Abnormalities of the extremities (clinodactyly, syndactyly, abnormally small or large hands or feet) are important to document as well in trying to define specific genetic syndromes (such as PWS) or clusters of dysmorphic features that may help determine the need for the type of further etiologic studies noted later.

A detailed neurologic examination should document asymmetries in tone or focal neurologic signs, in addition to fine and gross motor coordination abnormalities, generalized hypotonia or spasticity, oral motor coordination problems, cranial nerve abnormalities (seen in Moebius syndrome), and cerebellar dysfunction, including ataxia or tremor. Abnormalities in the neurologic examination, regression in developmental skills, significant birth trauma, significant dysmorphic features, or concern for possible CNS abnormality or malformation suggest the need for MRI. Abnormalities on the neurologic examination or on imaging indicate the need for referral to a pediatric neurologist, if one is not on the evaluation team.

During the medical examination the ability of the child to relate socially, communicate verbally and nonverbally, and engage in joint attention and pretend play can be assessed informally. Formal standardized assessments of these abilities are addressed in Chapter 3. The presence of stereotypies, motor or vocal tics, repetitive behaviors, compulsions, and rigidity in thinking and behavior should be documented. If tics are present, or described by history, it is important to establish their time of onset, pattern, course, and functional impairments. Tics, repetitive behaviors, or self-injurious behaviors that significantly interfere with daily activities and learning, or that result in physical injury that requires treatment, should be evaluated for behavioral intervention and/or medication.

Laboratory Studies

The decision to order further laboratory workup should be guided by the history and examination. Any concerns about hearing or visual impairment require referral to a specialist for thorough evaluation. The medical evaluation should routinely include high-resolution cytogenetic studies, with a particular focus on 15q and 7q (another "hot spot" suggested by molecular genetic studies), in addition to telomere deletions (Chudley et al. 1998; Cook et al. 1997; Filipek et al. 2000; Gillberg 1998; International Molecular Genetic Study of Autism Consortium 2001; Yu et al. 2002). Since duplications or deletions at 15q may not be detected microscopically with high-resolution studies, it is recommended that the molecular technique of FISH be carried out, which utilizes a fluorescent DNA probe for the region of interest. Because the 15q region can cause autism in 1%–4% of patients, we believe that FISH studies for this region should be routinely carried out in all patients with a diagnosis of autism. These patients usually have very subtle or no obvious dysmorphic features, and their IQ can range from normal to severely retarded, so they are difficult to distinguish clinically. Other FISH studies for microdeletion syndromes such as Williams syndrome (7q11), velocardio-facial syndrome (22q11), or Smith-Magenis syndrome (17p11), which almost always have atypical phenotypes, should be ordered only when clinically indicated. Although not yet widely available for clinical assessment, FISH for telomere deletions should be considered in children with ASD and mental retardation if there is a family history of mental retardation, history of intrauterine growth retardation, or the presence of two or more facial or nonfacial dysmorphic features (Baker et al. 2002; de Vries et al. 2001).

Another study that should be routinely ordered in the medical evaluation of children with autism is the *FMR1* DNA study, which detects the fragile X mutation. Since fragile X causes 2%–8% of autism, and many young children do not have the classical phenotype of a long face and prominent ears, this should be routinely tested. In the future, more DNA studies will be routinely available, particularly for critical regions at 7q such as the *FOXP2* gene, which causes severe apraxia and speech and language delays when mutated. It is likely that we will be searching for the interaction of multiple susceptibility alleles or mutations that cause the clinical picture of autism.

One can selectively order the DNA testing for a mutation in the *MECP2* gene that causes Rett disorder in girls and X-linked mental retardation in boys (Couvert et al. 2001). The DNA test involves sequencing of the *MECP2* gene to detect mutations that lead to an abnormal protein. In the past, clinicians have only looked for this mutation in females who presented with a downhill course after the first year, with loss of motor and language milestones and repetitive hand wringing. However, more recent studies of males with X-linked mental retardation have shown that approximately 2% have mutations in *MECP2*, which are not lethal in males and cause mild to moderate mental retardation (Couvert et al. 2001). It is not yet known what percentage of individuals with autism have a mutation in *MECP2*, so at this time it is not routinely studied, but this may change in the future. Phenotypes suggestive of Rett disorder in females and unexplained mental retardation consistent with X-linkage in boys are indicators for testing for a mutation of *MECP2*.

In the future, it is likely that a battery of molecular testing will be completed on a microarray chip that would cover all the alleles potentially related to ASD. Although these studies are carried out in a research format currently, they are not yet utilized clinically.

A complete blood count with differential to look for abnormalities of red and white blood cell indices that may reflect underlying disorders such as anemia or immunologic dysfunction is often obtained, but is rarely helpful without clinical concerns raised by history or examination. There is insufficient evidence to recommend obtaining extensive immunologic studies routinely at this point, although further research may eventually help to define clinical subgroups for which this may be important (see Chapter 8). A chemistry panel including liver and renal function tests that may reflect underlying metabolic disorders is often carried out, particularly in the context of suggestive history or examination.

Quantitative serum amino acid and urine organic acid studies are indicated if the chemistry panel is abnormal, or in cases with a history of cyclic vomiting, lethargy, failure to thrive, deteriorating developmental skills, coarse facial features, or dysmorphology suggesting storage disease, especially when mental retardation is present and when the results of newborn metabolic screening are unknown. Thyroid function studies are indicated if suggested by decelerating growth parameters and abnormalities on examination such as large tongue, dry skin and hair, hypotonia, and mental retardation. Research studies have shown that an identifiable metabolic disorder is seen in less than 5% of those with ASD (Dykens and Volkmar 1997; Filipek et al. 1999), although the yield is higher when there are clinical indications for testing. Serum lead testing is recommended in children with pica or who have persistent mouthing.

Conclusion

The pediatrician has a critical role as a member of the evaluation and treatment team. The routine medical workup includes high-resolution cytogenetic testing, FISH studies for 15q duplications, and *FMR1* DNA testing. Additional blood or urine testing and other studies, such as audiology and visual assessment, MRI, and EEG, are carried out when clinically indicated.

References

Asano E, Chugani DC, Muzik O, et al: Autism in tuberous sclerosis complex is related to both cortical and subcortical dysfunction. Neurology 57:1269–1277, 2001

American Psychiatric Association: Diagnostic and Statistical Manual of Mental Disorders, 4th Edition, Text Revision. Washington, DC, American Psychiatric Association, 2000

Bailey A, Bolton P, Butler L, et al: Prevalence of the fragile X anomaly amongst autistic twins and singletons. J Child Psychol Psychiatry 34:673–688, 1993

Bailey A, Palferman S, Heavey L, et al: Autism: the phenotype in relatives. J Autism Dev Disord 28:369–392, 1998

Bailey DB Jr, Hatton DD, Skinner M, et al: Autistic behavior, FMR1 protein, and developmental trajectories in young males with fragile X syndrome. J Autism Dev Disord 31:165–174, 2001a

Bailey DB Jr, Hatton DD, Tassone F, et al: Variability in FMRP and early development in males with fragile X syndrome. Am J Ment Retard 106:16–27, 2001b

Baker E, Hinton L, Callen DF, et al: Study of 250 children with idiopathic mental retardation reveals nine cryptic and diverse subtelomeric chromosome anomalies. Am J Med Genet 107:285–293, 2002

Bauman M, Kemper TL: Limbic and cerebellar abnormalities: consistent findings in infantile autism. J Neuropathol Exp Neurol, 47:369, 1988

Belser R, Sudhalter V: Conversational characteristics of children with fragile X syndrome: repetitive speech. Am J Ment Retard 106:28–38, 2001

Blomquist HK, Bohman M, Edvinsson SO, et al: Frequency of the fragile X syndrome in infantile autism: a Swedish multicenter study. Clin Genet 27:113–117, 1985

Bolton PF, Griffiths PD: Association of tuberous sclerosis of temporal lobes with autism and atypical autism. Lancet 349:392–395, 1997

Bolton PF, Dennis NR, Browne CE, et al: The phenotypic manifestations of interstitial duplications of proximal 15q with special reference to the autistic spectrum disorders. Am J Med Genet 105:675–685, 2001

Bourneville D: Sclerose tubereuse des circonvolutions cerebrales: idiotie et epilepsie hemiplegique. Arch Neurol (Paris) 1:81–91, 1880

Braden M: Academic interventions in fragile X, in Fragile X Syndrome: Diagnosis, Treatment, and Research, 3rd Edition. Edited by Hagerman RJ, Hagerman PJ. Baltimore, MD, Johns Hopkins University Press, 2002, pp 428–464

Brown WT, Jenkins EC, Cohen IL, et al: Fragile X and autism: a multicenter survey. Am J Med Genet 23:341–352, 1986

Browne CE, Dennis NR, Maher E, et al: Inherited interstitial duplications of proximal 15q: genotype-phenotype correlations. Am J Hum Genet 61:1342–1352, 1997

California Department of Developmental Services: Autistic Spectrum Disorders: Best Practice Guidelines for Screening, Diagnosis and Assessment. Sacramento, CA, California Department of Developmental Services, 2002

Cantú ES, Stone JW, Wing AA, et al: Cytogenetic survey for autistic fragile X carriers in a mental retardation center. Am J Ment Retard 94:442–447, 1990

Cassidy SB, Morris CA: Behavioral phenotypes in genetic syndromes: genetic clues to human behavior. Adv Pediatr 49:59–86, 2002

Christian SL, Fantes JA, Mewborn SK, et al: Large genomic duplicons map to sites of instability in the Prader-Willi/Angelman syndrome chromosome region (15q11–q13). Hum Mol Genet 8:1025–1037, 1999

Chudley AE, Gutierrez E, Jocelyn LJ, et al: Outcomes of genetic evaluation in children with pervasive developmental disorder. J Dev Behav Pediatr 19:321–325, 1998

Cook EH, Lindgren V, Leventhal BL, et al: Autism or atypical autism in maternally but not paternally derived proximal 15q duplication. Am J Hum Genet 60:928–934, 1997

Courchesne E: Abnormal early brain development in autism. Mol Psychiatry 7 (suppl 2):S21–S23, 2002

Couvert P, Bienvenu T, Aquaviva C, et al: MECP2 is highly mutated in X-linked mental retardation. Hum Mol Genet 10:941–946, 2001

Croen LA, Grether JK, Selvin S: Descriptive epidemiology of autism in a California population: who is at risk? J Autism Dev Disord 32:217–224, 2002

Curfs LM, Fryns JP: Prader-Willi syndrome: a review with special attention to the cognitive and behavioral profile. Birth Defects Orig Artic Ser 28:99–104, 1992

de Vries PJ, Bolton PF: Genotype-phenotype correlations in tuberous sclerosis. J Med Genet 37:E3, 2000

de Vries BB, White SM, Knight SJ, et al: Clinical studies on submicroscopic subtelomeric rearrangements: a checklist. J Med Genet 38:145–150, 2001

Dykens EM, Volkmar FR: Medical conditions associated with autism, in Handbook of Autism and Pervasive Developmental Disorders. Edited by Cohen DJ, Volkmar FR. New York, Wiley, 1997, pp 388–407

Elia M, Bergonzi P, Ferri R, et al: The etiology of autism in a group of mentally retarded subjects. Brain Dysfunction 3:228–240, 1991

Filipek PA, Accardo PJ, Ashwal S, et al: Practice parameter: screening and diagnosis of autism: report of the Quality Standards Subcommittee of the American Academy of Neurology and the Child Neurology Society. Neurology 55:468–479, 2000

Filipek PA, Accardo PJ, Baranek GT, et al: The screening and diagnosis of autistic spectrum disorders. J Autism Dev Disord 29:439–484, 1999

Gane L, Cronister A: Genetic counseling, in The Fragile X Syndrome: Diagnosis, Treatment, and Research, 3rd Edition. Edited by Hagerman RJ, Hagerman PJ. Baltimore, MD, Johns Hopkins University Press 2002, pp 251–286

Gillberg C: Autism and related behaviours. J Intellect Disabil Res 37:343–372, 1993

Gillberg C: Chromosomal disorders and autism. J Autism Dev Disord 28:415–425, 1998

Gillberg C, Coleman M: Autism and medical disorders: a review of the literature. Dev Med Child Neurol 38:181–202, 1996

Gillberg IC, Gillberg C, Ahlsen G: Autistic behaviour and attention deficits in tuberous sclerosis: a population-based study. Dev Med Child Neurol 36:50–56, 1994

Gomez M: Tuberous sclerosis complex, in Developmental Perspectives in Psychiatry. Edited by Harris J. New York, Oxford University Press, 1999, p 31

Goodlin-Jones BL, Bacalman S, Jardini T, et al: Fragile X and autism diagnosis by two standard methodologies. Paper presented at the 8th International Fragile X Conference, Chicago, IL, July 17–21, 2002

Hagerman RJ: Medical follow-up and pharmacotherapy, in Fragile X Syndrome; Diagnosis, Treatment, and Research, 2nd Edition. Edited by Hagerman RJ, Cronister A. Baltimore, MD, Johns Hopkins University Press, 1996, pp 283–331

Hagerman RJ: Angelman syndrome and Prader-Willi syndrome, in Neurodevelopmental Disorders: Diagnosis and Treatment. New York, Oxford University Press, 1999a, pp 243–290

Hagerman RJ: Fetal alcohol syndrome, in Neurodevelopmental Disorders: Diagnosis and Treatment. New York, Oxford University Press, 1999b, pp 3–59

Hagerman RJ: Medical follow-up and pharmacotherapy, in Fragile X Syndrome: Diagnosis, Treatment, and Research, 3rd Edition. Edited by Hagerman RJ, Hagerman PJ. Baltimore, MD, Johns Hopkins University Press, 2002a, pp 287–338

Hagerman RJ: The physical and behavioral phenotype, in Fragile X Syndrome: Diagnosis, Treatment and Research, 3rd Edition. Edited by Hagerman RJ, Hagerman PJ. Baltimore, MD, Johns Hopkins University Press, 2002b, pp 3–109

Hagerman RJ, Jackson AW III, Levitas A, et al: An analysis of autism in fifty males with the fragile X syndrome. Am J Med Genet 23:359–374, 1986

Hagerman RJ, Wilson P, Staley LW, et al: Evaluation of school children at high risk for fragile X syndrome utilizing buccal cell FMR-1 testing. Am J Med Genet 51:474–481, 1994

Hills-Epstein J, Riley K, Sobesky W: The treatment of emotional and behavioral problems, in Fragile X Syndrome: Diagnosis, Treatment, and Research, 3rd Edition. Edited by Hagerman RJ, Hagerman PJ. Baltimore, MD, Johns Hopkins University Press 2002, pp 339–362

Hunt A, Shepherd C: A prevalence study of autism in tuberous sclerosis. J Autism Dev Disord 23:323–339, 1993

International Molecular Genetic Study of Autism Consortium: A genomewide screen for autism: strong evidence for linkage to chromosomes 2q, 7q, and 16p. Am J Hum Genet 69:570–581, 2001

Kemper TL, Bauman ML: Neuropathology of infantile autism. Mol Psychiatry 7 (suppl 2):S12–S13, 2002

Lainhart JE, Piven J, Wzorek M, et al: Macrocephaly in children and adults with autism. J Am Acad Child Adolesc Psychiatry 36:282–290, 1997

Lauritsen MB, Mors O, Mortensen PB, et al: Medical disorders among inpatients with autism in Denmark according to ICD-8: a nationwide register-based study. J Autism Dev Disord 32:115–119, 2002

Li SY, Chen YC, Lai TJ, et al: Molecular and cytogenetic analyses of autism in Taiwan. Hum Genet 92:441–445, 1993

Lord C, Mulloy C, Wendelboe M, et al: Pre- and perinatal factors in high-functioning females and males with autism. J Autism Dev Disorder 21:197–209, 1991

Mao R, Jalal SM: Characteristics of two cases with dup(15)(q11.2–q12): one of maternal and one of paternal origin. Genet Med 2:131–135, 2000

Mignon C, Malzac P, Moncla A, et al: Clinical heterogeneity in 16 patients with inv dup 15 chromosome: cytogenetic and molecular studies, search for an imprinting effect. Eur J Hum Genet 4:88–100, 1996

Miles JH, Hillman RE: Value of a clinical morphology examination in autism. Am J Med Genet 91:245–253, 2000

Miller LJ, McIntosh DN, McGrath J, et al: Electrodermal responses to sensory stimuli in individuals with fragile X syndrome: a preliminary report. Am J Med Genet 83:268–279, 1999

Minshew NJ, Sweeney J, Bauman ML: Neurological aspects of autism, in Handbook of Autism and Pervasive Developmental Disorders. Edited by Cohen DJ, Volkmar F. New York, Wiley, 1997, pp 344–369

Nelson KB: Prenatal and perinatal factors in the etiology of autism. Pediatrics 87:761–766, 1991

Nelson KB, Grether JK, Croen LA, et al: Neuropeptides and neurotrophins in neonatal blood of children with autism or mental retardation. Ann Neurol 49:597–606, 2001

Nurmi EL, Bradford Y, Chen Y, et al: Linkage disequilibrium at the Angelman syndrome gene *UBE3A* in autism families. Genomics 77:105–113, 2001

O'Callaghan FJ: Tuberous sclerosis. Br Med J 318:1019–1020, 1999

Piven J, Simon J, Chase GA, et al: The etiology of autism: pre-, peri- and neonatal factors. J Am Acad Child Adolesc Psychiatry 32:1256–1263, 1993

Reiss AL, Freund L: Fragile X syndrome. Biol Psychiatry 27:223–240, 1990

Roach ES, Gomez MR, Northrup H: Tuberous sclerosis complex consensus conference: revised clinical diagnostic criteria. J Child Neurol 13:624–628, 1998

Roberts J, Mirrett P, Burchinal M: Receptive and expressive communication development of young males with fragile X syndrome. Am J Ment Retard 106:216–230, 2001

Rodier PM, Ingram JL, Tisdale B, et al: Embryological origin for autism: developmental anomalies of the cranial nerve motor nuclei. J Comp Neurol 370:247–261, 1996

Rodier PM, Ingram JL, Tisdale B, et al: Linking etiologies in humans and animal models: studies of autism. Reprod Toxicol 11:417–422, 1997

Rogers SJ, Wehner EA, Hagerman RJ: The behavioral phenotype in fragile X: symptoms of autism in very young children with fragile X syndrome, idiopathic autism, and other developmental disorders. J Dev Behav Pediatr 22:409–417, 2001

Rutter M, Bailey A, Bolton P, et al: Autism and known medical conditions: myth and substance. J Child Psychol Psychiatry 35:311–322, 1994

Scharfenaker S, O'Connor R, Stackhouse T, et al: An integrated approach to intervention, in Fragile X Syndrome: Diagnosis, Treatment, and Research, 3rd Edition. Edited by Hagerman RJ, Hagerman PJ. Baltimore, MD, Johns Hopkins University Press, 2002, pp 363–427

Schroer RJ, Phelan MC, Michaelis RC, et al: Autism and maternally derived aberrations of chromosome 15q. Am J Med Genet 76:327–336, 1998

Scott S: Mental retardation, in Child and Adolescent Psychiatry: Modern Approaches. Edited by Rutter M, Taylor E, Hersov L. Oxford, UK, Blackwell Scientific, 1994, pp 616–646

Smalley SL, Burger F, Smith M: Phenotypic variation of tuberous sclerosis in a single extended kindred. J Med Genet 31:761–765, 1994

Steffenburg S: Neuropsychiatric assessment of children with autism: a population-based study. Dev Med Child Neurol 33:495–511, 1991

Steffenburg S, Gillberg CL, Steffenburg U, et al: Autism in Angelman syndrome: a population-based study. Pediatr Neurol 14:131–136, 1996

Thomas JA, Johnson J, Peterson TL, et al: Genetic and clinical characterization of patients with an interstitial duplication 15q11–q13, emphasizing behavioral phenotype and response to treatment. Am J Med Genet (in press)

Turk J, Graham P: Fragile X syndrome, autism, and autistic features. Autism 1:175–197, 1997

Verkerk AJ, Pieretti M, Sutcliffe JS, et al: Identification of a gene (FMR-1) containing a CGG repeat coincident with a breakpoint cluster region exhibiting length variation in fragile X syndrome. Cell 65:905–914, 1991

Vogt H: Zur diagnostik der tuberosen sklerose. Erforsch Behandl jugendl Schwachsinns 2:1–12, 1908

Walker HA: Incidence of minor physical anomaly in autism. J Autism Child Schizophr 7:165–176, 1977

Wassink TH, Piven J, Patil SR: Chromosomal abnormalities in a clinic sample of individuals with autistic disorder. Psychiatr Genet 11:57–63, 2001

Yu CE, Dawson G, Munson J, et al: Presence of large deletions in kindreds with autism. Am J Hum Genet 71:100–115, 2002

Chapter 5

Contributions of Neurology

Barry R. Tharp, M.D.

Introduction

Autism is a neurologic syndrome with predominantly behavioral manifestations. It overlaps clinically with many static and progressive encephalopathies and psychiatric disorders. Many children with autism manifest neurologic symptoms and signs including seizures, dyspraxia, hypotonia, mental retardation, gait abnormalities, and macrocephaly. Children whose autistic behavior is associated with a severe or generalized disturbance of brain function, such as tuberous sclerosis or a chromosomal disorder, may have more striking neurologic deficits, including pyramidal tract findings and ataxia.

We assume that autism is a syndrome with many etiologies. The location of the pathology, rather than the pathology per se, is more than likely responsible for the clinical presentation. This lack of a single etiology behooves the physician to initiate a thorough neurologic and genetic evaluation after making the diagnosis of autism spectrum disorder. Approximately 10%–20% of children with autism spectrum disorders (ASD) have a definable neurodevelopmental genetic syndrome; this number is likely to increase as more sophisticated chromosomal analyses become clinically available (Shevell et al. 2001). These individuals are referred to

111

Table 5–1. Causes of syndromic autism

Chromosomal syndromes (e.g., fragile X, Angelman syndrome, 15q duplication, Down syndrome, del22q11, Ring 20, Rett disorder)

Neurocutaneous syndromes (e.g., tuberous sclerosis)

Syndromes without known chromosomal abnormality (e.g., Sotos, Smith-Lemli-Opitz, Moebius, CHARGE association)

Congenital/acquired infections (e.g., cytomegalovirus)

In utero drug exposure (e.g., thalidomide, valproic acid)

Inherited metabolic disorders

Miscellaneous, including hypoxic-ischemic encephalopathy

as having "syndromic" autism, the remainder as having "idiopathic" autism. The percentage of cases with a definable medical condition varies depending on 1) the year the study was performed (older studies lack the in-depth genetic and imaging capabilities provided in more recent surveys), 2) the criteria for ASD (recent studies are more likely to label children with a diagnosis of ASD who would have been omitted from earlier reports), 3) the ascertainment bias, and 4) the thoroughness of the neurologic assessment (Bertrand et al. 2001; Gillberg and Coleman 1996; Shevell et al. 2001). Large-population studies often rely on the clinical assessments of a wide range of physicians, many with limited or no neurologic or genetic training or expertise with autism. This results in inconsistent diagnostic practices and, consequently, a low incidence of cases identified with a definable syndrome. Smaller cohorts from academic centers with experienced clinicians tend to have a higher percentage of identified syndromes in their populations, which may be due to ascertainment biases. Table 5–1 contains a list of syndromes and medical conditions that appear to be associated with autism. This topic is further discussed later in this chapter and in Chapter 4.

This chapter addresses the more common neurologic etiologies of ASD, the current understanding of the pathological substrate, and the relationship between ASD and seizures. First, recent literature is reviewed, followed by a discussion of practice implications, including findings on neurologic examination and potential neurologic treatment approaches.

Neuroimaging Findings in ASD

Studies of patients with ASD have shown deviations from normal in the volume of the hippocampus and amygdala, cerebellum, brain stem, and neocortex, particularly the frontal and temporal lobes. Decreased volume of the cerebellar vermis, particularly lobules VI and VII, has received the most attention in the literature (Courchesne et al. 1988), although hyperplasia is also reported (Courchesne et al. 1994a). The same research group has shown that these cerebellar changes are age related, with larger cerebellar white matter volumes in childhood, smaller gray matter volumes at older ages, and the volumes of vermal lobules VI and VII diminished throughout life (Courchesne et al. 2001). The direction of the volume changes appears to be related to many factors, including IQ, age, and the control population with which the individuals with ASD were compared (Aylward et al. 1999; Courchesne et al. 1994b; Piven et al. 1992; Sparks et al. 2002). Cerebellar volume loss is more commonly seen in children with autism who also have mental retardation. Vermal hypoplasia is not specific to autism. Schaefer et al. (1996) described vermal atrophy in individuals with a wide variety of neurogenetic disorders, both those that have symptoms in common with autism (fragile X syndrome, Rett disorder) and those that do not (general mental retardation, Usher syndrome, neurofibromatosis).

Hippocampal and amygdala volumes, on the other hand, were found to be increased in children with ASD regardless of IQ (Sparks 2002), but smaller in older individuals. These age-related volumetric changes appear to mirror total brain volume changes, suggesting early brain overgrowth and later slowing of growth or perhaps loss of tissue as the individual ages (Courchesne et al. 2001). However, Saitoh et al. (2001) found that the area dentata (dentate gyrus and CA4) of the hippocampus was significantly smaller on the magnetic resonance imaging (MRI) results of children with autism than normal children, particularly in those of preschool age. In summary, MRI results are variable across studies and do not point to any signature abnormality that is diagnostic of ASD or readily apparent on routine MRI. Volumetric changes evident in group studies are usually not apparent on visual inspection of the MRI. For this reason, an MRI is not recommended as part of the routine workup (see the later section "Practice Parameters").

Neuropathology Findings in ASD

Routine Brain Pathology Studies

The pathology of autism is relatively unimpressive, particularly in the 80%–90% of children with idiopathic autism. The changes present in detailed autopsy studies of a limited number of individuals with autism (most of whom also had significant mental retardation) consist of increased neuronal density, particularly in the hippocampus; olivary dysplasia; scattered areas of cortical and white matter dysplasia, including neuronal ectopia; and other nonspecific developmental abnormalities in the brainstem and cerebellum (Bailey et al. 1998; Bauman 1996; Kemper and Bauman 1993). The amygdala differences reported by Bauman and Kemper (1988) that have received so much attention have not been replicated by other autopsy studies (Bailey et al. 1998).

In children with autism who have well-established syndromes, the pathology is quite ubiquitous; the location of the pathological changes appears to be the critical factor in determining the phenotype, and not the pathology per se. Weidenheim et al. (2001) describe two individuals with autism and neuroaxonal dystrophy, a rare, often familial neurodegenerative disorder. The hallmark pathology of this disorder, the swollen axonal terminal, rarely involves the limbic system, thalamus, and hypothalamus, but was strikingly present in these locations in both individuals. The authors speculated that the location of the pathology may have been responsible for the autistic behavior, which is not typical of the neuroaxonal dystrophy phenotype. Similarly, the location of the brain tubers in children with tuberous sclerosis appears to play a central role in determining which children develop autism. Bolton et al. (2002) found that the presence of tubers in the temporal lobes appeared to be necessary for development of ASD. Thus, the location of the major neuropathology appears critical to the ultimate behavioral phenotype.

Microcolumnar Studies

It is evident from this brief review of the pathology of autism that traditional pathological techniques are not likely to provide information regarding the underlying pathophysiology of this complex disorder. More sophisticated techniques, however, are beginning to yield some interesting results. Casanova and his colleagues have recently described subtle abnormalities of cortical architecture in the neocortex of a small group of autopsied brains (Buxhoeveden et al. 2002; Casanova et al. 2002a, 2002b, 2002c). The cytoarchitecture of the neocortex of most vertebrates and invertebrates is arranged in parallel vertical columns. In humans, the cortex consists of six horizontally oriented laminae and vertical chains of cells that link with the cells of neighboring laminae. The basic unit is the minicolumn, a chain of neurons oriented perpendicular to the cortical surface, surrounded by axons and dendrites coursing vertically to and from the cortical neurons (Mountcastle 1997). Casanova and colleagues (2002a) have utilized a computer imaging technique to quantify the size, density, and number of minicolumns and intervening neuropil per unit distance in sections of neocortex obtained from the superior and middle temporal gyrus and superior and middle frontal gyrus. They described significant changes in the size of the minicolumns, relative to normal controls, in the brains of nine patients with autism, two individuals with Asperger syndrome, and an adult with dyslexia. In the individuals with autism, the minicolumns were smaller and more numerous, their cellular columns were less compact, and the peripheral neuropil space was reduced relative to control subjects. Similar but less striking changes were also seen in the Asperger patients. The individual with dyslexia showed the opposite changes; the minicolumns were larger in area 22 from both hemispheres.

The neurophysiologic consequences of abnormal minicolumn size and function are purely speculative. One could hypothesize that the increased number of columns expands the receptor capabilities of the neocortex, which might explain the heightened sensory awareness and aroused state of some children with autism. For more detailed information on the minicolumn and its role in brain function, the reader is referred to a recent review by Buxhoeveden and Casanova (2002). If other investigators confirm these anatomic observations, it would add support to the hypothesis that autism is a congenital disorder with onset in early fetal life. Researchers are currently unraveling the genetic bases for normal cortical development, including minicolumn structure. Progenitor cell divisions early in gestation determine the size and number of minicolumns (Kornack and Rakic 1995). This knowledge may prove useful in discovering the genetic bases for autism in the future.

Association of ASD and Seizures

Clinical Semiology

Seizures occur more frequently in children with ASD than in typical children. Large epidemiologic studies have shown that approximately 1% of all children without autism will have an afebrile seizure before they reach 14 years of age (Hauser and Nelson 1986). The incidence of seizures in children with autism is clearly higher, but quite variable across studies. Low rates of 3% have been reported in large community-based studies (Bertrand et al. 2001), and much higher rates (over 30%) have been found in smaller selective populations, particularly from large academic referral centers (Rossi et al. 2000). There are a number of possible reasons for this variability, in addition to potential ascertainment biases. First, the diagnosis of seizures can be quite difficult in children with ASD because the repetitive stereotypic behaviors, periods of inattention ("staring spells"), and behavioral outbursts they often manifest may mimic epileptic seizures. The problem is compounded by the fact that electroencephalograms (EEGs) in the pediatric population are often "overread." Normal patterns, particularly during sleep, are often considered epileptiform and in the setting of paroxysmal abnormal behavior lead the clinician to the erroneous diagnosis of seizures. Additionally, nonepileptic children with ASD have an increased incidence of electroencephalographic abnormalities compared with the normal population, which leads to an erroneous diagnosis of epilepsy without a critical review of the behavior in question (Tuchman et al. 1991b). Approximately 5% of normal children have epileptiform activity on a routine EEG, particularly those with a history of febrile seizures or a family history of seizures (Okubo et al. 1994). In some situations, video/electroencephalographic monitoring is necessary to make a firm diagnosis of the events in question. Incidence figures will be higher when children with known neurologic disorders, e.g., tuberous sclerosis and fragile X syndrome, are included in samples along with children with idiopathic autism. For all these reasons, the true incidence of seizures in ASD is not known.

All seizure types have been reported in children with ASD. Simple and complex partial seizures with or without secondary generalization and generalized motor seizures are most common (Tuchman et al. 1991b). Less frequently, generalized nonconvulsive seizures (absences) and myoclonic and drop attacks have occurred. Seizures are more likely to occur in children with mental retardation and those who have significant motor abnormalities on neurologic examination. Our experience and that of others is that the onset of the seizures is most often in the first decade of life, though others have reported another peak in onset in early adolescence. For example, Rossi et al. (2000) found that seizure onset was after the age of 12 in two-thirds of their patients. They also reported that the prevalence of seizures was 38.3%. This high prevalence was probably due to selection bias, as all their patients had mental retardation and one-third had computed tomography (CT)/MRI abnormalities, suggesting a more neurologically compromised group of individuals.

Infantile spasms are frequently followed by a static encephalopathy that includes mental retardation and ASD. Infantile spasms (IMS) that occur as part of the phenotype of tuberous sclerosis (TS) are particularly associated with autism spectrum disorders. It has been reported, for example, that over 50% of infants with TS and IMS develop autism compared with 13% of children with IMS from other etiologies (Hunt and Dennis 1987; Riikonen and Amnell 1981). Asano et al. (2001) performed 2-deoxy-2-[^{18}F]fluoro-D-glucose (FDG) and α-[^{11}C]methyl-L-tryptophan (AMT; a measure of serotonin metabolism) positron emission tomography (PET) scans on 26 children with tuberous sclerosis and intractable epilepsy, 9 of whom had autism. The latter group, compared with TS children without autism, had decreased glucose metabolism in the lateral temporal gyri bilaterally, increased glucose uptake in the deep cerebellar nuclei bilaterally, and increased AMT uptake in the caudate nuclei bilaterally. This is consistent with a previous report by the same research group that approximately 10% of patients with infantile spasms and normal MRI scans had decreased glucose metabolism on PET scan bilaterally in the temporal lobes and were most likely to develop autism (Chugani et al. 1996).

Electroencephalography Findings

Electroencephalographic abnormalities in children with autism have been well chronicled. As with seizures, the reported incidence of epileptiform activity is quite variable across studies, from 15% to over 80% (Lewine et al. 1999), for many of the same reasons. Incidence is dependent on the age of the population studied (low or absent in the very young), the presence or absence of clinical seizures (much higher in children with seizures), the neurologic examination (more frequent in those with abnormal exams), and IQ (more frequent in mentally retarded individuals). Incidence rates of epileptiform activity also differ in syndromic versus idiopathic autism. Children with genetic neurologic disorders, such as fragile X syndrome, tuberous sclerosis, or Angelman syndrome, will have a much higher incidence of electroencephalographic epileptiform abnormalities, approaching 100% for Angelman syndrome (except for those children with the less frequent *UBE3A* mutation). The incidence appears much lower in children with idiopathic autism, particularly if they are high-functioning or have Asperger syndrome.

The EEG morphology of the epileptiform activity reported in children with autism is quite variable, but one of the most frequent patterns is spike or spike-wave discharges over the centrotemporal region (Rossi et al. 1995). These potentials closely resemble the spikes seen in the most common partial epileptic syndrome of childhood, benign rolandic epilepsy. It is also interesting to note that the same pattern is commonly seen in children with Rett disorder (Hagne et al. 1989; Robb et al. 1989), fragile X syndrome (Musumeci et al. 1999), and other rare chromosomal syndromes (Stern 1996; Sturm et al. 2000). Other studies of small numbers of children with purported autism have stressed a preponderance of epileptiform activity in the frontal (Hashimoto et al. 2001) and occipital (Nass et al. 1998) regions.

Magnetoencephalography Findings

Magnetoencephalography measures the magnetic fields of the brain and resembles an EEG. It has been used to record epileptic spikes in the presurgical assessment of patients with epilepsy and, more recently, to identify spikes in children with autism (Lewine et al. 1999). The magnetoencephalogram (MEG) has certain advantages over the conventional EEG; specifically, magnetic fields are less distorted by the scalp and skull, and the source of the spikes can be identified. Though this tool is gaining respect in the search for epileptic foci in individuals with intractable seizures, its value in screening for epileptiform activity (spikes and sharp waves) is more controversial, particularly when one does not know the source of abnormal activity before the recording. (In the presurgical assessment of epileptic patients, the routine EEG, imaging studies, and the semiology of the seizures allow one to select specific brain areas in which to focus the MEG and thus avoid many of the potential problems associated with this technology.)

Magnetoencephalography has disadvantages compared with the conventional EEG, most notably the lack of an established set of criteria for spike identification. The selection of spikes on the MEG is not straightforward, and identification parameters are still being established. It is beyond the scope of this chapter to discuss the many issues surrounding this new technique, particularly regarding the difficulty in the identification of epileptiform potentials. The interested reader is referred to a recent paper that discusses the problems of spike identification in simultaneous MEG and EEG recordings (Zijlmans et al. 2002).

This cautionary approach should be used in interpreting the results of a recent study published in a leading journal using magnetoencephalography in a group of children with autism. The authors reported that an astonishing 82% of 50 children with "regressive autism" had epileptiform abnormalities on the MEG (Lewine et al. 1999). They suggested that the regressive form of autism is more commonly associated with the presence of seizures or epileptiform activity on EEG or MEG than the nonregressive form (Lewine et al. 1999). However, this study had several methodologic limitations. The interpretation of the MEG was not done blind to group membership, and control recordings from an age-matched typical sample were not available. There is also the question of ascertainment bias; 15 children had clinical seizures, and many were referred because of physician concern that they had Landau-Kleffner syndrome (LKS), a rare nonfamilial epileptic syndrome characterized by a regression in development and acquired aphasia. LKS and its relationship to autism are discussed further in a later section of this chapter. Other concerns with the Lewine study are that diagnoses of ASD were not made by objective criteria or confirmed by experts, and no mention was made of other neurologic findings or level of cognitive development. Other problems with this particular study were outlined in a letter to the editor in a subsequent edition of the same journal (Kallen 2001). Other studies have failed to find convincing evidence of an etiologic relationship between regression and epileptiform activity (Tuchman and Rapin 1997; Tuchman et al. 1991b). Despite this, the term *epileptic regression* is sometimes incorrectly used in the autism literature.

The Neurologic Assessment

Early Neurologic Symptoms

Young children with autism are often neurologically normal with typical motor development, but some are characterized by mild motor delays, hypotonia, and toe-walking (Rapin 1996). Somewhat older children may be mildly ataxic, with other subtle signs of cerebellar dysfunction (Haas et al. 1996) and motor symptoms best described as dyspraxic (Weimer et al. 2001). Many of the older studies were undertaken on mixed samples that included children with tuberous sclerosis and other genetic syndromes known to have a high incidence of neurologic findings on examination. For example, Tuchman et al. (1991a) noted that sensorimotor signs and ataxia were more common in children with autism than in children with isolated dysphasia, but the group differences disappeared when girls with Rett disorder were excluded. Motor stereotypies also commonly appear as the child ages. Sensory processing abnormalities frequently appear in the preschool years and consist of an increased or decreased appreciation of a variety of sensory stimuli, paradoxical responses to stimuli, and preoccupation with sensory features of objects. Other, more complex sensory disturbances suggesting parietal lobe dysfunction have been reported, including disturbances in graphesthesia, stereognosis, somatosensory location, spatial orientation, and body posture (Carmody et al. 2001; Haas et al. 1996). Rapin (1996) provided a detailed summary of the components of the neurologic examination.

Megalencephaly

Excessive brain size is more common in children with autism than in those with typical development or other neurodevelopmental disorders (Davidovitch et al. 1996; Fidler et al. 2000). Approximately 10%–20% of children with autism have head circumference above the 97th percentile. Brain weight at autopsy may also be increased in children with autism. In an analysis of brain weight in 21 postmortem cases, Courchesne et al. (1999) found that 3 were megalencephalic and 1 microcephalic. The increase in brain size and weight does not seem to correlate with abnormalities in brain development or pathology on clinical MRI or with routine light microscopy at autopsy. Some of the discrepancies in the literature concerning head size may be related to the age at which the individual was examined. Courchesne et al. (2001) described serial MRI brain volume measurements in 60 autistic and 52 typical boys, ages 2 to 16 years. Head circumference records from birth were also obtained. Brain volume at birth was in the normal range, but 90% of the 2- to 4-year-olds had brain volumes larger than the normal average, and 37% had volumes above the 97th percentile. Cortical gray and white matter and cerebellar white matter volume means exceeded the control subjects' in the 2- to 4-year-old group. The older autistic children and adolescents did not have such enlarged gray and white matter volumes, however, suggesting that abnormal regulation of brain growth resulted in early overgrowth, followed by abnormally slowed growth. In summary, it is important to monitor head circumference in patients with autism, although the clinical significance of the changes and fluctuations is not yet understood.

Practice Parameters

The neurologic assessment of children with suspected autism should include many of the elements already reviewed in Chapters 3 and 4 (e.g., developmental and medical history, observation of the child, structured assessment of autistic symptoms). Here we focus on those aspects that are unique to the neurologic examination. As discussed in the previous chapter, there is debate over the necessity and extent of the laboratory assessment and other medical testing (e.g., immunologic assays, measurement of trace elements, and gastrointestinal surveys), particularly when a specific syndrome is not readily apparent. There is also no consensus on the need for imaging studies, particularly MRI, and electrophysiologic testing, such as electroencephalography. These issues are expanded on in the following discussion.

The recently published practice parameters of the American Academy of Neurology provide recommendations for the identification of the child with autism (Filipek et al. 2000). This section concentrates on recommendations for a level 2 evaluation, which are more relevant to the medical specialist, regardless of whether he or she is a neurologist, psychiatrist, or developmental pediatrician. The committee also provided criteria for level 1 assessment, which are more pertinent to the screening of children in the primary care physician's office. They include screening parameters for all children and particularly those who are at risk (e.g., the sibling of an autistic child). These guidelines included recommendations for screening for a list of specific behavioral milestones that, if not met, should prompt further evaluation. The guidelines also recommend evaluation of lead levels and audiologic assessment.

American Academy of Neurology Level 2 Testing Recommendations

Genetic testing is recommended, including high-resolution chromosome studies and DNA analysis for fragile X, particularly in individuals with mental retardation, family history of undiagnosed mental retardation, or dysmorphic features. The M.I.N.D. Institute Clinic policy is to obtain DNA for fragile X on all boys with ASD, including those who are high-functioning or have Asperger syndrome, and on girls with a family history suggesting fragile X or those with low or borderline intellectual function. We also routinely obtain a fluorescent in situ hybridization (FISH) analysis for 15q duplication on all children with autism. The threshold for more specific genetic testing should be low in evaluating children with ASD. Many clinics screen children for velocardiofacial syndrome, which is due to a 22q11 deletion and has an extremely variable phenotype, ranging from neonatal seizures with hypocalcemia to mental retardation with subtle facial dysmorphism (Roubertie et al. 2001). Another disorder that is sometimes associated with autism is Angelman syndrome, discussed in the previous chapter. It is also becoming increasingly apparent that many children, including males, with Rett disorder have atypical phenotypes that do not meet the criteria originally proposed for this disorder (Hammer et al. 2002; Hoffbuhr et al. 2001). Some appear to have autism, with and without mental retardation, so there should be a low threshold for obtaining the necessary studies for mutations of the *MECP2* gene as well. Genetic testing for many of these disorders is described in detail in Chapter 4.

Metabolic testing should be done if suspicious clinical and physical findings exist, such as "lethargy, cyclic vomiting and early seizures; dysmorphic features or coarse features; evidence of mental retardation or if mental retardation cannot be ruled out; or if occurrence or adequacy of newborn screening at birth is questionable" (Filipek et al. 2000, p. 474). In our experience, metabolic neurodegenerative disorders are usually evident through an inexorable albeit slow clinical progression, abnormalities on the physical examination (hepatosplenomegaly and hair and skin abnormalities), more extensive motor involvement, and progressive behavioral and language deterioration. Therefore, we do not routinely perform metabolic testing on all children with ASD.

The American Academy of Neurology practice parameters do not recommend EEGs for all children with autism. The committee recommends an adequate "sleep-deprived EEG with appropriate sampling of slow wave sleep" in individuals with seizures or suspicion of "subclinical seizures," or with a history of regression at any age (Filipek et al. 2000, p. 474). A definition of "subclinical seizures" was not provided and is controversial (see the earlier discussion of epileptiform activity and autism). In my opinion, this may lead to unnecessary electroencephalographic recordings, including expensive and stressful overnight monitoring. Indeed, it is not clear whether a sleep-deprived tracing is warranted. This activating procedure has been shown to increase the yield of tracings that contain definitive epileptiform discharges in individuals with the generalized epilepsies, but there is little evidence that it is effective in the assessment of the focal epilepsies of childhood, which are most common in autism. It is well known that interictal epileptiform activity is more likely to occur during the transition into light sleep than during deeper stages of sleep. Thus, a routine EEG with sleep is usually adequate to screen for sleep-activated epileptiform discharges. If the child does not sleep, a repeat recording after partial sleep deprivation is then warranted. An EEG obtained after heavy sedation (often needed in the child with autism) is usually much less informative than one obtained during transition into light natural sleep.

Abnormalities in the routine MRI are usually confined to children with known syndromes (e.g., tuberous sclerosis) and are uncommon in children with idiopathic autism. Criteria for determining which population of children with autism is more likely to have clinically relevant information on MRI are not established. The Quality Standards Subcommittee of the American Academy of Neurology states that "routine clinical neuroimaging in the diagnostic evaluation of autism, even in the presence of megalencephaly" is not indicated (Filipek et al. 2000, p. 474). In the M.I.N.D. Institute Clinic, we order an MRI if the child has dysmorphic features, seizures, a family history of developmental or neurologic problems, or abnormalities on the neurologic examination, particularly if they are focal or asymmetrical.

Neurologic Treatment Approaches for ASD

Over the past several decades some physicians and parent groups have endorsed treatment programs for autism that are similar to those used for

Landau-Kleffner syndrome (LKS). These include oral steroids, anticonvulsant medications, and neurosurgery. The pathophysiologic relationship between LKS and autism is tenuous at best, and the evidence supporting the use of these controversial therapies is purely anecdotal. The relationship between these two disorders, in this writer's opinion, is limited: 1) language regression can occur in both conditions, 2) some children with autism have epileptiform activity in the temporal regions, and 3) some children with LKS have some autistic features (although not full-blown ASD). There are no controlled studies that support these therapies for children with ASD.

Anticonvulsant Medication

It has been suggested that suppression of seizures or interictal epileptiform activity with antiepileptic drugs (AEDs) may lead to amelioration of aberrant behaviors, improved cognitive function, and reduction of symptoms of autism (Dulac 2001), but this is controversial. Several AEDs have therapeutic effects on behavior in addition to their anticonvulsant effect. If symptoms of autism improve with these medications, it is most likely from this mechanism rather than from an effect on the abnormal electrical activity (DiMartino and Tuchman 2001). The majority of currently used AEDs have little or no effect on the electroencephalographic interictal discharges, particularly those that are focal (the type typically seen in LKS and autism). Even though total seizure control may be attained, the frequency of focal spikes on the EEG is often unchanged. Generalized spike and wave discharges, commonly recorded in children with generalized nonconvulsive epilepsy (absence seizures), are the primary type of epileptiform activity typically reduced or eliminated with the antiabsence AEDs, such as ethosuximide and valproic acid. The idiopathic generalized epilepsy syndromes, however, are usually not associated with autism. Future studies attempting to show that AEDs improve behavioral symptoms primarily on the basis of the elimination of interictal epileptiform activity will require repeated prolonged EEGs during the treatment period, proper instruments to measure the autistic symptomatology, unbiased and blind raters of behavior, and parental input.

One of the problems inherent in many AED studies is the lack of age- and IQ-matched clinical control groups and unbiased observers. Two papers on the effect of lamotrigine and autistic symptoms illustrate this issue. Uvebrant and Bauziene (1994) reported excellent seizure control by lamotrigine in 45 children and adolescents with intractable epilepsy. In 8 of the 13 children with autism, the autistic symptoms decreased even in those with unchanged seizure frequency. They concluded that there was a "positive psychotropic effect of lamotrigine in mentally retarded and autistic children" (p. 284). However, a subsequent randomized, double-blind, placebo-controlled trial of lamotrigine with 28 nonepileptic children with autism found no evidence of efficacy utilizing a battery of standardized, objective rating instruments (Belsito et al. 2001).

Neurosurgical Approaches to Autism

There is no proven surgical approach to autism. There are anecdotal reports of improvement of autistic symptoms in children after surgery for various brain lesions, most accompanied by seizures. The goal of the surgery was the resection of the offending pathology, usually a tumor in the temporal lobes or an area of cortical dysplasia that was causing severe seizures or other neurologic dysfunction. The results of such lesional surgery are variable, and many children show no improvement in cognition or behavior even with cessation or improvement of the seizures; some may actually deteriorate (Szabo et al. 1999).

A surgical treatment that is being utilized more frequently in children with autism and epileptiform EEG abnormalities, with and without clinical seizures, is multiple subpial transection (MST; Nass et al. 1999; Patil and Andrews 1998). This technique was introduced in the late 1960s for the elimination of epileptiform activity in nonresectable cortex, usually in conjunction with a standard cortical resection or temporal lobectomy (Morrell and Hanbery 1969). The technique consists of multiple parallel linear incisions placed 5 mm apart below the pial surface of cortical gyri in epileptogenic regions. The incision is presumed to interrupt the short horizontal fibers that provide cortical-cortical interactions in the gray matter, the network primarily responsible for supporting the epileptic process. The vertical bundles entering and leaving the cortex, as well as the columns of cortical neurons, are presumed to be preserved. The latter are responsible for the normal function of the cortex and include the long cortico-subcortical connections. Using this technique, the surgeon can eliminate the epileptogenic process while preserving the normal function of the involved cortex. Though this technique is useful in epilepsy surgery, there is evidence that the mechanism of the epileptic suppression may not be as simple as initially proposed. Anatomic examination of specimens that were transected prior to a traditional temporal lobectomy and then removed en bloc for histologic examination showed that deep injury was present in many instances, in addition to interruption of the midcortical horizontal fibers

(Kaufmann et al. 1996). These authors concluded that in addition to horizontal desynchronization, "a deafferentation mechanism involving different fiber systems may contribute to the antiseizure effects of MST" (p. 342).

MST has also been introduced over the last few years to treat children with LKS when the epileptogenic process involves the language cortex (Morrell et al. 1995). Subpial transection of portions of the primary language cortex, the source of the abundant epileptiform activity during sleep, leads to marked clinical improvement in some children with LKS without a significant loss of function. The application of MST to autism is an extension of its use in LKS and is based on the totally unproven relationship between the epileptogenic process and autism, particularly the regressive form (see previous discussion). The clinical data provided in the literature are limited at best, and particularly in reference to the autistic symptomatology, the postoperative observations are inadequate (Nass et al. 1999; Patil and Andrews 1998). Even with the scant follow-up data provided, the improvements were limited and, in the authors' words, "temporary in most cases" (Nass et al. 1999, p. 464). One finds it intuitively difficult to accept the premise that elimination of one or several superficial cortical spike foci in a child without seizures would lead to major improvement in a syndrome that most likely involves diffuse brain pathology. This is an unsupported and potentially dangerous treatment for autism and is not recommended.

Vagal Nerve Stimulation

Stimulation of the left vagal nerve is now an accepted therapy for the treatment of intractable seizures in adults and children (Labar 2000; Murphy and Pediatric Vagal Nerve Stimulation Study Group 1999). Approximately 40% of children will have a significant reduction in seizure frequency, though the response may be delayed to the second postoperative year. The pulse generator is well tolerated and the surgery is relatively straightforward. Many children show an improvement in behavior and improvement in quality of life after implantation. This may be due to reduced seizure frequency, reduction of medication side effects from reduced or discontinued use of AEDs, and perhaps also other effects of the stimulation beyond those directly related to the seizure mechanism. The vagal nerve stimulation has not been implanted in nonepileptic children with autism, but anecdotal reports, lacking in follow-up details, suggest improvement in autistic behavior in some autistic children who also have epilepsy (Murphy et al. 2000).

Conclusion

The neurologic assessment of the child with ASD is essential in clarifying the diagnosis, as well as in examining possible etiologies. This review emphasizes that the patient should be approached, as should any child with an unexplained encephalopathy, with an open mind. A battery of diagnostic tests should be undertaken, dictated by the findings on examination, the family history, the presence of seizures, and the history of a possible significant neurologic insult before or after birth. The physician should be persistent in pursuing a genetic etiology, including consultation with a pediatric geneticist. It is becoming increasingly clear that the earlier the diagnosis is made and behavioral therapy initiated, the better the long-term outcome. The determination of a specific diagnosis is also critical in the determination of prognosis and for genetic counseling. In these roles, the neurologist can contribute significantly to the interdisciplinary assessment of the child.

References

Asano E, Chugani DC, Muzik O, et al: Autism in tuberous sclerosis complex is related to both cortical and subcortical dysfunction. Neurology 57:1269–1277, 2001

Aylward EH, Minshew NJ, Goldstein G, et al: MRI volumes of amygdala and hippocampus in non–mentally retarded autistic adolescents and adults. Neurology 53:2145–2150, 1999

Bailey A, Luthert P, Dean A, et al: A clinicopathologic study of autism. Brain 121:889–905, 1998

Bauman ML: Neuroanatomic observations of the brain in pervasive developmental disorders. J Autism Dev Disord 26:199–203, 1996

Bauman M, Kemper TL: Limbic and cerebellar abnormalities: consistent findings in infantile autism. J Neuropathol Exp Neurol 47:369, 1988

Belsito KM, Law, PA, Kirk KS, et al: Lamotrigine therapy for autistic disorders: a randomized, double-blind, placebo-controlled trial. J Autism Dev Disord 31:175–181, 2001

Bertrand J, Mars A, Boyle C, et al: Prevalence of autism in a United States population: the Brick Township, New Jersey, investigation. Pediatrics 108:1155–1161, 2001

Bolton PF, Park RJ, Higgins JN, et al: Neuro-epileptic determinants of autism spectrum disorders in tuberous sclerosis complex. Brain 125:1247–1255, 2002

Buxhoeveden DP, Casanova MF: The minicolumn hypothesis in neuroscience. Brain 125:935–951, 2002

Buxhoeveden D, Fobbs A, Roy E, et al: Quantitative comparison of radial cell columns in children with Down's syndrome and controls. J Intellect Disabil Res 46:76–81, 2002

Carmody DP, Kaplan M, Gaydos AM: Spatial orientation adjustments in children with autism in Hong Kong. Child Psychiatry Hum Dev 31:233–247, 2001

Casanova MF, Buxhoeveden DP, Switala AE, et al: Minicolumnar pathology in autism. Neurology 58:428–432, 2002a

Casanova MF, Buxhoeveden DP, Switala AE, et al: Asperger's syndrome and cortical neuropathology. J Child Neurol 17:142–145, 2002b

Casanova MF, Buxhoeveden DP, Cohen M, et al: Minicolumnar pathology in dyslexia. Ann Neurol 52:108–110, 2002c

Chugani HT, Da Silva E, Chugani DC: Infantile spasm, III: prognostic implications of bitemporal hypometabolism on positron emission tomography. Ann Neurol 39:643–649, 1996

Courchesne E, Yeung-Courchesne R, Press GA, et al: Hypoplasia of cerebellar vermal lobules VI and VII in autism. N Engl J Med 318:1349–1354, 1988

Courchesne E, Saitoh O, Yeung-Courchesne R, et al: Abnormality of cerebellar vermian lobules VI and VII in patients with infantile autism: identification of hypoplastic and hyperplastic subgroups with MR imaging. Am J Roentgenol 162:123–130, 1994a

Courchesne E, Townsend J, Saitoh O: The brain in infantile autism: posterior fossa structures are abnormal. Neurology 44:214–223, 1994b

Courchesne E, Muller R, Saitoh O: Brain weight in autism: normal in the majority of cases, megalencephalic in rare cases. Neurology 52:1057–1059, 1999

Courchesne E, Karns CM, Davis BS, et al: Unusual brain growth patterns in early life in patients with autistic disorder: an MRI study. Neurology 57:245–254, 2001

Davidovitch M, Patterson B, Gartside P: Head circumference measurements in children with autism. J Child Neurol 11:389–393, 1996

Di Martino A, Tuchman RF: Antiepileptic drugs: affective use in autism spectrum disorders. Pediatr Neurol 25:199–207, 2001

Dulac O: Epileptic encephalopathy. Epilepsia 42 (suppl 3):23–26, 2001

Fidler DJ, Bailey JN, Smalley SL: Macrocephaly in autism and other pervasive developmental disorders. Dev Med Child Neurol 42:737–740, 2000

Filipek PA, Accardo PJ, Ashwal S, et al: Practice parameter: screening and diagnosis of autism. Neurology 55:468–479, 2000

Gillberg C, Coleman M: Autism and medical disorders: a review of the literature. Dev Med Child Neurol 38:191–202, 1996

Haas RH, Townsend J, Courchesne E, et al: Neurologic abnormalities in infantile autism. J Child Neurol 11:84–92, 1996

Hagne I, Witt-Engerstrom I, Hagberg B: EEG development in Rett syndrome: a study of 30 cases. Electroencephalogr Clin Neurophysiol 72:1–6, 1989

Hammer S, Dorrani, N, Dragich J, et al: The phenotypic consequences of *MECP2* mutations extend beyond Rett syndrome. Ment Retard Dev Disabil Res Rev 8:94–98, 2002

Hashimoto T, Sasaki M, Sugai K, et al: Paroxysmal discharges on EEG in young autistic patients are more frequent in frontal regions. J Med Invest 48:175–180, 2001

Hauser WA, Nelson KB: Epidemiology of epilepsy in children. Cleve Clin J Med 56 (suppl 1, pt 2):S185–S194, 1986

Hoffbuhr K, Devaney JM, LaFleur B, et al: *MECP2* mutations in children with and without the phenotype of Rett syndrome. Neurology 56:1486–1495, 2001

Hunt A, Dennis J: Psychiatric disorders among children with tuberous sclerosis. Dev Med Child Neurol 29:190–198, 1987

Kallen RJ: A long letter and an even longer reply about autism magnetoencephalography and electroencephalography. Pediatrics 107:1232–1235, 2001

Kaufmann WE, Krauss GL, Uematsu S, et al: Treatment of epilepsy with multiple subpial transactions: an acute histologic analysis in human subjects. Epilepsia 37:342–352, 1996

Kemper TL, Bauman ML: The contribution of neuropathologic studies to the understanding of autism. Neurol Clin 11:175–187, 1993

Kornack DR, Rakic P: Radial and horizontal deployment of clonally related cells in the primate neocortex: relationship to distinct mitotic lineages. Neuron 15:311–321, 1995

Labar D: Vagus nerve stimulation for intractable epilepsy in children. Dev Med Child Neurol 42:496–499, 2000.

Lewine JD, Andrews R, Chez M, et al: Magnetoencephalographic patterns of epileptiform activity in children with regressive autism spectrum disorders. Pediatrics 104:405–418, 1999

Morrell F, Hanbery JW: A new surgical technique for the treatment of focal cortical epilepsy. Electroencephalogr Clin Neurophysiol 26:120, 1969

Morrell F, Whisler WW, Smith MC, et al: Landau-Kleffner syndrome: treatment with subpial intracortical transaction. Brain 118:1529–1546, 1995

Mountcastle VB: The columnar organization of the neocortex. Brain 120:701–722, 1997

Murphy JV, Pediatric Vagal Nerve Stimulation Study Group: Left vagal nerve stimulation in children with medically refractory epilepsy. J Pediatr 134:563–566, 1999

Murphy JV, Wheless JW, Schmoll CM: Left vagal nerve stimulation in six patients with hypothalamic hamartomas. Pediatr Neurol 23:167–168, 2000

Musumeci SA, Hagerman RJ, Ferri R, et al: Epilepsy and EEG findings in males with Fragile X syndrome. Epilepsia 40:1092–1099, 1999

Nass R, Gross A, Devinsky O: Autism and autistic epileptiform regression with occipital spikes. Dev Med Child Neurol 40:453–458, 1998

Nass R, Gross A, Wisoff J, et al: Outcome of multiple subpial transactions for autistic epileptiform regression. Pediatr Neurol 21:464–470, 1999

Okubo Y, Matsuura M, Asai T, et al: Epileptiform EEG discharges in healthy children: prevalence, emotional and behavioral correlates, and genetic influences. Epilepsia 35:832–841, 1994

Patil AA, Andrews R: Surgical treatment of autistic epileptiform regression. J Epilepsy 11:368–373, 1998

Piven J, Nehme E, Simon J, et al: Magnetic resonance imaging in autism: measurement of the cerebellum, pons, and fourth ventricle. Biol Psychiatry 31:491–504, 1992

Rapin I: Neurological examination, in Preschool Children With Inadequate Communication. Edited by Rapin I. London, Mac Keith Press, 1996, pp 98–122

Riikonen R, Amnell G: Psychiatric disorders in children with earlier infantile spasms. Dev Med Child Neurol 23:747–760, 1981

Robb SA, Harden A, Boyd SG: Rett syndrome: an EEG study in 52 girls. Neuropediatrics 20:192–195, 1989

Rossi PG, Parmeggiani A, Bach V, et al: EEG features and epilepsy in patients with autism. Brain Dev 17:169–174, 1995

Rossi PG, Posar A, Parmegiani A: Epilepsy in adolescents and young adults with autistic disorder. Brain Dev 22:102–106, 2000

Roubertie A, Semprino M, Chaze AM, et al: Neurological presentation of three patients with 22q11 deletion (CATCH 22 syndrome). Brain Dev 23:810–814, 2001

Saitoh O, Karns CM, Courchesne E: Development of the hippocampal formation from 2 to 42 years: MRI evidence of smaller area dentata in autism. Brain 124:1317–1324, 2001

Schaefer GB, Thompson JN, Bodensteiner JB, et al: Hypoplasia of the cerebellar vermis in neurogenetic syndromes. Ann Neurol 39:382–385, 1996

Shevell MI, Majnemer A, Rosenbaum P, et al: Etiologic yield of autistic spectrum disorders: a prospective study. J Child Neurol 16:509–512, 2001

Sparks BF, Friedman SD, Shaw DW, et al: Brain structure abnormalities in young children with autism spectrum disorder. Neurology 59:184–192, 2002

Stern JM: The epilepsy of trisomy 9p. Neurology 47:821–824, 1996

Sturm K, Knake S, Schomburg U, et al: Autonomic seizures versus syncope in 18q-deletion syndrome: a case report. Epilepsia 41:1039–1043, 2000

Szabo CA, Wyllie E, Dolske M, et al: Epilepsy surgery in children with pervasive developmental disorder. Pediatr Neurol 20:349–353, 1999

Tuchman RF, Rapin I: Regression in pervasive developmental disorders: seizures and epileptiform electroencephalogram correlates. Pediatrics 99:560–566, 1997

Tuchman RF, Rapin I, Shinnar S: Autistic and dysphasic children, I: clinical characteristics. Pediatrics 88:1211–1218, 1991a

Tuchman RF, Rapin I, Shinnar S: Autistic and dysphasic children, II: epilepsy. Pediatrics 88:1219–1225, 1991b

Uvebrant P, Bauziene R: Intractable epilepsy in children: the efficacy of lamotrigine treatment, including non-seizure-related benefits. Neuropediatrics 25:284–289, 1994

Weidenheim KM, Goodman L, Dickson DW, et al: Etiology and pathophysiology of autistic behavior: clue from two cases with an unusual variant of neuroaxonal dystrophy. J Child Neurol 16:809–819, 2001

Weimer AK, Schatz AM, Lincoln A, et al: "Motor" impairment in Asperger syndrome: evidence for a deficit in proprioception. J Dev Behav Pediatr 22:92–101, 2001

Zijlmans M, Huiskamp GM, Leijten SS, et al: Modality-specific spike identification in simultaneous magnetoencephalography/electroencephalograpy. J Clin Neurophysiol 19:183–191, 2002

Part III

Treatment

Chapter 6

Nonmedical Interventions for Autism Spectrum Disorders

Ann M. Mastergeorge, Ph.D.
Sally J. Rogers, Ph.D.
Blythe A. Corbett, Ph.D.
Marjorie Solomon, Ph.D.

Introduction

One of the many contradictions in autism is that, on the one hand, it is a disorder marked by severe and chronic impairments in multiple aspects of development and behavior, and on the other hand, hundreds of studies demonstrate the responsiveness of individuals with autism to carefully planned and implemented treatments. The purpose of this chapter is to give the practitioner a sense of the types and ranges of successful and efficacious nonmedical treatments for autism spectrum disorders (ASD). In small or rural communities, few of these treatments may be available, whereas in larger metropolitan areas, parents may face a plethora of choices. All intervention proponents and researchers emphasize that treatment intervention must begin early, be intensive, and actively involve families (e.g., Fenske et al. 1985; Prizant and Wetherby 1988; Rogers 1998). More recently, it has also been emphasized that treatments should be based on sound theoretical constructs, rigorous methodologies, and empirical studies of efficacy (Rogers 1998; Schreibman 2000). The goal of this chapter is to refer practitioners to treatment strategies that have been used successfully with children with ASD and help them decipher which of the treatments available in their community have some empirical support behind them.

The American Psychological Association has defined an empirically supported treatment as one that meets either of the following conditions: 1) significant group differences are apparent in well-designed and independently replicated studies involving random assignment to experimental and alternative treatment or community standard conditions, or 2) changes in targeted variables are evident across a series of independently replicated multiple-baseline-design studies involving three or more subjects (Lonigan et al. 1998). The autism treatment literature consists of many more of the latter designs than group studies, as well as many more short-term than long-term outcome investigations (for a review, see Matson et al. 1996). In this chapter, we review empirical support for the most widely used language, social, behavioral, and educational treatments for ASD. While motor and sensory integration interventions are also commonly used with children with autism, empirical support from controlled trials is limited (Baranek 2002), and thus they will not be discussed here. Practical implications of the research literature for clinical care of children with ASD are provided.

Language Interventions

Basic Language Skill Approaches

It is difficult to overemphasize the importance of language interventions for children with ASD. Language functioning is the strongest predictor of outcome in autism (Venter et al. 1992), and very limited language at age 5 is a powerful indicator of severe handicap in adulthood (Lotter 1974; Rutter 1984). For several decades, the clinical literature suggested that a large proportion of children with autism remained nonverbal. More recently, however, there is agreement from several different research groups, using very different approaches to language intervention, that 75%–95% of young children with autism can develop useful speech when provided with specific language interventions that are sufficiently intense. What are these effective interventions and how are they delivered? Several excellent reviews have recently been published, and the reader is referred to them for additional information (Goldstein 2002; Koegel 2000; National Research Council 2001). Three approaches for basic language skill acquisition are described next: discrete trial training interventions, naturalistic behavioral interventions, and developmental-pragmatic interventions.

Discrete Trial Training Interventions

Several different approaches have demonstrated success at teaching basic speech and language skills to children with autism. Probably the best-known approach at this time involves the use of behavioral techniques as described by Lovaas (1981, 1987) and commonly referred to as discrete trial training (DTT). Skills are taught through discrete teaching trials that consist of a trainer-provided antecedent (an instruction and/or stimulus), a behaviorally defined response from the child, and a consequence that rewards a correct response or marks an incorrect response. Complex behaviors are broken down into individual, teachable skills through a process known as task analysis. Techniques such as shaping, prompting, and chaining are then used to develop the new behavior. The DTT teaching style is highly directive. The teaching adult chooses which skill is to be taught, gives an instruction, requires the child to respond, provides consequences for the response, and repeats the sequence until the response is mastered. DTT can be used to teach many different kinds of skills; in this section, we focus on its application to language.

Relying on the child's imitation of adult speech, DTT uses prompting, shaping, and chaining strategies to build understanding and use of single words, and then various word combinations. For children who do not yet imitate speech, verbal imitation itself is taught. While early language lessons focus on naming and requesting objects, later lessons target a wide range of language functions (asking questions, conversing, describing, commenting, social greetings, etc.) (Lovaas 1981). Studies demonstrate that DTT approaches result in short-term language gains and, in Lovaas's studies (to be discussed later in this chapter), long-term effects on intelligence and behavior. Although the DTT approach results in acquisition of language abilities in many previously nonverbal children, it has been criticized for its dependence on extrinsic adult-delivered reinforcement and the rote and repetitive nature of the teaching sessions. Language learned in DTT teaching sessions may not readily generalize to other situations or people unless generalization is specifically considered and programmed through careful instructional strategies (Goldstein 2002).

Naturalistic Behavioral Interventions

Other approaches teach basic language skills within a more natural interactive exchange, while also relying upon behavioral techniques. For the purposes of this chapter, these will be referred to as naturalistic behavioral approaches (which are also used to teach a variety of other skills beyond language; see later discussion). Two models with several similarities fall within this category, pivotal response training (PRT; L.K. Koegel et al. 1998; Pierce and Schreibman 1997) and incidental teaching (McGee et al. 1983, 1985). Instead of teaching specific verbal responses (e.g., individual words), as is the focus in applied behavior analysis, PRT teaches "pivotal" communication behaviors that can have broad effects on language, such as requesting. Incidental teaching engineers the environment to motivate communication (e.g., by providing desirable toys and activities) and then uses any child-initiated communication as an opportunity to prompt for more elaborate communication. Both of these approaches grew out of Hart and Risley's (1975) work to improve language development in young children with language delays in preschool settings. Both approaches use discrete teaching episodes, but they are delivered quite differently from DTT. In the naturalistic approaches, the teaching episode begins with a child communication, generally a request. The teaching adult follows the child's request with a prompt for a more mature level of communication, and then delivers the item the child asked for after the response.

Key differences from DTT are 1) child initiation of communication, rather than adult directiveness, 2) use of intrinsic rather than extrinsic reinforcement, and 3) instruction in the natural context, rather than at a table using drill and practice. For these naturalistic approaches to work most effectively, there must be many opportunities for communication. Thus, the adult must set up the situation in such a way that the child will need to communicate spontaneously in some way. For example, enticing objects may be placed within sight but out of reach. Once the child has spontaneously initiated communication of any form, no matter how basic, the adult follows with a prompt or model, rather than directing the child to produce a specific response. Perhaps the child will reach for the object while crying. The teacher then prompts for a more mature form of communication, perhaps molding the hand into a pointer, and then gives the child the object. The child's attainment of his or her original goal is the reinforcement for the communication, rather than adult delivery of a reinforcer that is not part of the ongoing activity. Repetitions of the behavior for practice are delivered in the same naturalistic fashion. This kind of teaching is much closer to natural communicative exchanges than the DTT approach. Comparative data suggest that naturalistic paradigms lead to more rapid generalization of language skills and more spontaneous language use (see Delprato 2001 for a review). However, naturalistic approaches require that the child be motivated for objects and activities and spontaneously produce some type of communication. Some children, particularly those with very low rates of initiations, may need to begin with a more adult-directed DTT approach before they can make maximum use of naturalistic paradigms.

Developmental-Pragmatic Interventions

Treatment models based on the developmental-pragmatic approach adhere closely to principles of child development in their recognition that communicative and cognitive development typically occur through affective exchanges and social interactions. Thus, such approaches emphasize play, child-centered control of interactions, and sharing emotions with others (Prizant and Wetherby 1998). Following the child's lead and "tempting" communication by entering his or her world are central tenets of these models. The primary goals of developmental-pragmatic therapies are to foster warmth and pleasure in relationships, motivating the child to communicate by teaching that communication with others is satisfying and enjoyable.

The empirical literature supporting the efficacy of this approach is limited. Rogers et al. (1986, 1989, 1991) reported outcomes of a large group of children with autism enrolled in a daily group program that focused particularly on communication, affect, engagement, and development of social relationships. By age 5, 75% of the children used multiword speech in communicative fashion, including 50% of those who were nonverbal at the time they began the program. Similarly, Greenspan and Wieder (1997) described outcomes of their therapy approach, called the Developmental Individual-difference Relationship-based (DIR) model, using record reviews. They highlighted language and affective gains made by the children. While these reports are encouraging, the research designs do not unambiguously demonstrate treatment effects and do not meet the criteria set out by the American Psychological Association for empirically supported treatments. More research is needed to determine whether the developmental-pragmatic approaches to teaching language are as effective as behavioral models.

Complex Language Intervention Approaches

A number of creative approaches have been developed to improve the pragmatics of communication, including initiation of communication, use of gestures and body language, and turn taking. Initiation is a very significant problem for many children with autism. Some children have the ability to speak yet do so relatively infrequently, mostly in response to other people's initiations. Lack of initiation severely limits opportunities for communicative exchanges, social relationships, and learning from others. Krantz and McClannahan (1993) described a creative approach to increasing initiations that builds on the typically good visual skills of children with autism. They wrote instructions on cards that they embedded in the child's schedule in class. These instructions prompted the child to approach a peer and make a comment. Children followed the instructions, which were faded over time. The intervention increased not only conversational initiations, but also spontaneous comments to others. Koegel (2000) described other approaches that increase conversational initiations. Other complex communication skills that research demonstrates can be successfully taught include articulation and gestures. R. L. Koegel et al. (1998) published a single subject design study demonstrating the use of pivotal response training techniques to improve articulation. Buffington et al. (1998) reported a behavioral treatment targeted at increasing and normalizing conversational gestures in children with autism. Outcome data demonstrated that the children with autism had generalized the gestures to other contexts and were indistinguishable from typical peers in the form of the gestures.

For individuals who are not verbal, other kinds of communication systems need to be taught as early as possible. Lack of functional communication skills is thought to contribute significantly to the problematic behaviors that some children with ASD display. Current best practices for handling unwanted behaviors focus on teaching the child an alternative, acceptable communication strategy for meeting the goals that the unwanted behavior currently provides. For example, if a child is screaming or throwing things to communicate that he or she is frustrated, a more appropriate behavior, such as raising a hand, ringing a bell, or turning sideways in the seat, can be taught to signal the need for help. This approach uses the reinforcement strength of the child's internally motivated goal to support the newly taught communicative behavior rather than the previously used unwanted behavior. See O'Neill et al. (1996) for detailed information about using communication interventions to replace unwanted behaviors.

Functional communication skills for children who are not yet verbal involve visual systems. In the current zeitgeist of autism treatment, pictorial symbols are the strategies most often taught. Several studies have demonstrated the efficacy of using pictures as communication devices for requesting (Reichle et al. 1996). One of the most widely used approaches is the Picture Exchange Communication System (PECS) described by Bondy and Frost (1994). Unlike most picture systems, the PECS program teaches the child to *initiate* a picture request and persist with the communication until the partner responds. PECS has a detailed and straightforward treatment manual that lays out a clear step-by-step teaching process. Although there are no replicated studies to date demonstrating its effectiveness, the original article is convincing, and the methods and theoretical basis are quite strong. Variations of pictures used in other visual communication systems include drawings, photos, objects, and printed word cards (e.g., the Treatment and Education of Autistic and Related Communication-handicapped Children [TEACCH] model; Schopler et al. 1995).

In contrast to the use of picture systems, which are burgeoning in autism intervention, the use of sign language is much less common now than in past treatment programs. The special knowledge that the communicative partner must have to understand a child's signs makes it less effective as a general communication tool than speech, print, or pictures. And the difficulty that many nonverbal children have imitating other people's movements (Rogers et al. 1996) makes signing hard to teach. On the other hand, the strength of sign is its constant availability and the ease with which meaning can be elaborated. Goldstein (2002) reviews a number of studies that demonstrated success in using sign to teach nonverbal children with autism to communicate.

One issue that often presents itself to clinicians is parental resistance to the use of alternative communication systems (picture or sign), due to the worry that the child will have less motivation to speak if he or she can rely on nonspoken means. There are no data to support this position, however, and there are several studies (Bondy and Frost 1994; Layton 1988) and much clinical experience demonstrating that noncommunicative children will be more stimulated to learn speech if they already understand something about symbolic communication. For children for whom speech is difficult, these alternative systems provide a way of mapping meaning onto a symbol. Since the augmentative symbols are always accompanied by spoken words (or should always be), the meaning and power of spoken words may in fact be highlighted by the use of alternative symbols. For both cognitive and emotional development, it is crucial that children can communicate their wants and experiences and can understand the communications of other people in some way. Thus, it is an essential part of any treatment program to provide a symbolic communication system that is effective for the child and can be used spontaneously and independently.

Practitioner Implications

The studies on language interventions for children with autism reviewed in this section have some clear messages for practitioners. One is that virtually all children with autism can learn to use some type of symbolic communication system to express needs, wants, and preferences. Another message is that the majority of children with autism can learn to use multiword speech as a communication system. Use of speech is a predictor of outcome (Venter et al. 1992). Thus, it must be the expectation of all practitioners that children with autism in their care be provided with the types of interventions reviewed here that are known to be effective in teaching communication (National Research Council 2001). Communication intervention should begin immediately and be pursued systematically, generally involving daily teaching episodes. The focus on teaching initial skills has to be matched by a focus on maintenance and generalization of learned skills across environments and communicative partners. The practitioner needs to be aware of the details of the child's communication interventions across contexts (e.g., the Individualized Education Plan [IEP], other written treatment plans, at home) and how progress is being monitored and evaluated. Poor progress indicates ineffective teaching approaches and signals a need for an immediate reconsideration of the child's treatment plan (National Research Council 2001). Finally, there is only limited evidence that attending speech and language therapy sessions once or twice a week results in significant language gain (Stone and Yoder 2001). If the individual conducting the child's language treatment is not using approaches such as those described here or is not giving parents activities to continue treatment at home on a daily basis, then it is possible that the child is not receiving effective treatment.

Social Competency Interventions

The literature contains a wide range of creative and effective methods for helping children with ASD develop appropriate social behaviors. Available social interventions vary along a few important dimensions: who is initiating the social exchange (adult vs. peer), the context (individual vs. group teaching), and the specific social goal being taught (initiations vs. responses, play, etc.). Following are descriptions and empirical reviews of a number of teaching techniques for enhancing the social abilities of children with ASD.

Adult-Delivered Interventions

Social Skills Groups

Many researchers and clinicians believe that social behavior should be taught in social settings (e.g., groups) rather than in one-on-one teaching contexts. Consequently, group interventions are frequently included in treatment for persons with ASD, allowing practice of skills in a scaffolded and supportive social situation. Social skills groups may be diagnostically homogeneous, including only children with ASD, or may be diverse and inclusive in their membership. Models and empirical support exist for each approach. Most groups described in the literature have been developed for children with ASD who have language and are relatively high-functioning.

Topics that social skills groups often address include appropriate body language and eye contact, emotion recognition and understanding, perspective taking, and conversational skills. Basic behaviors important to interactions, such as introducing oneself, joining a group, giving compliments, negotiating, sharing, and taking turns, are also a typical focus of social skills groups. Additionally, they often address social problem-solving skills, such as handling teasing and being told "no," dealing with being left out, and regulating and expressing emotions in age-appropriate ways. Most social skills training groups consist of a fairly consistent set of activities, including didactic social "lessons," group games and activities, conversation periods, and food-related activities. Some groups also include "field trips" to practice newly acquired skills in the community. Several authors have outlined suggestions for social skills group schedules, activities, and participant composition, and the interested reader is referred to these for more detail (Gutstein and Sheely 2002; Krasny et al., in press; Mesibov 1986).

Several descriptive studies, without control groups for comparison, have been conducted to examine the outcome of this form of intervention (Howlin and Yates 1999; Marriage et al. 1995; Mesibov 1984; Williams 1989). These studies report high satisfaction with the intervention by participants and parents, but only relatively modest improvement in specific target skills (conversational reciprocity, eye contact, etc.). More recently, a few empirical studies have used control group designs to examine the efficacy of social skills groups. One found improvement on laboratory measures of perspective taking, but gains did not generalize to more naturalistic contexts or produce changes in teacher-reported social behavior (Ozonoff and Miller 1995). Two new controlled studies suggest that social skills groups may be efficacious in improving participants' moods and senses of atypicality and inadequacy (Ozonoff et al. 2002a; M. Solomon et al., under review).

Social skills groups often are implemented in school settings. A recent paper by Bauminger (2002) described a school-based social interaction curriculum for high-functioning children with ASD, age 8–16 years. Her approach combined twice-weekly school-based social groups with home interventions implemented by parents. Children demonstrated social growth in a number of different areas, and improvements were sustained into the following school year. The results of this study demonstrate both the effectiveness of carefully designed and implemented social skills groups and the level of intensity and follow-through needed to achieve positive outcomes. As with all other areas of treatment reported in this chapter, social interventions for children with autism require careful planning, sustained delivery, and measurement of outcomes in order to realize their positive potential.

Social Stories

Another adult-mediated intervention that is often used in schools, this one administered individually in a one-on-one teaching context, is Gray's social story technique. Social stories are written (sometimes illustrated) stories that teach social rules and appropriate social behavior (Gray and Garand 1993). The stories can be individualized to the needs of each child and have been used to teach dozens of social behaviors, such as taking turns, waiting in lines, greeting others, and sharing. Although the technique is widely discussed and recommended, little empirical work has been done to examine its efficacy. A few small studies have demonstrated the utility of social stories for increasing sharing, play, and appropriate initiations and reducing aggression (Kuttler et al. 1998; Norris and Dattilo 1999; Swaggert et al. 1995), but more investigation of this potentially promising intervention is clearly needed.

Visual Cuing

A very creative visual cuing system has been described with both preschoolers and older children by Krantz and McClannahan (1993), who used printed cues in the children's work schedules to stimulate social initiations to other peers with autism.

Social Games

Use of games to increase peer interactions has been described by two groups. Goldstein et al. (1988) taught socio-dramatic scripts to trios of preschool children consisting of two typical peers and a child with autism. Baker et al. (1998) created games that revolved around the special interests of a child with autism and then taught the game to the child and some typical peers during a playground period at school. Both techniques increased peer interactions in multiple ways.

Techniques for the Home Setting

Social skills must be practiced on a daily basis for generalization and maintenance of skills to occur. Thus, the development and implementation of techniques that can be used by parents at home is important. Ozonoff et al. (2002b) provide a number of recommendations for working on social skills at home. These techniques are most appropriate for verbal children with ASD and their parents:

- Write out and rehearse "scripts" for common social situations.
- Videotape conversations and interactions, review the tapes, and coach on appropriate behaviors.
- Arrange well-supervised, structured "play dates," where important skills like taking turns, sharing, and compromising can be practiced.
- Provide structured conversation times at home where children are encouraged to stay away from circumscribed interests and talk about other age-appropriate topics.
- Enroll the child in groups that revolve around his or her special interests so that there is an opportunity to meet like-minded others.

Others have provided suggestions for working on social and communication skills (Gutstein and Sheely 2002; McAfee 2002), some of which are appropriate for low verbal or nonverbal children with autism (Quill 1995). However, there have been no empirical studies of these approaches to date.

Video Modeling

Another approach to teaching social behavior (as well as many other skills) is video modeling (Dorwick and Jesdale 1991). In this technique, a "model" (adult or peer) demonstrates a behavior on videotape that can be imitated. Segments are typically quite short (5 to 15 seconds in length). An adult reviews the videotape with the child and then immediately prompts imitation of the behavior ("let's do that!"). The use of video appears to offer many advantages to individuals with ASD, as it capitalizes on their typically good visual skills and also their natural interest in television and video media (Krantz et al. 1991).Video modeling has been used successfully to teach children with ASD a number of different social and communication skills, including conversation (Charlop and Milstein 1989), affectionate statements (Charlop and Walsh 1986), toy play, receptive and expressive language, and emotion recognition and expression (Corbett et al. under review). It has also been used to teach adaptive behavior, such as shopping skills (Haring et al. 1995). In some studies, video modeling has yielded better skill acquisition, maintenance, and generalization of behavior than in vivo teaching techniques (Charlop-Christy et al. 2000; Haring et al. 1987). These interventions appear very promising, and more research on them is needed.

Peer-Mediated Techniques

The largest body of published work focuses on peer-mediated interventions for improving social behavior, perhaps because the current emphasis on inclusive school experiences for children with disabilities has made peer interaction such a focal issue. Progress in this area has been profoundly influenced by the work of Strain, Odom, Goldstein, and their associates, who have developed a number of successful peer-mediated strategies over the past 20 years (Goldstein and Strain 1988; Odom and Strain 1986; Strain et al. 1979). Their work has the strongest empirical support of any single social intervention for autism. Typical preschool peers are taught to initiate "play organizing" behaviors, such as sharing, helping, and giving affection and praise, with children with autism. Peers first role-play with adults until they have learned the strategies successfully. Then adults cue them to interact with the target children around typical play materials and activities. The peers are initially reinforced by adults for their efforts, but the reinforcements are systematically and carefully faded over time. These strategies are powerful at increasing social interactions of young children with autism. Both generalization and maintenance of social behaviors have been demonstrated in inclusive preschool classes, as reported in many multiple baseline studies (Goldstein et al. 1992; Hoyson et al. 1984; Odom and Strain 1986; Odom et al. 1999; Strain et al. 1977, 1979).

Over the years these researchers have carefully explored variables involved in achieving maximum effects, including generalization and maintenance. Variables have included characteristics of the peers, methods of prompting and reinforcing peers, fading reinforcers, ages of children, and characteristics of the setting. Various replications of these techniques have demonstrated the importance of using multiple peer trainers in achieving generalization across untrained peers (Brady et al. 1987) and of maintaining skills in the peer trainers (Sainato et al. 1992). Self-monitoring systems have been successfully used to maintain the interactions without adult reinforcement (Strain et al. 1994). Delivering these interventions in inclusive preschools rather than lab settings results in the most stable, generalized, and well-maintained increases in social interactions. Finally, Strain and colleagues demonstrated that parents could be taught to teach peer-mediated approaches to siblings at home, with resulting improvements in child-sibling interactions (Strain and Danko 1995; Strain et al. 1994).

Lord and colleagues have used group designs to examine the effects of typical peers on the social engagement of children with autism. They have demonstrated that daily exposure to untrained but motivated peers increases social engagement, social responsiveness, and constructive play, as well as decreases purposeless activity (Lord and Magill-Evans 1995). Lord and Hopkins (1986) demonstrated that daily exposure in play sessions with same-age untrained peers elicited more social behavior from children with autism than similar sessions with younger peers. Significant increases were found in a number of social behaviors, including proximity, appropriate play, time spent looking at peers, and time engaged socially with peers. These effects generalized to new peers who were introduced to the setting. Another study examined the effects of differing types of play materials on dyadic peer play with a typical child (Dewey et al. 1988). The study demonstrated that rule-governed games facilitated the most complex social interactions, were the most fun, and kept the children most involved with the peer. Construction materials were the next most effective in facilitating social interactions, with dramatic and functional play least helpful in promoting peer play.

Naturalistic Behavioral Techniques

Approaches similar to those described in the language intervention section have also been used to teach social behavior in peer-mediated teaching situations. McGee and colleagues have taught typical peers in inclusive classrooms to prompt social behavior using incidental teaching techniques (McGee et al. 1992). Results for three children with autism demonstrated long-term (5-month) increases in both reciprocal social behavior and social initiations, as well as higher peer acceptance. Typical peers maintained greatly increased rates of social initiations to the children with autism after the fading of adult prompts. However, gains generalized to other contexts for only one of the three children.

Schreibman and colleagues have trained typical peers to use pivotal response techniques (described earlier) to enhance peer interactions and increase the complexity of sociodramatic play (Pierce and Schreibman 1997; Thorp et al. 1995). Pivotal response training has also been used to increase symbolic play skills and positive responses to adult initiations (Stahmer 1995). Naturalistic techniques similar to PRT have been described for teaching minimally verbal children and teenagers to play catch and share objects (Coe et al. 1990).

Practitioner Implications

This review of social interventions for children with ASD contains several important messages for practitioners. The primary conclusion of this section is that the social impairments of autism are remediable. Many creative teaching techniques have been developed that are effective in improving the quality and frequency of the social repertoires of children with autism. Peer-mediated approaches appear to be particularly effective, as they eliminate the need to transfer learning from adult partners to peers. This is an important feature because studies have demonstrated that adult-directed training does not easily generalize to social interactions with peer partners. The most effective peer interventions involve trained peers but are complex to deliver. They require skilled typical peers and precise adult control of training, managing and fading reinforcement, and monitoring ongoing child interaction data. Fortunately, many of the approaches are now well described in manuals and publications (e.g., Danko et al. 1998).

As with communication interventions, explicit teaching of social behavior needs to be part of each child's treatment plan. Different techniques have been demonstrated to be effective for children with autism across wide age ranges and functioning levels. Lack of speech does not prevent development of increased social skills. However, social interactions do require communication, further underscoring the need for all children with autism to be taught symbolic communication systems that they can use to initiate interactions and respond to others. As stated earlier, poor progress indicates ineffective teaching approaches and signals a need for a reexamination of the treatment plan (National Research Council 2001).

Interventions for Unwanted Behaviors

Functional Analysis and Positive Behavioral Support

The treatment of unwanted behaviors, particularly self-injury, aggression, and stereotyped behavior, is a critical component for practitioners working with individuals with autism, as these behavioral excesses are highly concerning to families and teachers and can significantly affect the success of other interventions. Left untreated, they can drastically limit a child's access to available treatments, activities, interactions with others, and community experiences. While medication is often the first treatment considered for these problem behaviors (see Chapter 7), behavioral treatments also have a well-established history as empirically validated treatments for unwanted behaviors and should be the first intervention applied.

The technique of functional behavior analysis underlies most well-designed behavioral treatment. It rests on the assumption that behaviors exist in a person's repertoire because they serve an adaptive function, resulting in some kind of gain. Functions of problem behaviors include attainment of positive reinforcement (a desired object or activity) and escape from undesired events. Because these behaviors are supported by their consequences, they will not go away on their own. There is no point to waiting them out. In the absence of treatment, unwanted behaviors are very likely to worsen rather than improve. They need to be treated, and the earlier they are treated, the more rapid and successful the improvement. In a functional analysis, the target behavior is first carefully defined, and then the frequency and intensity of the behavior are measured across several days and situations to get a baseline against which to measure improvement. The selected target needs to be an observable, definable, measurable behavior (e.g., "hits self with hand") rather than an inference about the cause of the behavior (e.g., "gets frustrated when asked to complete work").

The second step of a functional analysis involves determining the antecedent events that immediately precede the behavior and the consequences or gains that the person receives from carrying out the behavior. Positive events that the person may attain include attention (even negative attention), desired objects, or desired sensations (e.g., self-stimulation). Negative reinforcers generally involve escape or avoidance of disliked tasks, people, environments, or stimuli, or escape from pain or events that were in the past associated with discomfort. Identifying the gains that the behavior provides determines the *function* of the behavior.

One of the biggest changes in behavioral treatment over the past two decades is the replacement of punishment procedures with more positive behavioral approaches. Studies have demonstrated that punishment procedures are less effective than reinforcement approaches and may result in avoidance of adults, negative affect on the part of both children and adults, lack of maintenance and generalization, and lack of replacement of the unwanted behavior with more desirable behaviors. Some punishment approaches used in the past are now considered inhumane and unethical.

Positive behavioral approaches begin by requiring the treatment team to answer the following question: What do you want the child to do instead of what he is now doing to receive the reward he seeks? This simple but pivotal question reveals two fundamental values in this approach. First, the goal is not to eliminate a behavior from a child's repertoire or to end a child's desire for a certain consequence. Children like what they like and want what they want. They are entitled to their choices and preferences, as are all of us. Thus, there is an underlying respect for the child and a recognition of the right to goals (including the right to say no). The second value in this approach is that the focus is now on teaching the child a substitute behavior rather than on eliminating an unwanted behavior from an already limited behavioral repertoire. Several recent reviews of this literature are available to the interested reader (Didden et al. 1997; Horner et al., in press; Koegel et al. 1996; O'Neill et al. 1996).

Finally, functional analysis can be used to prevent behavior problems from developing, in addition to treating them once they occur. This involves careful control of the antecedents that may precede problem behavior. Environments are carefully examined to determine if the curriculum, social milieu, scheduling of activities, and access to reinforcers are appropriate and support positive experiences, learning, and relationships for children with autism, thus minimizing the power of unwanted behaviors (Carr et al. 1998; Dunlap et al. 1991). By changing the antecedents in a behavioral chain, we can prevent the unwanted behaviors from occurring.

Self-Management Approaches

Self-management approaches teach individuals to monitor their own behavior and reinforce themselves. Koegel et al. (1992) used such an approach to increase appropriate verbal responses to others' social initiations. Children were taught to distinguish appropriate from inappropriate verbal responses. They then were taught to use a wrist counter to keep track of their verbal responses. The frequencies they recorded were converted to points and exchanged at intervals for small rewards, mainly edibles. Reinforcement was thinned quickly within the first few training sessions. Each of the four children reported in the study demonstrated rapid improvement in appropriate responding that remained at high levels across the rest of the study; there were also collateral decreases in inappropriate language and disruptive behavior. However, withdrawal of the procedure resulted in decreases in responding for two of the four children. Koegel and Frea (1993) reported a similar self-management approach to improving conversational skills in two high-functioning teenagers with autism. The children rapidly learned the desired behavior, achieving 100% on the first day of intervention. Careful fading of reinforcers resulted in conversational behaviors maintained for 30-minute intervals between reinforcement, with generalization of conversational skills to new situations and improvements in other social-communication skills. Thus, self-management programs demonstrate promise for children with ASD.

Educational Interventions

Comprehensive Preschool Interventions

The interventions reviewed thus far are focused on fairly specific target skills. An additional body of intervention studies examines "comprehensive" treatment programs. Such interventions target multiple areas of development (language, cognition, social behavior, motor and self-help skills, etc.), are delivered many hours per week, and extend over long periods of time, from 1 to 2 or more years. In contrast to the studies reviewed thus far, investigations of comprehensive treatment programs generally involve pooled group data, and change is often measured by rise in standardized test scores over time.

Comprehensive preschool treatment models arise from a variety of theoretical backgrounds, including behavioral and developmental approaches. They are delivered in various ways, including specialized, center-based, group preschool programs; inclusive preschool programs; and individual teaching. In the past 15 years, outcome studies of different models have demonstrated significant enhancement in the development of young children with autism. Parents who have just received a diagnosis of autism for their young child ask professionals for guidance to the best treatment approaches. Unfortunately, there are very few studies that have used controlled group designs and no studies that have directly compared different approaches. Several excellent reviews of this literature exist (Dawson and Osterling 1997; National Research Council 2001; Rogers 1998). Handleman and Harris (2001) have written a text appropriate for both professionals and parents that describes many of the best-known preschool education models in detail, along with their supporting data.

The best designed of the preschool outcome studies, and the only replicated intervention, is the applied behavior analysis (ABA) method developed by Lovaas and colleagues. Both the original study (Lovaas 1987; McEachin et al. 1993) and two replication studies that used random group assignment (Smith et al. 1997, 2000) demonstrated significant change in intelligence and behavior in children receiving one-on-one home-based ABA at least 27 hours a week for 2 years. The original study reported that a substantial proportion of participants, close to 50%, were symptom-free after the intervention (Lovaas 1987; McEachin et al. 1993), but the two replications have not found the same magnitude of IQ and language gain (Smith et al. 1997, 2000). Far less developmental gain was realized by children who met full criteria for autistic disorder than those diagnosed with pervasive developmental disorder not otherwise specified (PDDNOS)

(Smith et al. 1998). These points notwithstanding, the group data support an overall enhancement of developmental rate for children who receive ABA delivered by well-trained and supervised staff for 27 or more hours per week.

Several other comprehensive preschool models have published outcome studies, most using retrospective designs without control groups or random assignment. Some approaches, such as the Princeton Child Development Institute (McClannahan and Krantz 2001) and the Douglass Developmental Disabilities Center (Harris et al. 2001), employ discrete trial behavioral methods, but, unlike Lovaas's model, deliver them in group settings rather than individually in homes. Several programs use the naturalistic behavioral approaches and peer-mediated models described earlier, including pivotal response training (Koegel et al. 1999), the Walden Preschool (McGee et al. 2001), and the LEAP program (Strain and Cordisco 1994). Developmental-pragmatic approaches that emphasize relationships, affect, and play, in addition to language and other developmental skills, include the Denver Model (Rogers et al. 2001) and Developmental Individual-Difference Relationship-Based Treatment (DIR; Greenspan and Wieder 1997). An approach that utilizes visual structure and organization of the environment and learning materials is the TEACCH program, which is also generally characterized as a developmental approach, with considerable focus on learning cognitive, adaptive behavior, and independence skills (Marcus et al. 2001; Schopler et al. 1995). The differences among these approaches are often less marked than they might seem, given that they all focus on intensive teaching of developmentally necessary skills. Prizant and Wetherby (1998) have provided a helpful way of comparing these approaches on a continuum of characteristics (structure, child choice, etc.) rather than seeing them as distinct and unrelated to each other.

Most comprehensive programs available to young children with autism come from community sources, as opposed to these "brand-name" intervention programs. Thus, most practitioners will be in the situation of helping families evaluate various local choices, rather than selecting a model delivered by experts in the field. Several sources have distilled the essential elements of effective early intervention programs for individuals with autism (Dawson and Osterling 1997; National Research Council 2001; Prizant and Wetherby 1998; Rogers 1998):

- Intervention must begin early, as soon as children are identified as being at risk for autism, rather than being deferred for a definitive diagnosis.
- Intervention must be intensive, 25 or more hours per week, 52 weeks per year, with a low ratio of students to teachers.

- Intervention must involve family participation in the development of goals, priorities, and treatment plans and provide ongoing parent support, training, and consultation.
- Intervention must be individualized to the specific needs, strengths, interests, and challenges of the child.
- Intervention must be designed and delivered by experienced, professional interdisciplinary teams.
- Intervention objectives should target the development of social attention, peer interaction, functional spontaneous language, and appropriate toy play, and decrease problem behaviors using positive behavioral approaches.
- Progress must be evaluated frequently and adjusted or redesigned as needed when it is not adequate.

Educational Interventions for School-Age Children With ASD

As with comprehensive preschool programs, educational intervention for older children with ASD involves assessment of existing skills, definition of goals and objectives, selection and implementation of appropriate techniques, assessment of progress, and adaptation of teaching strategies so that students acquire target skills (Cipani and Spooner 1994). Every educational placement for individuals with autism, regardless of their age, should document this process.

Many educational interventions for school-age students with ASD rely on techniques described in earlier sections, including discrete trial and naturalistic behavioral principles, peer mediation, visual cuing, and careful organization and structuring of the environment. Children may be educated in a variety of different settings or placements, including regular classrooms and special classes for children with disabilities. Children of any functioning level (not just those who are verbal or of average intelligence) can be educated in inclusive settings, but significant supports and accommodations are necessary to make these placements work. For children who are eligible for special education services, the educational program is laid out in the IEP. Most children with ASD, whether they receive special education or not, benefit from a variety of accommodations in the school setting. An accommodation is an alteration in presentation format, response format, or setting in which education takes place. Accommodations do not substantially change level, content, or performance, but rather make equitable both instruction and testing formats for the learner. They may include consistent rules and routines, visual schedules, written directions, reduced workload, access to a keyboard for writing tasks, and alternative formats for assignments and tests (see Myles and Adreon 2001 and Ozonoff et al. 2002b for more educational accommodations and practical recommendations).

Special Education Law and Issues

The final topic for this chapter involves the laws that underlie special education and rehabilitation services for children with autism. It is important that all practitioners be aware of the educational rights of the children for whom they provide care. The existing laws provide protection for children and assert their right to the least restrictive environment that is effective in educating them. Practitioners need to understand what these laws entail (and what they do not) and communicate this to families to ensure the delivery of an appropriate education.

Public Law 94-142 and the Individuals With Disabilities Education Act

In 1975 Public Law 94-142 (PL 94-142) was instituted. It required schools to assess children to determine eligibility for special education services, design individualized educational plans to meet the needs of each child, and deliver education in the least restrictive environment possible. This law was reauthorized in 1997 as the Individuals With Disabilities Education Act (IDEA). The law serves a dual purpose: 1) it is a grants program that provides funds to states to serve students with disabilities in need of special education, and 2) it extends the constitutional right to equitable educational opportunities to all students, regardless of disability. IDEA mandates that an IEP be set up for all eligible children. Eligibility guidelines vary from state to state, but generally require a discrepancy between a child's IQ and his or her academic or other functional skills to qualify for special education. IDEA mandates that a team develop, review, and revise the IEP. The IEP team consists of teachers, other school personnel providing services to the child (e.g., speech or occupational therapist), school administrators, and parents. The IEP is best thought of as a contract between parents and schools that outlines what the team agrees is an appropriate education for the child, how it will be delivered, and how it will be evaluated to see if it is working. The IEP specifies long-term goals and short-term objectives for the child's education.

Section 504 of the Rehabilitation Act of 1973

If a child is not eligible for special education, school districts still have a legal obligation to serve students with disabilities under civil rights law statutes, one of which is Section 504 of the Rehabilitation Act of 1973. Section 504 states that districts must provide a free and appropriate education to school-age children regardless of the nature and severity of their disability. Disabilities are broadly defined in this legislation (more broadly than in IDEA) as any limit in any major life activity, including "learning." At first, this law was interpreted as an obligation to provide *physical* access to education for people with disabilities (e.g., curb cuts, elevators, sign language interpreters). More recently, however, the meaning of "access" to an appropriate education has been expanded. Section 504 has increasingly been used to secure services for children with disabilities who do not qualify for special education but still have educational needs. As such, it is ideal for children with high-functioning autism spectrum disorders, who may not display educational delays but still require classroom accommodations or special services such as social skills groups. All school districts have a "504 coordinator," who plans and manages such programs. If a child is not eligible for special education, practitioners should steer the parents toward the school's 504 coordinator to see what other types of accommodations can be offered.

National and state parent education and advocacy groups can provide further help to parents regarding their child's educational rights according to these laws. The Appendix contains a list of many of these groups. The most effective treatment that exists for autism is educational intervention, and the law assures each child's right to an appropriate educational program. Practitioners must help parents attain appropriate services for their children with autism. Existing educational systems do not always have the necessary expertise to provide an appropriate education, but they must take the steps necessary to uphold the laws that mandate this. Lack of resources at a school district level is not an excuse for inadequate education for children with autism. Practitioners can play an important role in advocating for educational rights and in helping parents evaluate whether the services being offered to their child are appropriate.

Conclusion

Parents of children with autism often seek out professionals to help them make decisions about appropriate interventions and educational choices for their children. The practitioner who agrees to take on this role is responsible for learning about empirically supported practices and sharing relevant information with families. Making intervention decisions requires ongoing evaluation of children's current strengths and needs. There is no one intervention that is right for all children with autism or that treats all their developmental needs. Children with autism are a very heterogeneous group and interventions must be fitted to the specific child, in the specific family and community context, at a specific point in time. Although all parents share a long-term goal of the best possible outcome, they differ greatly in immediate and short-term objectives. Thus, practitioners in a guidance role must frequently update their knowledge of the child's current needs, the family's current goals, and the current educational plan, as well as current empirical findings in the autism treatment literature. Clearly, this takes time, energy, and commitment to a child and family unlike that required in much other clinical work, and sometimes over many years. The rewards for this work lie in the progress that a child with autism can make over time and the hope and resilience families can maintain as they raise a child with autism.

References

Baker MJ, Koegel RL, Koegel LK: Increasing the social behavior of young children with autism using their obsessive behaviors. J Assoc Pers Sev Handicaps 23:300–308, 1998

Baranek G: Efficacy of sensory and motor interventions for children with autism. J Autism Dev Disord 32:397–422, 2002

Bauminger N: The facilitation of social-emotional understanding and social interaction in high-functioning children with autism: intervention outcomes. J Autism Dev Disord 32:283–298, 2002

Bondy AS, Frost LA: The Picture Exchange Communication System. Focus on Autistic Behavior 9:1–19, 1994

Brady MP, Shores RE, McEvoy MA, et al: Increasing social interactions of severely handicapped autistic children. J Autism Dev Disord 17:375–390, 1987

Buffington D, Krantz P, McClannahan L, et al: Procedures for teaching appropriate gestural communication skills to children with autism. J Autism Dev Disord 28:535–545, 1998

Carr EG, Carlson JI, Langdon NA, et al: Two perspectives on antecedent control, in Antecedent Control: Innovative Approaches to Behavior Support. Edited by Luiselli JK, Cameron J. Baltimore, MD, Brookes, 1998

Charlop MH, Milstein JP: Teaching autistic children conversational speech using video modeling. J Appl Behav Anal 22:275–285, 1989

Charlop MH, Walsh ME: Increasing autistic children's spontaneous verbalizations of affection: an assessment of time delay and peer modeling procedures. J Appl Behav Anal 19:307–314, 1986

Charlop-Christy MH, Le L, Freeman KA: A comparison of video modeling with in vivo modeling for teaching children with autism. J Autism Dev Disord 30:537–552, 2000

Cipani E, Spooner F: Curricular and Instructional Approaches for Persons With Severe Disabilities. Boston, MA, Allyn and Bacon, 1994

Coe D, Matson J, Fee V, et al: Training nonverbal and verbal play skills to mentally retarded and autistic children. J Autism Dev Disord 20:177–187, 1990

Corbett BA: Video modeling interventions to treat children with autism. J Am Acad Child Adolesc Psychiatry 41:73–74, 2002

Danko CD, Lawry J, Strain PS: Social Skills Intervention Manual. Denver, CO, University of Colorado, Center for Collaborative Leadership, 1998

Dawson G, Osterling J: Early intervention in autism, in The Effectiveness of Early Intervention: Second Generation Research. Edited by Guralnick MJ. Baltimore, MD, Brookes, 1997, pp 307–326

Delprato DJ: Comparisons of discrete-trial and normalized behavioral language interventions for young children with autism. J Autism Dev Disord 31:315–325, 2001

Dewey D, Lord C, Magill J: Qualitative assessment of the effect of play materials in dyadic peer interactions of children with autism. Can J Psychol 42:242–260, 1988

Didden R, Duker PC, Korzilius H: Meta-analytic study of treatment effectiveness for problem behaviors with individuals who have mental retardation. Am J Ment Retard 101:387–399, 1997

Dorwick PW, Jesdale DC: Practical Guide to Using Video in the Behavioral Sciences. New York, Wiley, 1991

Dunlap G, Kern-Dunlap L, Clarke S, et al: Functional assessment, curricular revision, and severe problem behaviors. J Appl Behav Anal 24:387–397, 1991

Fenske EC, Zalenski PJ, Krantz PJ, et al: Age at intervention and treatment outcome for autistic children in a comprehensive intervention program. Analysis and Intervention in Developmental Disabilities 5:49–58, 1985

Goldstein H: Communication intervention for children with autism: a review of treatment efficacy. J Autism Dev Disord 32:373–396, 2002

Goldstein H, Strain PS: Peers as communication intervention agents: some new strategies and research findings. Topics in Language Disorders 9:44–57, 1988

Goldstein H, Wickstrom S, Hoyson M, et al: Effects of sociodramatic play training on social and communicative interaction. Education and Treatment of Children 11:97–117, 1988

Goldstein H, Kaczmarek L, Pennington R, et al: Peer-mediated intervention: attending to, commenting on, and acknowledging the behavior of preschoolers with autism. J Appl Behav Anal 25:289–305, 1992

Gray C, Garand J: Social stories: improving responses of students with autism with accurate social information. Focus on Autistic Behavior 8:1–10, 1993

Greenspan SI, Weider S: Developmental patterns and outcomes in infants and children with disorders in relating and communicating: a chart review of 200 cases of children with autistic spectrum diagnoses. Journal of Developmental and Learning Disorders 1:87–141, 1997

Gutstein SG, Sheely RK: Relationship Development Intervention With Young Children: Social and Emotional Development Activities for Asperger Syndrome, Autism, PDD, and NLD. London, Jessica Kingsley, 2002

Handleman JS, Harris SL (eds): Preschool Education Programs for Children With Autism, 2nd Edition. Austin, TX, Pro-Ed, 2001

Haring TG, Kennedy CH, Adams MJ, et al: Teaching generalization of purchasing skills across community settings to autistic youth using videotape modeling. J Appl Behav Anal 20:89–96, 1987

Haring TG, Breen CG, Weiner J, et al: Using videotape modeling to facilitate generalized purchasing skills. Journal of Behavioral Education 5:29–53, 1995

Harris SL, Handleman JS, Arnold MS, et al: The Douglass developmental disabilities center: two models of service delivery, in Preschool Education Programs for Children With Autism, 2nd Edition. Edited by Handleman JS, Harris SL. Austin, TX, Pro-Ed, 2001, pp 233–260

Hart B, Risley TR: Incidental teaching of language in the preschool. J Appl Behav Anal 8:411–420, 1975

Horner R, Strain P, Carr E: Problem behavior interventions for young children with autism: a research synthesis. J Autism Dev Disord 32:423–446, 2002

Howlin P, Yates P: The potential effectiveness of social skills groups for adults with autism. Autism 3:299–307, 1999

Hoyson M, Jamieson B, Strain PS: Individualized group instruction of normally developing and autistic-like children: the LEAP curriculum model. Journal of the Division of Early Childhood 8:157–172, 1984

Koegel LK: Interventions to facilitate communication in autism. J Autism Dev Disord 30:383–391, 2000

Koegel LK, Koegel RL, Hurley C, et al: Improving social skills and disruptive behavior in children with autism through self-management. J Appl Behav Anal 25:341–353, 1992

Koegel LK, Koegel RL, Dunlap G: Positive Behavioral Support. Baltimore, MD, Brookes, 1996

Koegel LK, Koegel RL, Carter CM: Pivotal responses and the natural language teaching paradigm. Semin Speech Lang 19:355–371, 1998

Koegel, LK, Koegel RL, Harrower JK, et al: Pivotal response intervention: overview of approach. J Assoc Pers Sev Handicaps 24:174–185, 1999

Koegel RL, Camarata S, Koegel L, et al: Increasing speech intelligibility in children with autism. J Autism Dev Disord 28:241–251, 1998

Koegel RL, Frea WD: Treatment of social behavior in autism through the modification of pivotal social skills. J Appl Behav Anal 26:369–377, 1993

Krantz PJ, McClannahan LE: Teaching children with autism to initiate to peers: effects of a script-fading procedure. J Appl Behav Anal 26:121–132, 1993

Krantz PJ, MacDuff GS, Wadstrom O, et al: Using video with developmentally disabled learners, in Practical Guide to Using Video in the Behavioral Sciences. Edited by Dorwick PW. New York, Wiley, 1991, pp 256–266

Krasny L, Williams BJ, Provencal S, et al: Social skills interventions for the autism spectrum: essential ingredients and a model curriculum. Child Adolesc Psychiat Clin N Am 12:107–122, 2003

Kuttler S, Myles BS, Carlson JK: The use of social stories to reduce precursors to tantrum behavior in a student with autism. Focus on Autism and Other Developmental Disabilities 13:176–182, 1998

Layton TL: Language training with autistic children using four different modes of presentation. J Commun Disord 21:333–350, 1988

Lonigan, CJ, Elbert JC, Johnson SB: Empirically supported psychosocial interventions for children: an overview. Journal of Clinical Child Psychiatry 27:138–145, 1998

Lord C, Hopkins JM: The social behavior of autistic children with younger and same-age nonhandicapped peers. J Autism Dev Disord 16:249–262, 1986

Lord C, Magill-Evans J: Peer interactions of autistic children and adolescents. Dev Psychopathol 7:611–626, 1995

Lotter V: Factors related to outcome in autistic children. J Autism Child Schizophr 4:263–277, 1974

Lovaas OI: Teaching Developmentally Disabled Children: The "Me" Book. Baltimore, MD, University Park Press, 1981

Lovaas OI: Behavioral treatment and normal educational and intellectual functioning in young autistic children. J Consult Clin Psychol 55:3–9, 1987

Marcus L, Schopler E, Lord C: TEACCH services for preschool children, in Preschool Education Programs for Children With Autism, 2nd Edition. Edited by Handleman JS, Harris SL. Austin, TX, Pro-Ed, 2001, pp 215–232

Marriage KJ, Gordon V, Brand L, et al: A social skills group for boys with Asperger's syndrome. Aust N Z J Psychiatry 29:58–62, 1995

Matson JL, Benavidez DA, Compton LS, et al: Behavioral treatment of autistic persons: A review of research 1980 to the present. Res Dev Disabil 17:433–465, 1996

McAfee J: Navigating the Social World. Arlington, TX, Future Horizons, 2002

McClannahan LE, Krantz PJ: Behavior analysis and intervention for preschoolers at the Princeton Child Development Institute, in Preschool Education Programs for Children With Autism, 2nd Edition. Edited by Handleman JS, Harris SL. Austin, TX, Pro-Ed, 2001, pp 191–214

McEachin JJ, Smith T, Lovaas OI: Long-term outcome for children with autism who received early intensive behavioral treatment. Am J Ment Retard 97:359–372, 1993

McGee GG, Almeida MC, Sulzer-Azaroff B, et al: Promoting reciprocal interactions via peer incidental teaching. J Appl Behav Anal 25:117–126, 1992

McGee GG, Krantz PJ, Mason D, et al: A modified incidental-teaching procedure for autistic youth: acquisition and generalization of receptive object labels. J Appl Behav Anal 16:329–338, 1983

McGee GG, Krantz PJ, McClannahan LE: The facilitative effects of incidental-teaching on preposition use by autistic children. J Appl Behav Anal 18:17–32, 1985

McGee GG, Daly T, Jacobs HA: The Walden early childhood programs, in Preschool Education Programs for Children With Autism, 2nd Edition. Edited by Handleman JS, Harris SL. Austin, TX, Pro-Ed, 2001, pp 157–190

Mesibov GB: Social skills training with verbal autistic adolescents and adults: a program model. J Autism Dev Disord 14:395–404, 1984

Mesibov GB: A cognitive program for teaching social behaviors to verbal autistic adolescents and adults, in Social Behavior in Autism. Edited by Schopler E, Mesibov GB, Kunce JT. New York, Plenum, 1986, pp 265–283

Myles BS, Adreon D: Asperger Syndrome and Adolescence: Practical Solutions for School Success. Shawnee Mission, KS, Autism Asperger, 2001

National Research Council: Educating Children With Autism. Washington, DC, National Academy Press, 2001

Norris C, Dattilo J: Evaluating effects of a social story intervention on a young girl with autism. Focus on Autism and Other Developmental Disabilities 14:180–186, 1999

Odom SL, Strain PS: A comparison of peer-initiation and teacher-antecedent interventions for promoting reciprocal social interaction of autistic preschoolers. J Appl Behav Anal 19:59–71, 1986

Odom SL, McConnell SR, McEvoy MA, et al: Relative effects of interventions for supporting the social competence of young children with disabilities. Topics in Early Childhood Special Education 19:75–92, 1999

O'Neill R, Horner R, Albin R, et al: Functional Assessment and Program Development for Problem Behavior: A Practical Handbook. Pacific Grove, CA, Brookes/Cole, 1996

Ozonoff S, Miller JN: Teaching theory of mind: a new approach to social skills training for individuals with autism. J Autism Dev Disord 25:415–433, 1995

Ozonoff S, Provencal S, Solomon M: The effectiveness of social skills training programs for autism spectrum disorders. Paper presented at the annual meeting of the American Academy of Child and Adolescent Psychiatry, San Francisco, CA, 2002a

Ozonoff S, Dawson G, McPartland J: A Parent's Guide to Asperger Syndrome and High Functioning Autism. New York, Guilford, 2002b

Pierce K, Schreibman L: Multiple peer use of pivotal response training to increase social behaviors of classmates with autism: results from trained and untrained peers. J Appl Behav Anal 30:157–160, 1997

Prizant B, Wetherby A: Providing services to children with autism (0–2 years) and their families. Topics in Language Disorders 9:1–23, 1988

Prizant B, Wetherby A: Understanding the continuum of discrete-trial traditional behavioral to social-pragmatic developmental approaches in communication enhancement for young children with autism/PDD. Semin Speech Lang 19:329–353, 1998

Quill KA: Teaching Children With Autism: Strategies to Enhance Communication and Socialization. Albany, NY, Delmar, 1995

Reichle J, McEvoy M, Davis C, et al: Coordinating preservice and in-service training of early interventionists to serve preschoolers who engage in challenging behavior, in Positive Behavioral Support. Edited by Koegel LK, Koegel RL, Dunlap G. Baltimore, MD, Brookes, 1996, pp 227–264

Rogers SJ: Empirically supported comprehensive treatments for young children with autism. J Clin Child Psychol 27:168–179, 1998

Rogers SJ, DiLalla D: A comparative study of a developmentally based preschool curriculum on young children with autism and young children with other disorders of behavior and development. Topics in Early Childhood Special Education 11:29–48, 1991

Rogers SJ, Lewis H: An effective day treatment model for young children with pervasive developmental disorders. J Am Acad Child Adolesc Psychiatry 28:207–214, 1989

Rogers SJ, Herbison J, Lewis H, et al: An approach for enhancing the symbolic, communicative, and interpersonal functioning of young children with autism and severe emotional handicaps. Journal of the Division of Early Childhood 10:135–148, 1986

Rogers SJ, Bennetto L, McEvoy R, et al: Imitation and pantomime in high functioning adolescents with autism spectrum disorders. Child Dev 67:2060–2073, 1996

Rogers SJ, Hall T, Osaki D, et al: The Denver Model: a comprehensive integrated educational approach to young children with autism and their families, in Preschool Education Programs for Children With Autism, 2nd Edition. Edited by Handleman JS, Harris SL. Austin, TX, Pro-Ed, 2001, pp 95–134

Rutter M: Autistic children growing up. Dev Med Child Neurol 26:122–129, 1984

Sainato DM, Goldstein H, Strain PS: Effects of self-evaluation on preschool children's use of social interaction strategies with their classmates with autism. J Appl Behav Anal 25:127–141, 1992

Schopler E, Mesibov GB, Hearsey K: Structured teaching in the TEACCH system, in Learning and Cognition in Autism. Edited by Schopler E, Mesibov GB. New York, Plenum, 1995, pp 243–268

Schreibman L: Intensive behavioral/psychoeducational treatments for autism: research needs and future directions. J Autism Dev Disord 30:373–378, 2000

Smith T, Lovaas OI: Intensive and early behavioral intervention with autism: the UCLA Young Autism Project. Infants and Young Children 10:67–78, 1998

Smith T, Eikeseth S, Klevstrand M, et al: Intensive behavioral treatment for preschoolers with severe mental retardation and pervasive developmental disorder. Am J Ment Retard 102:238–249, 1997

Smith T, Groen AD, Wynn JW: Randomized trial of intensive early intervention for children with pervasive developmental disorder. Am J Ment Retard 105:269–285, 2000

Stahmer AC: Teaching symbolic play skills to children with autism using pivotal response training. J Autism Dev Disord 25:123–142, 1995

Stone WL, Yoder PJ: Predicting spoken language level in children with autism spectrum disorders. Autism 5:341–361, 2001

Strain PS, Cordisco LK: LEAP preschool, in Preschool Education Programs for Children With Autism. Austin, TX, Pro-Ed, 1994, pp 225–244

Strain PS, Danko CD: Caregivers' encouragement of positive interaction between preschoolers with autism and their siblings. Journal of Emotional and Behavioral Disorders 3:2–12, 1995

Strain PS, Shores RE, Timm MA: Effects of peer social initiations on the behavior of withdrawn preschool children. J Appl Behav Anal 10:289–298, 1977

Strain PS, Kerr MM, Ragland EU: Effects of peer-mediated social initiations and prompting/reinforcement procedures on the social behavior of autistic children. J Autism Dev Disord 9:41–54, 1979

Strain PS, Kohler FW, Storey K, et al: Teaching preschoolers with autism to self-monitor their social interactions: an analysis of results in home and school settings. Journal Emotional and Behavioral Disorders 2:78–88, 1994

Swaggert BL, Gagnon E, Bock SJ, et al: Using social stories to teach social and behavioral skills to children with autism. Focus on Autism and Other Developmental Disabilities 10:1–16, 1995

Thorp DM, Stahmer AC, Schreibman L: Effects of sociodramatic play training on children with autism. J Autism Dev Disord 25:265–282, 1995

Venter A, Lord C, Schopler E: A follow-up study of high-functioning autistic children. J Child Psychol Psychiatry 33:489–507, 1992

Williams TI: A social skills group for autistic children. J Autism Dev Disord 19:143–155, 1989

Chapter 7

Pharmacotherapy

Vincent des Portes, M.D., Ph.D.
Randi J. Hagerman, M.D.
Robert L. Hendren, D.O.

Introduction

Autism is a neurodevelopmental disorder characterized by a spectrum of abnormal behaviors that include marked impairment in social interaction and communication, along with restricted, repetitive, and stereotyped patterns of interests and activities (American Psychiatric Association 1994). As summarized in the previous chapter, treatment of autism spectrum disorders (ASD) requires psychological and social approaches including special education, speech and language therapy, and occupational and behavioral therapies (Campbell et al. 1996). Nevertheless, many individuals with ASD remain severely impaired, both from the primary deficits central to the disorder and from the often associated symptoms of aggression, self-injury, hyperactivity, hyperarousal, and anxiety. These behaviors constitute target symptoms for psychopharmacologic interventions.

A tremendous increase in psychotropic pharmacologic agents available for the treatment of ASD has taken place in the past 10 years. Since the late 1970s, researchers have wrestled with the respective efficacy of and interaction between behavior therapy and medications in the treatment of ASD, beginning with Campbell et al. (1978), who studied the efficacy of haloperidol. Following this pioneering study, several pharmacologic classes of psychotropic agents have been successively examined, depending on the dominant pathophysiologic theory of autism at the time: naltrexone, following the opioid dysregulation hypothesis (Sahley and Panksepp 1987); antipsychotics, following the controversial dopaminergic dysfunction hypothesis of autism (Gillberg and Srendsen 1987; McDougle et al. 2000 for review); and fenfluramine and selective serotonin reuptake inhibitors (SSRIs), following findings that serotoninergic pathways are involved in autism (Chugani et al. 1999; McDougle et al. 2000). Fenfluramine, which offered exciting promise in the 1980s, was withdrawn from the U.S. market in 1997 because of lack of consistent efficacy, possible neurotoxic effects of the drug on 5-HT (serotonin) neurons in animals (Schuster et al. 1986), and occasional severe adverse effects, most notably cardiac valvulopathy. The disappointing trajectory of this serotoninergic agent points out a rule of thumb in pediatric psychopharmacology: because medications interfering with a developing brain may have unpredictable deleterious long-term consequences, controlled studies are warranted for every psychotropic agent prescribed in children with ASD. Nevertheless, as described in this chapter, double-blind, placebo-controlled studies in children with autism are scarce and difficult to implement. Many medications, such as SSRIs, are currently widely prescribed despite a lack of controlled studies in childhood and U.S. Food and Drug Administration (FDA) approval in this age group (Aman et al. 1995; Martin et al. 1999; Vitiello and Jensen 1997). This dearth of information forces clinicians to extrapolate dosages for their young patients from the existing adult literature. Despite these critical safety and medico-legal issues, in the face of severely incapacitating illness, clinicians are often compelled to treat ASD with newer and less understood pharmacologic agents in the hopes that these youngsters will be able to live to their fullest potentials. In a review of 109 children with a diagnosis of ASD (Martin et al. 1999a), 55% had been given a psychotropic agent and 29.3% were on two or more medications concurrently. The medications were mainly antidepressants in high-functioning children, and neuroleptics in those with a low IQ.

In this chapter, we discuss general issues encountered in the pediatric psychopharmacology of autism, issues that may explain the difficulty of implementing cogent double-blind placebo-controlled trials; we then provide a review of the psychopharmacologic research literature; and finally, we discuss the practical implications of these research findings and propose an approach to psychopharmacologic treatment of target symptoms.

Psychopharmacology in Children With ASD: General Rules

Psychotropic Agents in the Developing Brain: Ethical Aspects and Safety Issues

During the past decade, the expansion of pediatric psychopharmacology has been enhanced by the availability of safer medications with better *short-term* benefit/risk ratios. For instance, the SSRIs do not have the cardiac toxicity of the older tricyclic antidepressants, and the new atypical neuroleptics have fewer extrapyramidal effects than the typical neuroleptics. Nevertheless, with the exception of the stimulants, whose effects have been extensively evaluated in children with attention-deficit/hyperactivity disorder (ADHD), *long-term* consequences of the interaction between psychotropic agents and the developing brain have not been investigated in humans. Scientific and health institutions have already recognized the tremendous public health relevance of the pediatric use of psychotropic agents. In 1995 a conference organized by the National Institute of Mental Health and the Food and Drug Administration gathered more than 100 experts from the lay and professional communities to identify the major obstacles to research in pediatric psychopharmacology and to propose feasible solutions (Vitiello and Jensen 1997). Among multiple recommendations, the Research Units of Pediatric Psychopharmacology (RUPP) Autism Network was established. One of the first fruits of this collaborative work was recently published in the *New England Journal of Medicine* (Research Units of Pediatric Psychopharmacology Autism Network 2002). This study clearly demonstrated the short-term safety and efficacy of risperidone in children with autism and severe behavior problems. However, the long-term effect of this medication remains to be studied. We know from animal studies that developing neurotransmitter systems can be very sensitive to early inhibition or stimulation by pharmacologic agents and can lead to permanent changes in adult life. As an example, and to emphasize the consequences of interfering with developmentally regulated neurotransmitter systems, we briefly illustrate the critical role of serotonin in the developing brain.

Serotonergic Neurons: Model of a Critically Regulated System in the Developing Brain

Dysregulation of the serotonin system in children with autism is likely to contribute not only to some aspects of abnormal behavior, anxiety, or mood instability, but also to core autistic features and cognitive impairment (Chugani et al. 1999; McDougle et al. 2000). Consequently, many medications targeting this pathway, such as atypical neuroleptic agents and SSRIs, are currently used and appear helpful in treating ASD.

There is evidence that serotonin acts as a trophic or differentiation factor, in addition to its role as a neurotransmitter. D'Amato et al. (1987) demonstrated a transient serotonergic innervation of primary sensory cortex between postnatal days 2 and 14 during the period of synaptogenesis in the rat cortex. Furthermore, this transient innervation actually represents transient expression of the high-affinity serotonin transporter (5HTT) and vesicular monoamine transporter by glutamatergic thalamocortical neurons (Bennett-Clarke et al. 1996; Lebrand et al. 1996), leading to the differentiation of thalamocortical neurons via 5-HT$_{1B}$ receptors (Lieske et al. 1999). Elegant and cogent experiments using knockout mice demonstrated that inactivation of the *5HTT* gene profoundly disturbs formation of the somatosensory cortex, with altered cytoarchitecture of cortical layer IV, the layer that contains synapses between thalamocortical terminals and their postsynaptic target neurons (Persico et al. 2001). In the cerebellum, 5-HT receptor expression is also developmentally regulated. For example, in rat pups, there is high expression of the serotonin 5-HT$_{1A}$ receptor in the Purkinje cell layer between postnatal days 2 and 9, but this receptor is not detectable in the cerebellum of adults (Miquel et al. 1994).

Developmental changes in brain serotonin content and serotonin receptor binding have also been demonstrated in nonhuman primates (Goldman-Rakic et al. 1982; Lidow et al. 1991). There is a rise in serotonin content in the cortex beginning before birth and reaching a peak at 2 months of age, followed by a slow decline until 3 years of age (Goldman-Rakic et al. 1982). Expression of serotonin receptors showed a similar developmental time course (Lidow et al. 1991). Furthermore, in humans, measures of the serotonin metabolite 5-hydroxyindoleacetic acid (5-HIAA) in cerebrospinal fluid (CSF) show higher values in children compared with adults (Hedner et al. 1986; Seifer et al. 1980). Also, serotonin synthesis capacity measured at different ages using [^{11}C]-alpha-methyl-L-tryptophan ([^{11}C]AMT) and positron emission tomography (PET) is more than 200% of adult values until the age of 5 years, after which it declines toward adult values (Chugani et al. 1999).

Manipulations of serotonin levels in developing animals cause disruption in neuronal differentiation (Lauder and Krebs 1978; Whitaker-Azmitia et al. 1987). For example, treatment of pregnant rats with *p*-chlorophenylalanine to deplete serotonin caused prolongation of the period of cell division in the pups in brain regions with dense serotonergic innervation, resulting in increased neuronal cell numbers in the hippocampus, superior colliculus, and several thalamic nuclei (Lauder and Krebs 1978). This is consistent with Bauman and Kemper's (1985) report of reduced neuronal cell size and increased cell number in the hippocampus of brains of individuals with autism. Depletion of serotonin in neonatal rat pups resulted in large decreases in the number of dendritic spines in the hippocampus (Yan et al. 1997), consistent with Bauman and Kemper's (1985) findings of decreased complexity and extent of dendritic arbors in the hippocampus of the brain of individuals with autism. Finally, decreased or increased brain serotonin during the prenatal and early postnatal periods are likely to lead to significant disruption of synaptic connectivity in sensory cortices, as demonstrated by Bennett-Clarke et al. (1994) in a rat model and by Cases et al. (1996) in monoamine oxidase A–deficient mice. Depletion of serotonin delays the development of the "barrel fields" of the mouse somatosensory cortex (Osterheld-Haas and Hornung 1996) and decreases the size of the barrel fields (Cases et al. 1996). Such findings might help explain the abnormal sensory perception reported in many subjects with autism (O'Neill and Jones 1997).

In summary, there is increasing evidence that serotonin system homeostasis is critical to the genesis, differentiation, and maturation of neuronal cells and networks in brain regions controlling sensory inputs, stimulus processing, and motor output (see Lesch 2001 for review). Interfering with the dysfunctional serotonergic system with medications represents a challenge that requires more research evaluation of long-term benefits and risks.

Medications Currently Available and Previously Studied for Efficacy and Safety

Here we review only medications currently available that have demonstrated efficacy through large open-label studies or placebo-controlled trials. Three major classes of psychotropic agents are reviewed: neuroleptics (or antipsychotics), antidepressants, and psychostimulants. Agents such as fenfluramine, which was taken off the market by the FDA, naltrexone, lamotrigine, and amantadine, all of which demonstrate only weak or equivocal efficacy, will be discussed later in the framework of a practical approach to specific target symptoms.

Antipsychotics (Classical/Atypical)

During the 1970s, almost all of the typical neuroleptics available were studied in individuals with autism, including children. They were shown to be beneficial in treating symptoms of aggression, social withdrawal, hyperactivity, stereotypies, self-injurious behavior, and sleep disturbances. Low-potency neuroleptics, such as chlorpromazine, were avoided because of sedation and adverse cognitive effects. Haloperidol, a dopamine D_2 receptor antagonist with high-potency neuroleptic properties, was the most studied and widely prescribed medication in autism treatment at the time. Campbell et al. (1978) published a study of 40 inpatient children with autistic disorder, ranging from 2 to 7 years old. The children were randomly assigned to one of four groups receiving treatment with 1) haloperidol and behavioral language therapy, 2) haloperidol alone, 3) placebo and behavioral language therapy, and 4) placebo alone. The children were followed over a 12-week period with the mean dose of haloperidol at 1.65 mg/day. Though the group on haloperidol showed more improvement than the placebo group, the group that received both haloperidol and behavioral language therapy made the most significant gains. Moreover, long-term efficacy of haloperidol over 6 months was observed in 56% of 60 patients who had been responders in a previous short-term trial (Perry et al. 1989).

Pimozide, another high-potency typical neuroleptic, was compared with haloperidol in a multicenter, double-blind, placebo-controlled crossover study (Naruse et al. 1982) that involved 87 subjects (age 6–13 years) with behavioral problems, 34 of whom had autism. Pimozide and haloperidol were both more effective than placebo in controlling aggression. Nevertheless, a major concern with typical neuroleptics is the frequent occurrence of extrapyramidal signs. Indeed, Campbell et al. (1997) observed tardive or withdrawal dyskinesia in 34% of 118 children (2–8 years old) with autism during a 6-month prospective, longitudinal study.

The atypical neuroleptic medications (clozapine, risperidone, quetiapine, olanzapine, and ziprasidone) are increasingly used to treat people with ASD due to their favorable side-effect profile, particularly their very rare extrapyramidal effects compared with typical neuroleptics (Biederman et al. 1997). In addition to dopaminergic antagonist action, these agents also exhibit serotonergic antagonistic properties.

Clozapine was the first atypical antipsychotic to be introduced in the United States, in 1991. Two reports exist regarding its use in autism, for a total of four patients (Chen et al. 2001; Zuddas et al. 1996). Three of the patients had a sustained response. However, because of the risk for agranulocytosis or seizures and the frequent blood tests needed to monitor for agranulocytosis, clozapine is not a commonly used treatment.

Quetiapine has clozapine-like activity, but without the hematologic or seizure side effects. It was used in an open trial in six males with autism (mean age 10.9 ± 3.3 years) for a 16-week period with doses ranging from 100 to 350 mg/day (Martin et al. 1999b). There was no significant improvement in behavioral rating scales, but two children were considered clinical responders.

Risperidone is the most investigated atypical agent in the treatment of ASD. McDougle et al. (1998a) carried out a double-blind, placebo-controlled study of risperidone in adults with ASD. Their study consisted of 31 adults randomly placed on either risperidone or placebo treatment for 12 weeks. In contrast with the placebo group, the risperidone group exhibited improvement in repetitive behavior, aggression, anxiety, depression, and irritability symptoms. Open-trial studies of risperidone in children and adolescents with ASD have also yielded encouraging results (Findling et al. 1997; McDougle et al. 1997; Nicolson et al. 1998). Mean dosing in these studies ranged from 1.1 to 1.8 mg/day.

Recently, the RUPP Autism Network (2002) published a multisite, randomized, double-blind trial of risperidone compared with placebo in 101 children (5 to 17 years old) with autism who also exhibited severe tantrums, aggression, and/or self-injurious behavior. All subjects enrolled in the study met DSM-IV (American Psychiatric Association 1994) diagnostic criteria for autistic disorder, corroborated by the Autism Diagnostic Interview–Revised (ADI-R). Inclusion criteria also required clinically significant behavioral problems, defined as ratings of "moderate" or higher on the Clinical Global Impressions (CGI) scale and as scores of 18 or higher on the Irritability subscale of the Aberrant Behavior Checklist (ABC; Aman et al. 1985). The mean daily dose of risperidone was 1.8 ± 0.7 mg (range 0.5 to 3.5). Positive response was defined as at least a 25% improvement in the score on the Irritability subscale and a rating of "much improved" or "very much improved" on the CGI scale at 8 weeks. Positive response was seen in 69% of the risperidone group but only 12% of the placebo group. Improvement was significant on the Irritability, Stereotypies, and Hyperactivity subscales of the ABC, but not the Social Withdrawal subscale. The degree of improvement in the risperidone group was very significant: 57% reduction in the Irritability score, compared with only a 14% decrease in the placebo group. Interestingly, these gains in the risperidone group were maintained for 6 months in 68% of the children who had a positive response in the double-blind phase of the study. Most adverse effects (fatigue, drowsiness, dizziness, tremor, and drooling) were mild and self-limited, and no children were withdrawn from the study because of an adverse effect. Weight gain associated with mild to moderate increased appetite was significantly greater in the risperidone group than in the placebo group (mean 2.7 kg vs. 0.8 kg). No extrapyramidal symptoms were observed, but the short period of this trial limits inferences about adverse effects such as tardive dyskinesia. In conclusion, the RUPP authors state that risperidone is an effective and well-tolerated medication for the treatment of tantrums, aggression, and self-injurious behavior in children with autism.

Case reports of olanzapine treatment of ASD are also promising and warrant systematic trials to further assess their efficacy in this population (Krishnamoorthy and King 1998; Potenza et al. 1999). Malone et al. (2001) carried out a 6-week open-label treatment that randomized 12 children with autism to receive either olanzapine or haloperidol. Five of 6 patients treated with olanzapine (mean dose 7.9 ± 2.5 mg) and 3 of 6 patients treated with haloperidol (mean dose 1.4 ± 0.7 mg) were rated as responders. However, significant weight gain occurred in the olanzapine group (9.0 ± 3.5 lb) compared with the haloperidol group (3.2 ± 4.9 lb).

McDougle et al. (2002) carried out a 6- to 30-week open-label study of ziprasidone in 12 children (mean age 11.6 ± 4.4 years) with autism or pervasive developmental disorder not otherwise specified (PDDNOS). Fifty percent responded well (dose range 20–120 mg/day), demonstrating significant improvement on the CGI and in symptoms of aggression, agitation, and irritability. Weight loss was seen in 5 patients and weight gain in only 1 patient. Sedation was the most common side effect. In general, ziprasidone was well tolerated and worthy of further controlled studies.

Antidepressants (Classical/SSRI)

In response to cumulative data suggesting disruption in serotonergic mechanisms during early development in children with autism, several interventions to modulate the serotonin system have been attempted. Short-term dietary depletion of the 5-HT precursor tryptophan has been associated with an exacerbation of behavioral symptoms in adults with autism (McDougle et al. 1996a). Conversely, clomipramine, a nonspecific serotonin reuptake inhibitor, has shown efficacy for certain symptoms (anger, hyperactivity, and repetitive behavior) in children, adolescents, and young adults with ASD (Gordon et al. 1993), but it has also been associated with seizures and cardiac effects. Significant adverse effects were also observed in a large prospective clomipramine open-label study of 35 adults with ASD (Brodkin et al. 1997). Furthermore, there is some evidence that clomipramine is even less tolerated and less effective for young children than for adolescents and adults (Brasic et al. 1997; Sanchez et al. 1996).

SSRIs have increasingly become the preferred medication treatment for many mood and anxiety disorders, because of their better side-effect profiles compared with tricyclics. SSRIs have received increased attention as a treatment for ASD, but only one double-blind, placebo-controlled study in patients with ASD has been published. McDougle et al. (1996b) demonstrated the effectiveness of fluvoxamine in 30 adults with autism. Eight of the 15 patients in the fluvoxamine group (compared with none in the placebo group) were categorized as "much improved" or "very much improved" on the CGI scale. Fluvoxamine significantly reduced repetitive behavior, maladaptive behavior, and aggression, with minimal adverse effects. In addition, fluvoxamine increased the communicative use of language. However, an unpublished fluvoxamine double-blind, placebo-controlled trial in children and adolescents was less encouraging (McDougle et al., unpublished data, reviewed by Posey and McDougle 2000). Only 1 of the 18 fluvoxamine-treated children (25–250 mg/day) demonstrated significant clinical improvement with the drug, and adverse effects were seen in 14, including insomnia, hyperactivity, agitation, aggression, anxiety, and anorexia. In two independent open-label trials of fluoxetine, this potential "behavior-activating" side effect was cited as a frequent cause of discontinuation, especially in children (Cook et al. 1992; DeLong et al. 1998). This adverse behavior activation might be related to SSRI-induced manic symptoms reported in some patients with ASD (Damore et al. 1998).

Sertraline is another SSRI of potential utility, and it seems less activating in our clinical experience. In a 28-day open-label trial of sertraline (at doses of 25–150 mg daily) in nine adults with mental retardation (five with autism), a significant decrease in aggression and self-injury occurred in eight (Hellings et al. 1996). Another large prospective 12-week open-label study of 42 adult patients with ASD found sertraline (mean dosage 122 mg/day) effective in improving aggression and repetitive behavior, but not social relatedness (McDougle et al. 1998b). Treatment response was not associated with the degree of mental retardation. Only 3 of the 42 patients experienced intolerable activation effects, such as agitation or anxiety. In pediatric populations, only one case series of nine children (ages 6–12 years) with autism is reported (Steingard et al. 1997). On sertraline (25–50 mg daily), eight showed significant improvement in anxiety, irritability, and "transition-induced behavior deterioration" or "need for sameness." Three of the responders demonstrated a return of symptoms after 3 to 7 months. Two children experienced agitation when the dose was raised to 75 mg daily. In view of these preliminary data, further placebo-controlled studies are warranted to address the issue of safety and efficacy of SSRIs in autistic children.

Psychostimulants and Alpha-Adrenergic Agonists

Early studies of the use of stimulants in ASD found an increase in irritability and stereotypic movements, which led to their underutilization. A review by Aman (1982) stated that stimulant medication was contraindicated in this group of children, particularly when mental retardation was also present. However, later case reports and open-label studies suggested their benefit in children with autism who were also hyperactive or had ADHD symptoms (Birmaher et al. 1988; Geller et al. 1981; Strayhorn et al. 1988; Vitriol and Farber 1981). More recently Quintana et al. (1995) carried out a double-blind crossover study of methylphenidate at two doses (10 mg or 20 mg bid) in 10 children (ages 7 to 11 years) with autism. The study lasted 6 weeks, and significant improvement relative to placebo was seen in hyperactivity and irritability. There was no significant effect of developmental level or dose of methylphenidate on the outcome variables or response. Five of the study patients were continued on methylphenidate long term. The authors concluded that stimulants should be tried before neuroleptics in children with autism who have significant ADHD symptoms, because they have fewer side effects and a worthwhile response rate. Subsequent work by Handen et al. (2000) that included 13 children with autism and ADHD in a double-blind controlled trial of methyphenidate demonstrated substantial benefit, with at least a 50% reduction of hyperactivity and inattention in 8 patients. Although ADHD symptoms decreased, no improvements were seen in autistic symptoms, and higher doses of methylphenidate (0.6 mg/kg) led to social withdrawal and irritability in some children. The use of stimulants in ASD is reviewed by Aman and Langworthy (2000), who reach the consensus that a subgroup of children with ASD who have ADHD symptoms are likely to benefit from this class of medications. They note, however, that the response rate (50%–60%) is lower than what is seen in nonautistic, normal-IQ children with ADHD, who respond in 80% to 90% of cases.

In the last 2 years a variety of long-acting stimulant preparations have become available, including Concerta, Adderall XR, Ritalin LA, Metadate CD, and Methylin ER. These are typically given only once in the morning and maintain a more consistent blood level throughout the day (Wender 2002). This effect can decrease rebound hyperactivity or irritability with smoother tapering in the late afternoon and evening. Many of these preparations have demonstrated efficacy in children with ADHD, but they have not yet been studied in a controlled trial of children with ASD and ADHD. However, our clinical experience suggests that they are as effective in children with ASD as the short-acting preparations.

In the subgroup of children with ADHD who have hyperarousal, the alpha-adrenergic agonists, including clonidine and guanfacine (Tenex), often have a calming effect, in addition to improving ADHD and facilitating sleep at bedtime (Hunt et al. 1995; Wilens 1999; Wilens et al. 1994). Only limited studies are available regarding their use in autism, however. Two controlled studies have demonstrated efficacy with autism samples, including Frankhauser et al. (1991), who studied the clonidine transdermal patch, and Jaselskis et al. (1992), who studied the clonidine pill.

One subgroup of patients who experience severe hyperarousal and ADHD symptoms are children who have both fragile X syndrome and autism. Typically these children respond well to clonidine. In a retrospective study of 35 children with fragile X (approximately 30% with autism), two-thirds of the mothers said that clonidine was very beneficial and improved ADHD symptoms, tantrums, and aggression (Hagerman et al. 1995). The side effects of clonidine include sedation, lowering of blood pressure, and rare prolongation of conduction, so a follow-up electrocardiogram is recommended after dosage changes, particularly when clonidine is combined with a stimulant (Wilens et al. 1999). Clonidine should be tapered when discontinued because headaches can occur with abrupt discontinuation. The clonidine patch can also cause skin irritation, which responds well to use of beclomethasone (Vancenase AQ) nasal spray to the back before placement of the patch (Hagerman 2002). One should avoid using the clonidine patch in young children, who have the potential to rip it off and eat it, which can cause coma (Hagerman et al. 1998). The use of clonidine and guanfacine in children and adolescents is reviewed by Riddle et al. (1999) and Aman and Langworthy (2000).

Practical Implications: An Approach to Targeting Behavioral Problems

Which Medication for Which Behavioral Symptom?

Table 7–1 lists potential agents for target symptoms common in ASD.

Mood Instability

Affective instability, including rapid cycling, rages, aggression, and euphoria, may be good indications for the use of mood stabilizers, including lithium, carbamazepine, valproate, and neurontin. Studies suggest that children

Table 7–1. Potential psychopharmacologic agents for common target symptoms

Target symptoms	Potential medications
Aggression, agitation, irritability	Neuroleptics
	Mood stabilizers
	Alpha-adrenergic agonists
Repetitive/impulsive behavior	SSRIs
	Opioid antagonists
	Alpha-adrenergic agonists
Disruptive behavior	Alpha-adrenergic agonists
	Neuroleptics
	Stimulants
Affective instability	Mood stabilizers
	SSRIs
Social withdrawal	Neuroleptics
Anxiety, hyperarousal	SSRIs
	Alpha-adrenergic agonists
	Buspirone
Insomnia	Antihistamines
	Trazodone
	Tricyclic antidepressants
	Melatonin

Note. SSRIs = selective serotonin reuptake inhibitors.

with ASD who have a family history of bipolar disorder (DeLong and Dwyer 1988; Delong and Nohria 1994) and display aggression and irritability may benefit from these agents (Steingard and Biederman 1987). Some patients with ASD also have seizures (see Chapter 5), which may exacerbate behavioral problems. The behavior of children with both ASD and seizures often improves with anticonvulsant-type mood stabilizers.

Sleep Disturbances

Sleep problems are common in young children with autism. A variety of medications have been used to treat sleep difficulties, including clonidine, described previously, and trazodone, an antidepressant. Trazodone selectively blocks reuptake of serotonin but is also a potent antagonist of the 5-HT$_2$ receptor (Preskorn 1993a, 1993b). Trazodone has strong sedative effects and is often utilized at bedtime to counteract sleep disturbances, but no published information is available concerning its efficacy in autism.

Melatonin is a sleep hormone that is produced in the pineal gland from metabolism of serotonin. Melatonin production is stimulated by darkness and is important for the induction and maintenance of sleep (Jan et al. 1994). This agent has been synthesized and is available in oral form through health food stores in the United States. It has been shown to be effective for the treatment of chronic insomnia (MacFarlane et al. 1991), sleep problems related to jet lag (Arendt and Broadway 1987), and delayed sleep phase syndrome (Dahlitz et al. 1991). Jan and O'Donnell (1996) and Jan et al. (1994) showed that 1 to 3 mg of melatonin given at bedtime improved sleep disturbances in 82% of more than 100 children with developmental disabilities. No significant side effects were reported, even after continuous use for more than 4 years (Jan and O'Donnell 1996). Other studies with neurologically disabled children showed a noticeable improvement in nighttime sleeping with the administration of melatonin at bedtime (Gordon et al 1993; Palm et al. 1997), although lack of efficacy has also been reported (Camfield et al. 1996). Sadeh et al. (1995) suggested that melatonin might also improve aggressive behavior, as seen in their case study of a blind boy with severe mental retardation. Two anecdotal articles mention contradictory effects of melatonin in autism (Hayashi et al. 2000; Jan and Espezel 1995), so further studies are warranted in autism. A double-blind placebo-controlled crossover study of children (2 to 18 years old) with autism and/or fragile X syndrome is currently ongoing at the M.I.N.D. Institute, and preliminary data suggest that 50% show significant improvement in sleep (S. Jacquemont, personal communication, May 2002).

Practical Information for Clinicians: Choosing and Combining Agents

Because autism is etiologically and clinically heterogeneous, there are many potential target symptoms to treat. It can be difficult to know what to target first. The general principles of using the least toxic medication first and only changing one medication at a time are important to remember. For example, if a child with ASD presents with significant hyperactivity and aggression, it is worthwhile to try a stimulant first, since it has relatively few side effects and may improve both symptoms. For children with significant hyperarousal, clonidine or guanfacine should be considered. If significant problems with anxiety or obsessive-compulsive behavior are present, then an SSRI should be considered, with a careful look for too much activation. Citalopram is perhaps the least activating of the SSRIs, but experience in children is still limited. In some children, activating effects may help language and socialization, so fluoxetine, which may be the most activating, may help this subgroup. If activation leads to aggression or mania, then consideration of a mood stabilizer or an atypical neuroleptic such as risperidone is often helpful. Although the dramatic benefits of risperidone from the Research Units on Pediatric Psychopharmacology Autism Network (2002) study should not be forgotten, the clinician may want to try an SSRI or even a stimulant first because of the fewer side effects. Generally speaking, all children with ASD should be tried on an SSRI at some point because of possible benefits to socialization, language, obsessive-compulsive behavior, and anxiety.

There has been an emerging trend in psychopharmacology over the past decade to combine medications to treat multiple target symptoms or multiple diagnoses in a child with comorbid conditions (Jensen et al. 1999a; Wilens et al. 1995). For example, in a study of 109 subjects with "high-functioning" ASD, 29.3% were on two or more medications simultaneously (Martin et al. 1999a). The benefit of such a practice is that each specific target symptom can be treated with the most effective medication, but the pitfalls include deleterious effects of medication combinations, which are not predictable from knowledge of the individual medications or their additive effects (Woolston 1999). There is a lack of controlled research on individual medications in childhood, much less on combined pharmacologic effects, so it will take some time for research to document the benefits that an experienced clinician may discover in practice (Jensen et al. 1999b). To date, clear combination medication strategies are not available, and the choice of the "best" combination for one child depends on the target symptoms and the experience of the clinician. The general strategy is to first prescribe a medication to address the most pressing problem and then add another drug to enhance or widen its effect. Prescription of combined medications should follow the basic rules laid out in Table 7–2. If drug interaction is the major pitfall of combined psychopharmacology, the risk of side effects might be reduced by using lower doses of all drugs.

Table 7–2. Combination psychopharmacology: underlying rationale and corresponding rule

Rationale	Rule
Multiple target symptoms	Identify and monitor target symptoms
Different mechanisms of action	Maximize dose before adding or discontinuing
Possible drug–drug synergy	Change and adjust one drug at a time
Possible drug interactions	Discontinue drugs of least benefit
Confusing symptoms and side effects	Monitor side effects

Can We Treat the Core Symptoms of Autism?

The preceding review focused on treating symptoms that are not core to autism (e.g., mood instability, hyperactivity, aggression). The ultimate goal of psychopharmacology is to treat the core symptoms of autism, improving social skills, language, and cognitive functions with the use of nootropic medications. This name, derived from *noos* (mind) and *tropin* (toward), can be used for any psychotropic agent that improves higher cerebral functions. In this section, nootropic effects of current medications in autism will first be discussed. Then a new research area, the α-amino-3-hydroxy-5-methyl-4-isoxazole propionate (AMPA) receptors of the glutamatergic system, will be reviewed and recent neurobiologic and clinical pharmacologic data will be discussed.

History of Transient Hope and Disappointments of Current Medications

Fascinating case reports have been published during the last 30 years documenting unexpected expressive language onset or dramatic social relatedness improvement in a few children with autism. The most recent excitement was generated by the fortuitous effect of secretin on language and social interaction in three patients with ASD given secretin for a gastrointestinal investigation (Horvath et al. 1998). As described in Chapter 8, however, these encouraging data were not confirmed by multiple placebo-controlled studies. Aside from spectacular, intriguing case reports, the effects of secretin and other psychotropics on cognitive and social skills, when thoroughly assessed during open-label and controlled studies, have not revealed improvements in core symptoms of ASD, although it is difficult to fully address this issue through short-term trials.

Long before secretin became popular, other medications went through the same cycle of initial excitement and later disappointment. Naltrexone, an opioid-receptor antagonist, was touted as improving core autism symptoms, but ultimately proved to have little effect. Controlled studies have demonstrated that stimulants are efficacious in decreasing hyperactivity, but rarely is any improvement in learning abilities shown (Bouvard et al. 1995; Kolmen et al. 1995; Willemsen-Swinkels et al. 1995). Concerning haloperidol, the most studied typical neuroleptic in autism, interesting effects on cognitive functions were observed in young children (ages 2 to 7) in the areas of language, relatedness, and discrimination learning in initial studies (Anderson et al. 1984; Campbell et al. 1978) but were not confirmed in later controlled investigations (Anderson et al. 1989). Propranolol, a beta-blocker, was prescribed in an open-label study in eight adults with autism (Ratey et al. 1987a, 1987b). Improvements in speech and socialization were reported but not confirmed by further controlled studies, and may have been due to a decrease of hyperarousal. Eight among 13 children and adolescents with autism who were given lamotrigine for intractable epilepsy demonstrated a decrease in autistic symptoms (Uvebrant et al. 1994), but again these results were not confirmed in a double-blind controlled trial (Belsito et al. 2001). Even in the recent excellent multisite placebo-controlled trial using risperidone in 101 autistic children, no improvement of social skills or cognition was observed after 8 weeks, despite a dramatic improvement of abnormal behavior (Research Units on Pediatric Psychopharmacology Autism Network 2002). An open-label study using olanzapine in seven autistic children and adults demonstrated significant improvements in language usage and social relatedness (Potenza et al. 1999). Since olanzapine seems to be more efficient than risperidone in alleviating the negative symptoms of schizophrenia (Tran et al. 1997), this medication may be more effective in diminishing social withdrawal in autism (McDougle et al. 2000) than risperidone, and further controlled studies are warranted. In summary, however, the nootropic effects of most medications used for ASD are not convincing.

Encouraging but Still Controversial: SSRIs

The putative ability of SSRIs to improve not only anxiety and repetitive behavior, but also expressive language and social interaction, has been reported by different authors, but findings have not always been replicated. McDougle et al. (1996b), using fluvoxamine (Luvox) in 30 adults in a placebo-controlled trial, found an increase in communicative language. Preliminary unpublished results of an open study in children were less encouraging, however (Posey and McDougle 2000). DeLong et al. (1998) noted marked improvements in behavioral, cognitive, affective, and social areas and language acquisition in children (2 to 8 years old) with autism over several years of treatment in an open-label study of fluoxetine (Prozac). However, no standardized outcome measures were used and there was no control for other interventions the child was receiving. In the absence of a control group, it is difficult to determine what role fluoxetine played in the improvement.

The recent report of Buchsbaum et al. (2001) coupled a fluoxetine trial in six adults with autism with PET–magnetic resonance imaging (MRI) and found that fluoxetine significantly increased metabolic rates in the right frontal lobe, especially in the cingulate gyrus and orbitofrontal cortex. Fifty percent of the patients had a clinical response to fluoxetine; these patients had the highest metabolic rates in the medial frontal region and cingulate when unmedicated. In the future, controlled trials of SSRIs in children with autism, coupled with functional MRI or PET studies, should yield helpful information regarding developmental changes in the brain in autism, which children may respond to SSRIs, and the metabolic changes that occur with a positive response to medication.

New Nootropic Medications

Several lines of study suggest that the glutamatergic system is an important pathway related to autism. First, brain regions implicated in autism on the basis of neuropathologic and brain imaging studies, such as the medial temporal lobe and related structures (Bauman 1991; Bauman and Kemper 1985; Raymond et al. 1996) and frontal and parietal cortex (Courchesne et al. 1993; Minshew 1991; Zilbovicius et al. 1995), are rich in glutamate receptors. A second line of evidence comes from the genomic approach called expression profiling, which has identified differences in gene expression between autism and control postmortem cerebellum (Purcell et al. 2001). Among the 9,000+ genes studied, the most striking abnormality was a group of five genes coding for glutamate receptors (*AMPA1, GLUR2, GLUR3,* and *NMDA*) and a glutamate transporter (*EEAT1*). All of these genes had elevated mRNA and protein. In the same study, autoradiography performed on cerebellum, prefrontal cortex, caudate, and putamen (six patients and nine control subjects) revealed that the cerebellum had a significant decrease in the density of AMPA receptors. The density of *N*-methyl-D-asparate (NMDA) receptors was not significantly different. The elevated gene activity and decreased AMPA receptor density reflect a general disturbance of the glutamate system occurring in autism. Third, symptoms produced by NMDA antagonists (ketamine, phencyclidine) in healthy subjects resemble those seen in autism (Hansen et al. 1988; Krystal et al. 1994; Muir and Lees 1995).

This research, in aggregate, suggests a deficiency of glutamatergic transmission in autism. Thus, enhancement of activation-dependent AMPA receptor activity might be helpful in managing the cognitive and behavioral symptoms of ASD. New agents, still in a development phase, may open new avenues for the nootropic treatment of ASD. Among these new agents is CX516, an AMPA-receptor modulator or ampakine, which binds to the AMPA receptor-channel complex and produces an allosteric increase in glutamate-induced ion conductance by slowing receptor deactivation, resulting in a longer open time and slower decay (Arai et al. 1994, 1996a). CX516 has been shown to increase excitatory activity at hippocampal synapses and facilitate long-term potentiation (Arai et al. 1996b).

Facilitatory effects are amplified across multisynaptic circuits, suggesting potential usefulness in facilitating complex brain operations. In rats, CX516 has been shown to enhance memory and speed of performance during spatial learning tasks, as well as enhance response in a conditioned eye-blink task and decrease methamphetamine-induced hyperactivity (Granger et al. 1993; Hampson et al. 1998a, 1998b; Larson et al. 1996; Rogan et al. 1997; Staubli et al. 1994).

Three Phase I studies in humans involved single doses of CX516 of two consecutive doses (Ingvar et al. 1997; Lynch et al. 1996, 1997). All three studies demonstrated clear enhancement on memory tasks. Three Phase II studies have also been performed—one in elderly Alzheimer's disease patients and two in schizophrenia patients. Both patient groups showed improvement in cognitive function. To explore the benefits and safety of CX516 for ASD, a randomized double-blind 4-week trial of CX516 in 100 adult patients with cognitive impairment and fragile X syndrome or ASD is under way at two sites (M.I.N.D. Institute in Sacramento, California, and Rush-Presbyterian Hospital in Chicago, Illinois).

Future Prospects: The Challenge of Subgrouping Patients to Identify Responders

Thorough clinical subtyping of children with autism will likely lead to the identification of subgroups who differ in terms of response, adverse effects, and long-term tolerance to medications. For this reason, future psychopharmacologic research should concentrate on subtyping, examining familial mood disorder, etiology of autism, age, cognitive level, and so on. As one example, DeLong et al. (1998) noticed that children from families with affective disorders are better responders to SSRIs. As another example, genetic polymorphisms might contribute to variations in medication response, as suggested by recent work on the serotonin transporter gene (*5HTT*). Tordjman et al. (2001) examined parent-to-offspring transmission of the "long" and "short" alleles of the polymorphism in the *5HTT* promoter region in families of 71 children with autism. The "short" allele, which is known to be less efficiently transcribed (Heils et al. 1996), had demonstrated a high prevalence in autistic individuals and their families in a previous study (Cook et al. 1997) but did not convey risk for autism in Tordjman's study. However, allelic transmission in probands was dependent on severity of impairments in the social and communication domains, with greater short allele transmission in severely impaired individuals (Tordjman et al. 2001). These data suggest that *5HTT* promoter alleles modify the severity of autistic behaviors and, by extension, may also modify the efficacy of SSRIs and other medications. This illustrates the importance of careful phenotype description in future medication studies.

Pharmacologic treatment is bringing about exciting new interventions for and understanding of ASD. Recently studied agents offer symptomatic improvement without apparent significant adverse events, although not all children and adolescents with ASD respond favorably. Additional research in phenotyping the spectrum of ASD will help us better match agents to particular children and particular target symptoms while minimizing adverse effects.

References

Aman MG: Stimulant drug effects in developmental disorders and hyperactivity: toward a resolution of disparate findings. J Autism Dev Disord 12:385–398, 1982

Aman MG, Langworthy KS: Pharmacotherapy for hyperactivity in children with autism and other pervasive developmental disorders. J Autism Dev Disord 30:451–459, 2000

Aman MG, Singh N, Stewart A, et al: The Aberrant Behavior Checklist: a behavior rating scale for the assessment of treatment effects. Am J Ment Defic 89:485–491, 1985

Aman MG, Van Bourgondien ME, Wolford PL, et al: Psychotropic and anticonvulsant drugs in subjects with autism: prevalence and patterns of use. J Am Acad Child Adolesc Psychiatry 34:1672–1681, 1995

American Psychiatric Association: Diagnostic and Statistical Manual of Mental Disorders, 4th Edition. Washington, DC, American Psychiatric Association, 1994

Anderson L, Campbell M, Grega D, et al: Haloperidol in the treatment of infantile autism: effects on learning and behavioral symptoms. Am J Psychiatry 141:1195–1202, 1984

Anderson L, Campbell M, Adams P, et al: The effects of haloperiodol on discrimination learning and behavioral symptoms in autistic children. J Autism Dev Disord 19:227–239, 1989

Arai A, Kessler M, Xiao P, et al: A centrally active drug that modulates AMPA receptor gated currents. Brain Res 638:343–346, 1994

Arai A, Kessler M, Ambrose-Ingerson J, et al: Effects of a centrally active benzoylpyrrolidine drug on AMPA receptor kinetics. Neuroscience 75:573–585, 1996a

Arai A, Kessler M, Rogers G, et al: Effects of a memory-enhancing drug on DL-α-amino-3-hydroxy-5-methyl-4-isoxazolepropionic acid receptor currents and synaptic transmission in hippocampus. J Pharmacol Exp Ther 278:627–638, 1996b

Arendt J, Broadway J: Light and melatonin as zeitgebers in man. Chronobiol Int 4:273–282, 1987

Bauman M, Kemper TL: Histoanatomic observations of the brain in early infantile autism. Neurology 35:866–875, 1985

Bauman ML: Microscopic neuroanatomic abnormalities in autism. Pediatrics 7:791–796, 1991

Belsito KM, Law PA, Kirk KS, et al: Lamotrigine therapy for autistic disorder: a randomized, double-blind, placebo-controlled trial. J Autism Dev Disord 31:175–81, 2001

Bennett-Clarke CA, Leslie MJ, Lane RD, et al: Effect of serotonin depletion on vibrissae-related patterns in the rat's somatosensory cortex. J Neurosci 14:7594–7607, 1994

Bennett-Clarke CA, Chiaia NL, Rhoades RW: Thalamocortical afferents in rat transiently express high-affinity serotonin uptake sites. Brain Res 733:301–306, 1996

Biederman J, Spencer T, Wilens T: Psychopharmacology, in Textbook of Child and Adolescent Psychiatry. Edited by Wiener JM. Washington, DC, American Psychiatric Press, 1997

Birmaher B, Quintana H, Greenhill LL: Methylphenidate treatment of hyperactive autistic children. J Am Acad Child Adolesc Psychiatry 27:248–251, 1988

Bouvard MP, Leboyer M, Launay JM, et al: Low-dose naltrexone effects on plasma chemistries and clinical symptoms in autism: a double-blind, placebo-controlled study. Psychiatry Res 58:191–201, 1995

Brasic JR, Barnett JY, Sheitman BB, et al: Adverse effects of clomipramine. J Am Acad Child Adolesc Psychiatry 36:1165–1166, 1997

Brodkin ES, McDougle CJ, Naylor ST, et al: Clomipramine in adults with pervasive developmental disorders: a prospective open-label investigation. J Child Adolesc Psychopharmacol 7:109–121, 1997

Buchsbaum MS, Hollander E, Haznedar MM, et al: Effect of fluoxetine on regional cerebral metabolism in autistic spectrum disorders: a pilot study. Int J Neuropsychopharmacol 4:119–125, 2001

Camfield P, Gordon K, Dooley J, et al: Melatonin appears ineffective in children with intellectual deficits and fragmented sleep: six "N of 1" trials. J Child Neurol 11:341–343, 1996

Campbell M, Anderson LT, Meier M, et al: A comparison of haloperidol and behavior therapy and their interaction in autistic children. J Am Acad Child Adolesc Psychiatry 17:640–655, 1978

Campbell M, Schopler E, Cueva JE, et al: Treatment of autistic disorder. J Am Acad Child Adolesc Psychiatry 35:134–143, 1996

Campbell M, Armenteros J, Malone R, et al: Neuroleptic-related dyskinesias in autistic children: a prospective, longitudinal study. J Am Acad Child Adolesc Psychiatry 36:835–843, 1997

Cases O, Vitalis T, Seif I, et al: Lack of barrels in the somatosensory cortex of monoamine oxidase A–deficient mice: role of a serotonin excess during the critical period. Neuron 16:297–307, 1996

Chen NC, Bedair HS, McKay B, et al: Clozapine in the treatment of aggression in an adolescent with autistic disorder. J Clin Psychiatry 62:479–480, 2001

Chugani D, Muzik O, Behen M, et al: Developmental changes in brain serotonin synthesis capacity in autistic and nonautistic children. Ann Neurol 45:287–295, 1999

Cook EH, Rowlett R, Jaselskis C, et al: Fluoxetine treatment of children and adults with autistic disorder and mental retardation. J Am Acad Child Adolesc Psychiatry 31:739–745, 1992

Cook EH, Courchesne R, Lord C, et al: Evidence of linkage between the serotonin transporter and autistic disorder. Mol Psychiatry 2:247–250, 1997

Courchesne E, Press GA, Yeung-Courchesne R: Parietal lobe abnormalities detected with MR in patients with infantile autism. AJR Am J Roentgenol 160:387–393, 1993

Dahlitz M, Alvarez B, Vignau J, et al: Delayed sleep phase syndrome response to melatonin. Lancet 337:1121–1124, 1991

D'Amato RJ, Blue ME, Largent BL, et al: Ontogeny of the serotonergic projection to rat neocortex: transient expression of a dense innervation to primary sensory areas. Proc Natl Acad Sci USA 84:4322–4326, 1987

Damore J, Stine J, Brody L: Medication-induced hypomania in Asperger's disorder. J Am Acad Child Adolesc Psychiatry 37:248–249, 1998

DeLong G, Dwyer J: Correlation of family history with specific autistic subgroups: Asperger's syndrome and bipolar affective disease. J Autism Dev Disord 18:593–600, 1988

DeLong G, Nohria C: Psychiatric family history and neurological disease in autistic spectrum disorders. Dev Med Child Neurol 36:441–448, 1994

DeLong GR, Teague LA, McSwain-Kamran M: Effects of fluoxetine treatment in young children with idiopathic autism. Dev Med Child Neurol 40:551–562, 1998

Findling RL, Maxwell K, Wiznitzer M: An open clinical trial of risperidone monotherapy in young children with autistic disorders. Psychopharmacology Bulletin 33:155–159, 1997

Frankhauser MP, Karumanchi VC, German ML, et al: A double-blind, placebo-controlled study of the efficacy of trasdermal clonidine in autism. J Clin Psychiatry 53:77–82, 1991

Geller B, Guttmacher LB, Bleeg M: Coexistence of childhood onset pervasive developmental disorder and attention deficit disorder with hyperactivity. Am J Psychiatry 138:388–389, 1981

Gillberg C, Srendsen P: CSF monoamines in autistic syndromes and other pervasive developmental disorders of early childhood. Br J Psychiatry 151:89–94, 1987

Goldman-Rakic PS, Brown RM: Postnatal development of monoamine content and synthesis in the cerebral cortex of rhesus monkeys. Dev Brain Res 4:339–349, 1982

Gordon CT, State RC, Nelson JE, et al: A double-blind comparison of clomipramine, desipramine, and placebo in the treatment of autistic disorder. Arch Gen Psychiatry 50:441–447, 1993

Granger R, Staubli U, Davis M, et al: A drug that facilitates glutaminergic transmission reduces exploratory activity and improves performance in a learning-dependent task. Synapse 15:326–329, 1993

Hagerman RJ: Medical follow-up and pharmacotherapy, in Fragile X Syndrome: Diagnosis, Treatment and Research, 3rd Edition. Edited by Hagerman RJ, Hagerman PJ. Baltimore, MD, Johns Hopkins University Press, 2002, pp 287–338

Hagerman RJ, Riddle JE, Roberts LS, et al: A survey of the efficacy of clonidine in Fragile X syndrome. Developmental Brain Dysfunction 8:336–344, 1995

Hagerman RJ, Bregman JD, Tirosh E: Clonidine, in Psychotropic Medication and Developmental Disabilities: The International Consensus Handbook. Edited by Reiss S, Aman MG. Columbus, OH, Ohio State University Nisonger Center, 1998, pp 259–269

Hampson RE, Rogers G, Lynch G, et al: Facilitative effects of the ampakine CX516 on short term memory in rats: correlations with hippocampal neuronal activity. J Neurosci 18:2748–2763, 1998a

Hampson RE, Rogers G, Lynch G, et al: Facilitative effects of the ampakine CX516 on short term memory in rats: enhancement of delayed-nonmatch-to-sample performance. J Neurosci 18:2740–2747, 1998b

Handen BL, Johnson CR, Lubetsky M: Efficacy of methylphenidate among children with autism and symptoms of attention-deficit hyperactivity disorder. J Autism Dev Disord 30:245–255, 2000

Hansen G, Jensen SB, Chandresh L, et al: The psychotropic effect of ketamine. J Psychoactive Drugs 20:419–425, 1988

Hayashi E: Effect of melatonin on sleep-wake rhythm: the sleep diary of an autistic male. Psychiatry Clin Neurosci 54:383–384, 2000

Hedner J, Lundell KH, Breese GR, et al: Developmental variations in CSF monoamine metabolites during childhood. Biol Neonate 49:190–197, 1986

Heils A, Teufel A, Petri S, et al: Allelic variation of human serotonin transporter gene expression. J Neurochem 66:2621–2624, 1996

Hellings JA, Kelley LA, Gabrielli WF, et al: Sertraline response in adults with mental retardation and autistic disorder. J Clin Psychiatry 57:333–336, 1996

Horvath K, Stefanatos G, Sokolski KN, et al: Improved social and language skills after secretin administration in patients with autistic spectrum disorders. J Assoc Acad Minor Phys 9:9–15, 1998

Hunt RD, Arnsten AFT, Asbell MD: An open trial of guanfacine in treatment of attention deficit hyperactivity disorder. J Am Acad Child Adolesc Psychiatry 34:50–54, 1995

Ingvar M, Ambros-Ingerson J, Davis M, et al: Enhancement by an ampakine of memory encoding in humans. Exp Neurol 146:553–559, 1997

Jan JE, Espezel H: Melatonin treatment of chronic sleep disorders. Dev Med Child Neurol 37:279–280, 1995

Jan JE, O'Donnell ME: Use of melatonin in the treatment of paediatric sleep disorders. J Pineal Res 21:193–199, 1996

Jan JE, Espezel H, Appleton RE: The treatment of sleep disorders with melatonin. Dev Med Child Neurol 36:97–107, 1994

Jaselskis CA, Cook EH Jr, Fletcher KE, et al: Clonidine treatment of hyperactive and impulsive children with autistic disorder. J Clin Psychopharmacol 12:322–327, 1992

Jensen PS, Kettle L, Roper MT, et al: Are stimulants overprescribed? Treatment of ADHD in four U.S. communities. J Am Acad Child Adolesc Psychiatry 38:797–804, 1999a

Jensen PS, Bhatara VS, Vitiello B, et al: Psychoactive medication prescribing practices for U.S. children: gaps between research and clinical practice. J Am Acad Child Adolesc Psychiatry 38:557–565, 1999b

Kolmen BK, Feldman HM, Handen BL, et al: Naltrexone in young autistic children: a double-blind, placebo-controlled crossover study. J Am Acad Child Adolesc Psychiatry 34:223–231, 1995

Krishnamoorthy J, King BH: Open-label olanzapine treatment in five preadolescent children. J Child Adolesc Psychopharmacol 8:107–113, 1998

Krystal JH, Karper LP, Seibyl JP: Subanesthetic effects of the noncompetitive NMDA antagonist, ketamine, in humans: psychotomimetic, perceptual, cognitive, and neuroendocrine responses. Arch Gen Psychiatry 51:199–214, 1994

Larson J, Quach CN, LeDuc BQ, et al: Effects of an AMPA receptor modulator on methamphetamine-induced hyperactivity in rats. Brain Res 738:353–356, 1996

Lauder JM, Krebs H: Serotonin as a differentiation signal in early embryogenesis. Dev Neurosci 1:15–30, 1978

Lebrand C, Cases O, Adelbrecht C, et al: Transient uptake and storage of serotonin in developing thalamic neurons. Neuron 17:823–835, 1996

Lesch KP: Variation of serotonergic gene expression: neurodevelopment and the complexity of response to psychopharmacologic drugs. Eur Neuropsychopharmacol 11:457–474, 2001

Lidow MS, Goldman-Rakic PS, Rakic P: Synchronized overproduction of neurotransmitter receptors in diverse regions of the primate cerebral cortex. Proc Natl Acad Sci U S A 88:10218–10221, 1991

Lieske V, Bennett-Clarke CA, Rhoades RW: Effects of serotonin on neurite outgrowth from thalamic neurons in vitro. Neuroscience 90:967–974, 1999

Lynch G, Kessler M, Rogers G et al: Psychological effects of a drug that facilitates brain AMPA receptors. Int Clin Psychopharmacol 11:13–19, 1996

Lynch G, Granger R, Ambros-Ingerson J, et al: Evidence that a positive modulator of AMPA-type glutamate receptors improves delayed recall in aged humans. Exp Neurol 145:89–92, 1997

MacFarlane JG, Cleghorn JM, Brown GM, et al: The effects of exogenous melatonin on the total sleep time and daytime alertness of chronic insomniacs: a preliminary study. Biol Psychiatry 30:371–376, 1991

Malone R, Cater J, Sheikh R, et al: Olanzapine versus haloperidol in children with autistic disorder: an open pilot study. J Am Acad Child Adolesc Psychiatry 40:887–894, 2001

Martin A, Scahill L, Klin A, et al: Higher-functioning pervasive developmental disorders: rates and patterns of psychotropic drug use. J Am Acad Child Adolesc Psychiatry 38:923–931, 1999a

Martin A, Koenig K, Scahill L, et al: Open-label quetiapine in the treatment of children and adolescents with autistic disorder. J Child Adolesc Psychopharmacol 9:99–107, 1999b

McDougle CJ, Naylor ST, Cohen DJ, et al: Effects of tryptophan depletion in drug-free adults with autistic disorder. Arch Gen Psychiatry 53:993–1000, 1996a

McDougle CJ, Naylor ST, Cohen DJ, et al: A double-blind, placebo-controlled study of fluvoxamine in adults with autistic disorder. Arch Gen Psychiatry 53:1001–1008, 1996b

McDougle C, Holmes J, Bronson M, et al: Risperdone treatment of children and adolescents with pervasive developmental disorders: a prospective, open-label study. J Am Acad Child Adolesc Psychiatry 36:685–693, 1997

McDougle CJ, Holmes JP, Carlson DC, et al: A double-blind, placebo-controlled study of risperidone in adults with autistic disorder and other pervasive developmental disorders. Arch Gen Psychiatry 55:633–641, 1998a

McDougle CJ, Brodkin ES, Naylor ST, et al: Sertraline in adults with pervasive developmental disorders: a prospective open-label investigation. J Clin Psychopharmacol 18:62–66, 1998b

McDougle CJ, Scahill L, McCracken JT: Research Units on Pediatric Psychopharmacology (RUPP) Autism Network: background and rationale for an initial controlled study of risperidone. Child Adolesc Psychiatr Clin N Am 9:201–224, 2000

McDougle C, Kem D, Posey D: Case series: use of ziprasidone for maladaptive symptoms in youths with autism. J Am Acad Child Adolesc Psychiatry 41:921–927, 2002

Minshew NJ: Indices of neural function in autism: clinical and biologic implications. Pediatrics 87:774–780, 1991

Miquel MC, Kia HK, Boni C, et al: Postnatal development and localization of 5-HT$_{1A}$ receptor mRNA in rat forebrain and cerebellum. Dev Brain Res 80:149–157, 1994

Muir KW, Lees KR: Clinical experience with excitatory amino acid antagonist drugs. Stroke 26:503–513, 1995

Naruse H, Nagahata M, Nakane Y, et al: A multicenter double-blind trial of pimozide, haloperidol, and placebo in children with behavioral disorders using crossover design. Acta Paedopsychiatrica 48:173–184, 1982

Nicolson R, Avad G, Sloman L: An open trial of risperidone in young autistic children. J Am Acad Child Adolesc Psychiatry 37:372–376, 1998

O'Neill M, Jones RS: Sensory-perceptual abnormalities in autism: a case for more research? J Autism Dev Disord 27:283–293, 1997

Osterheld-Haas MC, Hornung JP: Laminar development of the mouse barrel cortex: effects of neurotoxins against monoamines. Exp Brain Res 110:183–195, 1996

Palm L, Blennow G, Wetterberg L: Long-term melatonin treatment in blind children and young adults with circadian sleep-wake disturbances. Dev Med Child Neurol 39:319–325, 1997

Perry R, Campbell M, Adams P, et al: Long-term efficacy of haloperidol in autistic children: continuous versus discontinuous drug administration. J Am Acad Child Adolesc Psychiatry 28:87–92, 1989

Persico AM, Mengual E, Moessner R: Barrel pattern formation requires serotonin uptake by thalamocortical afferents, and not vesicular monoamine release. J Neurosci 21:6862–6873, 2001

Posey DJ, McDougle CJ: The pharmacotherapy of target symptoms associated with autistic disorder and other pervasive developmental disorders. Harv Rev Psychiatry 8:45–63, 2000

Potenza MN, Holmes JP, Kanes SJ, et al: Olanzapine treatment of children, adolescents, and adults with pervasive developmental disorders: an open-label pilot study. J Clin Psychopharmacol 19:37–44, 1999

Preskorn SH: Dose-effect and concentration-effect relationships with new antidepressants. Psychopharmacol Ser 10:174–189, 1993a

Preskorn SH: Pharmacokinetics of antidepressants: why and how they are relevant to treatment. J Clin Psychiatry 54 (suppl):55–56, 1993b

Purcell AE, Jeon OH, Zimmerman AW, et al: Postmortem brain abnormalities of the glutamate neurotransmitter system in autism. Neurology 57:1618–1628, 2001

Quintana H, Birmaher B, Stedge D, et al: Use of methylphenidate in the treatment of children with autistic disorders. J Autism Dev Disord 25:283–294, 1995

Ratey JJ, Bemporad J, Sorgi P, et al: Open trial effects of beta-blockers on speech and social behaviors in 8 autistic adults. J Autism Dev Disord 17:439–446, 1987a

Ratey JJ, Mikkelsen E, Sorgi P, et al: Autism: the treatment of aggressive behaviors. J Clin Psychopharmacol 7:35–41, 1987b

Raymond GV, Bauman ML, Kemper TL: Hippocampus in autism: a Golgi analysis. Acta Neuropathol (Berl) 91(1):117–119, 1996

Research Units on Pediatric Psychopharmacology Autism Network: Risperidone in children with autism and serious behavioral problems. N Engl J Med 347:314–321, 2002

Riddle MA, Bernstein GA, Cook EH, et al: Anxiolytics, adrenergic agents, and naltrexone. J Am Acad Child Adolesc Psychiatry 38:546–556, 1999

Rogan MT, Staubli UV, LeDoux JE: AMPA receptor facilitation accelerates fear learning without altering the level of conditioned fear acquired. J Neurosci 17:5928–5935, 1997

Sadeh A, Klitzke M, Anders TF, et al: Case study: sleep and aggressive behavior in a blind, retarded adolescent: a concomitant schedule disorder? J Am Acad Child Adolesc Psychiatry 34:820–824, 1995

Sahley TL, Panksepp J: Brain opioids and autism: an updated analysis of possible linkages. J Autism Dev Disord 17:201–216, 1987

Sanchez LE, Campbell M, Small AM, et al: A pilot study of clomipramine in young autistic children. J Am Acad Child Adolesc Psychiatry 35:537–544, 1996

Schuster CR, Lewis M, Seiden LS: Fenfluramine: neurotoxicity. Psychopharmacology Bulletin 22:148–151, 1986

Seifer WE Jr, Foxx JL, Butler IJ: Age effect on dopamine and serotonin metabolite levels in cerebrospinal fluid. Ann Neurol 8:38–42, 1980

Staubli U, Rogers G, Lynch G: Facilitation of glutamate receptors enhances memory. Proc Natl Acad Sci U S A 91:777–781, 1994

Steingard R, Biederman J: Lithium responsive manic-like symptoms in two individuals with autism and mental retardation. J Am Acad Child Adolesc Psychiatry 26:932–935, 1987

Steingard RJ, Zimnitzky B, DeMaso DR, et al: Sertraline treatment of transition-associated anxiety and agitation in children with autistic disorder. J Child Adolesc Psychopharmacol 7:9–15, 1997

Strayhorn JM Jr, Rapp N, Donina W, et al: Randomized trial of methylphenidate for an autistic child. J Am Acad Child Adolesc Psychiatry 27:244–247, 1988

Tordjman S, Gutknecht L, Carlier M: Role of the serotonin transporter gene in the behavioral expression of autism. Mol Psychiatry 6:434–439, 2001

Tran PV, Hamilton SH, Kuntz AJ, et al: Double-blind comparison of olanzapine versus risperidone in the treatment of schizophrenia and other psychotic disorders. J Clin Psychopharmacol 17:407–418, 1997

Uvebrant P, Bauziene R: Intractable epilepsy in children. The efficacy of lamotrigine treatment, including non-seizure-related benefits. Neuropediatrics 25:284–289, 1994

Vitiello B, Jensen PS: Medication development and testing in children and adolescents: current problems, future directions. Arch Gen Psychiatry 54:871–876, 1997

Vitriol C, Farber B: Stimulant medication in certain childhood disorders. Am J Psychiatry 138:1517–1518, 1981

Wender EH: Managing stimulant medication for attention-deficit/hyperactivity disorder: an update. Pediatr Rev 23:234–236, 2002

Whitaker-Azmitia PM, Lauder JM, Shemmer A, et al: Postnatal changes in serotonin$_1$ receptors following prenatal alterations in serotonin levels: further evidence for functional fetal serotonin$_1$ receptors. Dev Brain Res 33:285–289, 1987

Wilens TE: Straight Talk About Psychiatric Medications for Kids. New York, Guilford, 1999

Wilens TE, Biederman J, Spencer T: Clonidine for sleep disturbances associated with attention deficit hyperactivity disorder. J Am Acad Child Adolesc Psychiatry 33:424–426, 1994

Wilens TE, Spencer T, Biederman J, et al: Combined pharmacotherapy: an emerging trend in pediatric psychopharmacology. J Am Acad Child Adolesc Psychiatry 34:110–112, 1995

Wilens TE, Spencer TJ, Swanson JM, et al: Combining methylphenidate and clonidine: a clinically sound medication option [comments]. J Am Acad Child Adolesc Psychiatry 38:614–619; discussion 619–622, 1999

Willemsen-Swinkels SH, Buitelaar JK, Weijnen FG, et al: Placebo-controlled acute dosage naltrexone study in young autistic children. Psychiatry Res 58:203–215, 1995

Woolston JL: Combined pharmacotherapy: pitfalls of treatment. J Am Acad Child Adolesc Psychiatry 38:1455–1457, 1999

Yan W, Wilson CC, Haring JH: Effects of neonatal serotonin depletion on the development of rat dentate granule cells. Dev Brain Res 98:177–184, 1997

Zilbovicius M, Garreau B, Samson Y, et al: Delayed maturation of the frontal cortex in childhood autism. Am J Psychiatry 152:248–252, 1995

Zuddas A, Ledda MG, Fratta A, et al: Clinical effects of clozapine on autistic disorder. Am J Psychiatry 153:738, 1996

Chapter 8

Alternative Theories

Assessment and Therapy Options

Robin L. Hansen, M.D.
Sally Ozonoff, Ph.D.

Introduction

The number of children being diagnosed with autism spectrum disorders appears to be rising precipitously, as described in Chapter 1. The prevalence rate of strictly defined autism was estimated to be between 2 and 4 in 10,000 three decades ago but was found to be 16.8 in 10,000 today (Chakrabarti and Fombonne 2001). This increase has heightened concerns about the etiology of autism. Research suggests that autism spectrum disorders (ASD) are heavily influenced by genetic factors, as discussed in Chapter 1. The rapid increase in prevalence is difficult to explain from a purely genetic standpoint, however, as the frequency of the genes putatively involved would change little in the population over a 30-year time frame. This has led to the suggestion that exposure to unknown substances in the environment, particularly ones that are more common now than 30 years ago, may interact with genetic susceptibility to trigger autism, cause it alone, or mediate the expression and severity of the disorder (Hornig and Lipkin 2001). The list of possible suspects currently includes immunizations, heavy metals, infectious agents, and toxic chemicals. This list is likely to expand until the causes of and treatments for autism are known. This chapter reviews these alternative theories, explains the biological mechanisms proposed to be at work, and outlines practical applications for the clinician involved in evaluation and treatment.

The Need for Professional Involvement and Collaboration

The theories reviewed in this chapter are not (at least currently) "mainstream" and are dismissed by many medical professionals. However, it is important that those who work with families affected by autism be acquainted with these theories and therapies. The media and Internet contain much information about these approaches (not all of it reliable), and parents are quite likely to be aware of and ask questions about these topics. A recent study of preschool children enrolled in early intensive behavioral therapy found that over 50% had also tried at least one "alternative" treatment (Smith et al. 2000). Therefore, from a purely practical standpoint, clinicians need to understand these theories and their evaluation and treatment implications.

It is widely accepted that autism spectrum disorders are both etiologically and clinically heterogeneous. Subgroups of children with ASD with different phenotypes and different etiologies are likely. It is not inconceivable that some of the potential risks reviewed in this chapter may one day be shown to be associated with a subgroup of children with autism. Autism is a syndrome or collection of multiple symptoms that tend to co-occur. Multiple treatments may be needed for multiple target symptoms. Gastrointestinal or immune symptoms, when present, are not likely to be improved by appropriate educational and social interventions for autism, for example.

It is important to the therapeutic alliance with parents to be aware of and keep an open mind about the alternative approaches reviewed in this chapter. Therapy outcome research clearly shows that the quality of the bond between patient and professional strongly influences improvement. Simple acts such as listening empathically, valuing patients' ideas, and responding compassionately to their concerns improve outcome (Adler and Hammett 1973; Thomas 1994). These practitioner behaviors are thought to underlie the strong response to placebo seen in many drug studies (Rabkin et al. 1990). It has been speculated that the patient–practitioner relationship has an even more powerful effect on outcome in alternative medicine, since providers are often very enthusiastic and optimistic about the treatments they proffer and the patient's experience is rarely devalued or brushed aside (Kaptchuk 2002). Thus, collaborating with parents who seek an appropriate balance between conventional and alternative therapies is one important component of the "family-centered" approach that underlies the chapters in this book.

If professionals are able to establish an open dialogue with families about alternative treatments they have chosen to explore, they can play a very important role in counseling parents about the possible risks of these treatments, as well as observing and quantifying the intervention's positive and negative medical and behavioral effects. Practitioners can identify target behaviors for treatment and objectively assess pre- and post-intervention function. Ideally, the process would involve referral for testing by another professional who is unaware of the intervention, using standardized instruments such as those described in Chapter 3. Professionals can also solicit data from others (e.g., teachers, care providers, relatives) who do not know about the treatment. Clinicians can also be of immense utility in monitoring potential side effects of alternative treatments. But these useful roles can be played only if lines of communication are open, even when the professional does not agree with the treatment. A very helpful discussion of this topic is provided by Levy and Hyman (2002).

While being open to alternative approaches, it is of paramount importance to maintain the health and safety of the child and ensure that families do not forgo treatments of proven value in favor of alternative treatments of undetermined efficacy. It is important to help families find agencies or professionals qualified to provide the services they desire. Practitioners should encourage parents to ask about professional credentials, experience, and references. This chapter provides some guidelines for maintaining this delicate balance between conservative scientific standards and open-minded encouragement. Finally, we advise professionals to empirically scrutinize *all* potential therapies they consider for their patients, not just the alternative biomedical interventions covered here. As reviewed in Chapters 6 and 7, there are also behavioral and pharmacological interventions being used for children with ASD for which there is little empirical evidence of efficacy. Be as careful about these as about the alternative approaches we review here.

Alternative Theories of Causation

The Bowel–Brain Connection

Many parents report gastrointestinal (GI) disturbances in their children with autism, such as persistent diarrhea, constipation, and abdominal distension or pain. Melmed et al. (2000) reported clinically significant gastrointestinal symptoms in 46% of a clinical sample of American children with autism, compared with 10% of normal control subjects, based on parent report. However, Black et al. (2002) found no differences in the incidence of chronic inflammation of the GI tract, celiac disease, food intolerance, or recurrent gastrointestinal symptoms between children with and without autism, matched by age, sex, and medical practice, in a population-based, nested case-control study. In both groups, 9% reported symptoms of GI disturbance to their primary medical practitioner. We do not yet have consensus about whether GI symptoms are etiologically related to autism symptoms. In this section, we describe multiple theories for the origin of GI pathology in autism—immunizations, food allergies, metabolic problems, disruption of gut flora due to antibiotic overuse, among others—and the implications for practice.

The MMR Theory

Wakefield et al. (1998) described a case series of 12 children with gastrointestinal disturbances, including chronic constipation with overflow, pain, bloating, and esophageal reflux, often starting around the time that autistic behaviors became evident. Endoscopy revealed lymphonodular hyperplasia and macroscopic evidence of colitis, which Wakefield designated "autistic enterocolitis." He postulated that these children had a new subtype of "regressive autism" that was induced by the MMR (measles, mumps, and rubella) vaccination. He has more recently postulated that the onset of MMR-induced autism requires additional risk factors, such as an intercurrent infection at the time of vaccination, exposure to multiple vaccines concurrently, a history of atopy, and a strong family history of autoimmune disease (Wakefield 2002).

The postulated mechanism of the pathogenic interaction between the bowel disturbance and autistic symptomatology is a persistent measles virus infection resulting in mucosal damage, increased intestinal permeability, and gastrointestinal absorption of toxic neuropeptides causing central nervous system dysfunction and behavioral regression. Measles virus persistence in intestinal lymphoid tissues of the general population or developmentally normal children with gastrointestinal symptoms is not known. Measles virus RNA was detected in the bowel biopsies of 73 of 77 children (94.8%) with regressive autism, but only 5 of 44 control subjects (11.4%; Martin et al. 2002). Replication of these findings in other labs has not been successful, and concerns about contamination of samples with material that was used as a positive assay control have been raised (Afzal and Minor 2002). To clarify the differences found between laboratories and establish cross-lab reliability, the National Institute for Biological Standards and Control in the United Kingdom is coordinating an international collaborative study in which measles virus samples and control samples will be supplied to various independent laboratories for in-house evaluation and identification.

Epidemiologic data from three recent studies do not support an association between regressive autism, GI symptoms, and the MMR vaccine.

Taylor et al. (1999) identified 498 children with autism born since 1979 and linked clinical records to independently recorded immunization data. There was no evidence of a change in trend in incidence or age at diagnosis associated with the introduction of MMR vaccination in 1988. De-Wilde et al. (2001) confirmed these negative findings. In a repeat survey, Taylor et al. (2002) found that between 1979 and 1999, the proportion of children with regression (25%) or bowel symptoms (17%) did not change. No significant differences were seen in rates of bowel problems or developmental regression in children who received the MMR vaccine before their parents became concerned about their development, compared with those who received it only after such concern and those who had not received the MMR vaccine at all (Taylor et al. 2002). Fombonne and Chakrabati (2001) found a similar proportion of bowel problems (19%) in a well-validated sample of children with autism in the United Kingdom. And the most recent study, which followed all children born in Denmark between 1991 and 1998, strongly supported the findings of Taylor and colleagues, again failing to find any increase in vaccinated relative to unvaccinated children or any temporal clustering of cases of autism after immunization. Although it is possible that a small subgroup of susceptible children affected by immunization could be missed in large epidemiologic studies, these investigations indicate that MMR vaccination is not a significant contributor to the increased recognition of ASD.

Clinical Implications. As part of a complete medical history, practitioners need to ask about GI symptoms. However, the presence of GI symptoms is not currently a contraindication for vaccination unless the practitioner determines the child has an acute GI infection that requires treatment prior to vaccination. Contraindications to giving the MMR include anaphylaxis to egg ingestion, anaphylactic allergy to neomycin, and severe congenital or acquired immunodeficiencies (American Academy of Pediatrics 2000). Recent administration of immune globulin is also a contraindication because the serologic response to the vaccine will be attenuated by the immune globulin for several months. Monovalent vaccines are manufactured, although their availability is variable. However, there is no evidence to suggest that monovalent live virus vaccines are less likely to alter immune function than combined vaccines, and their use may result in delayed or missed immunizations (Halsey and Hyman 2001). The success of wide-scale public vaccination programs has eradicated or significantly reduced the risk of morbidity and mortality related to many childhood diseases, so that most parents and practitioners have not experienced the potentially fatal results of preventable infectious diseases in young children. Because of this, the perceived risk/benefit ratio of vaccines has been skewed, particularly as parents consider individual risks and benefits to their child based on personal experience and anecdotal information. Practitioners need to review carefully the indications, documented contraindications, established risks, and benefits of immunization with families in helping them make vaccine decisions, while we await the results of further research.

The Food Allergy Theory

Gastrointestinal symptoms as a result of food allergies to casein and gluten have been proposed as possible etiologic contributors to ASD. Several studies have reported increased levels of urinary peptides in children with autism (Le Couteur et al. 1988; Pedersen et al. 1999; Reichelt 1997). It has been postulated that this increase in urinary peptides is the result of increased gut permeability related to transulphation and/or peptidase defects (Alberti et al. 1999). Due to these metabolic abnormalities, peptides with opioid activity enter the central nervous system, cross-react with brain receptors, and alter neurotransmission (Reichelt 1997; Whiteley and Shattock 2002). The mammalian opioid system modulates social-affective processes. Since casein-containing milk, both breast and formula, and gluten-containing cereal are the primary sources of nutrition for infants, early and prolonged exposure is common in many children. Most children with milk or gluten intolerance (celiac disease) or other malabsorption disorders have GI symptoms of chronic diarrhea, abdominal pain, distension or gaseousness, and frequent failure to thrive. However, Horvath and Perman (2002) tested the sera of 420 children with autism and found no serologic or histologic signs of celiac disease on upper gastrointestinal endoscopies.

Clinical Implications.   As noted previously, a careful history related to GI symptoms is important, as well as a family history of GI disorders such as celiac disease, Crohn's disease, ulcerative colitis, and irritable bowel syndrome. Children with persistent GI symptoms or family history should be evaluated for treatable disorders. Stool pH and reducing substances reflect carbohydrate malabsorption, and stool alpha-1-antitrypsin is a measure of protein malabsorption. Stool blood can be seen with diarrhea, malabsorption, or infection. Serum for anti-endomysium antibodies (IgA EMA) and total IgA is a highly sensitive and specific screen for celiac disease in normal populations (Rossi and Tjota 1998).

The treatment proposed for gluten and casein intolerance is an elimination diet (LeBreton 2001), also known as the gluten-free casein-free (GFCF) diet. Anecdotal information suggesting improvement in behavior on such diets abounds on the Internet and in parent support groups. Several studies of restricted diets have been conducted, and most report beneficial results for some children (Knivsberg et al. 2001; Reichelt 1997; Whiteley et al. 1999), but few have used control groups, accounted for other interventions, or conducted standardized pre- and posttesting blind to intervention status. Recently, a single-blind, randomized, controlled study reported significant behavioral and developmental improvements in 10 children with autism placed on a gluten/casein-free diet for a year, compared with 10 children matched for severity of autistic behaviors, age, and cognitive level who were not on the diet (Knivsberg et al. 2002). All subjects also had abnormal urinary peptide metabolites, analyzed by HPLC using reverse phase c-18 columns. Parents were not blind to intervention status, although pre- and posttreatment evaluators reportedly were. Further research is needed in this area. If children are placed on GFCF diets, they need to be monitored for iron status, calcium, and protein intake. Nutritional consultation is recommended, with careful monitoring of the child's growth and health by the practitioner.

Secretin

Secretin is a hormone secreted by the GI tract to aid in digestion; it is also administered exogenously for radiologic imaging of the GI system. An initial case report described significant improvement in autistic symptoms following a single injection of secretin in three preschool-aged children with ASD and GI symptoms (Horvath et al. 1998). This and other media reports created widespread interest in the potential use of secretin for treating autism. Thousands of children received secretin treatment before formal studies were conducted. Initial controlled clinical trials failed to document significant treatment effects 1 to 4 weeks after a single administration of either porcine or human secretin (Coniglio et al. 2001; Dunn-Geier et al. 2000; Owley et al. 2001; Roberts et al. 2001; Sandler et al. 1999). A recent double-blind, multidose study using synthetic human secretin (C. Schneider et al. under review) suggested that a subgroup of children might be responders, however. In their sample of children 3–7 years of age with autism and GI symptoms, indicators of response to treatment included younger age and the absence of abnormal biomarkers of GI inflammation or pancreatic dysfunction. Significant improvements were found in reciprocal social interaction, as measured by the Autism Diagnostic Observation Schedule (ADOS); behavior, as measured by the Clinical Global Impression of Change (CGI-C) scale; and vocabulary. Testing and ratings were done blind to intervention status. This study differed from previously reported studies in that it evaluated three doses of secretin over an 8-week period, enrolled a younger group of children with autism who also had pronounced gastrointestinal symptoms at the time of entry, and studied a large sample ($n=129$). A replication study enrolling larger numbers of young subjects is currently in progress.

Clinical Implications.　At this point there is little indication from controlled studies that secretin has a significant effect on behavior or learning in the majority of children with autism. Intravenous use of secretin as a treatment for autism is not approved by the Food and Drug Administration, and it has become difficult to obtain. However, further research with a double-blind placebo-controlled methodology is needed to establish whether there are subgroups of children who respond positively to this intervention.

Immune and Infectious Theories

It has also been suggested that autoimmunity, other immune dysfunction, or infectious agents may play a role in triggering autism, either de novo or in genetically susceptible individuals. These theories are not mutually exclusive of the bowel-brain connection theories just reviewed, as immune dysfunction may cause gastrointestinal disorder. However, some immune and infectious theories propose a mechanism of action directly on the brain, independent of bowel involvement, so we discuss them separately here.

There are a few reports that children with ASD experience a disproportionate number of infections (Konstantareas and Homatidis 1987), consistent with the hypothesis that a subgroup of children with autism have immune system deficiencies. Mason-Brothers et al. (1993) examined the incidence of recurrent infections in an epidemiologic sample from Utah. They found that children with autism experienced significantly more otitis media, upper respiratory, and other infections than their nonautistic siblings. Other studies have found elevated rates of infections in children with other neurodevelopmental disorders such as learning disabilities and attention-deficit/hyperactivity disorder (ADHD) (Bishop and Edmundson 1986; Hagerman and Falkenstein 1987; Secord et al. 1988), and it is not clear if such infections thus pose a specific risk for autism or a more general risk for CNS-related dysfunction.

A wide variety of immunologic abnormalities have been postulated to be related to ASD, although there is tremendous variability in the differences found across studies and the hypothesized causal mechanisms. Most of the studies lack sufficient sample size, adequate diagnostic specificity, appropriate comparison groups, and controls for potential environmental triggers. The immune abnormalities most frequently reported in ASD include imbalance of serum immunoglobulins (selective IgA deficiency, increased IgE and IgG levels) and cytokines (increased IL-12 and IFN-gamma). Decreased T-cell response, reductions in natural killer-cell activity, and alterations of Th1 and Th2 cell subsets have also been reported, although no systematic studies have been completed (Korvatska et al. 2002). However, expected associations between altered serologic findings and clinical presentations of immune dysfunction (e.g., increased susceptibility to infection) have not been reported in most studies (Korvatska et al. 2002).

Antibiotic Overuse Hypotheses

One theory suggests the possibility that recurrent oral antibiotic use results in alterations in the normal bacterial flora of the GI tract, resulting in yeast overgrowth and production of toxins, bacterial overgrowth of other pathogenic organisms, and increased gut permeability. Proponents of the yeast overgrowth theory suggest that treatment with antifungal medications such as Nystatin or Diflucan are indicated to reduce yeast in the gut (Shaw et al. 1995). However, studies have not demonstrated the presence of yeast in small-intestine biopsy samples in children with GI symptoms and autism undergoing endoscopy (Horvath et al. 1999), and the presence of yeast in normal stool samples makes evidence for this theory difficult to substantiate. Antifungal medications have possible toxicity effects including seizures, liver damage, and leukopenia, particularly after the lengthy courses proposed for treatment of autism.

Sandler et al. (2000) proposed that repeated antibiotic use may disrupt the protective effect of indigenous intestinal organisms and allow colonization with one or more neurotoxin-producing species, such as clostridium. Based on this conjecture, he and colleagues studied 11 children with ASD and a history of antibiotic use, persistent diarrhea, and regression. The children were treated for 8 weeks with vancomycin, an antibiotic usually reserved for life-threatening, antibiotic-resistant bacterial infections. Improvements were noted in 8 of 10 children on paired videotapes pre- and posttreatment. Improvements were noted to wane after cessation of treatment. This was a small, open-label trial without controls and without identification of an offending organism in the GI system. Vancomycin is a very powerful antibiotic, and its use is carefully monitored to prevent the evolution of bacteria resistant to it. It also has serious side effects including colitis, ototoxicity, and renal damage (Benitz and Tatro 1995). Its use as a treatment for ASD cannot be recommended at this time, although further studies regarding the hypothesized overgrowth of neurotoxin-producing organisms in children with persistent diarrhea and regression are warranted.

Autoimmune Theories

Antibodies to CNS proteins have been found in significantly higher numbers in children and adults with ASD than in controls, including autoantibodies to a serotonin receptor (Todd and Ciaranello 1985), myelin basic protein (Singh et al. 1993), neuron-axon filament protein (Singh et al. 1997), and nerve growth factor (Kozlovskaia et al. 2000). Vojdani et al. (2002) measured autoantibodies against nine neuron-specific antigens in the serum of 40 children with autism and 40 age- and sex-matched control subjects using enzyme-linked immunosorbent assay (ELISA). Specimens were elevated in 27.5% of children with autism for IgA, 35% for IgG, and 50% for IgM compared with 2.5%, 5%, and 10%, respectively, of the controls. This study also found significantly elevated autoantibodies to three cross-reactive peptides for *Chlamydia pneumoniae*, streptococcal M protein, and milk butyrophilin in children with autism compared with controls. The authors postulated that infectious agents, as well as environmental agents, can induce alterations or overexpression of genes involved in structural differentiation of astrocytes and other neuronal cells, resulting in autoantibody production. The role of milk peptides and other factors in the induction of autoantibodies to neuronal antigens needs to be further studied. However, there are no signs of demyelination in individuals with ASD, either on neuroimaging or neuropathologic examination (Bauman and Kemper 1994), that would be expected in such an autoimmune process. The presence of antineuronal autoantibodies in the serum of normally developing control children raises further questions about the pathogenic role of these antibodies. They may, in fact, be secondary phenomena.

Comi et al. (1999) found an increased incidence of autoimmune disorders in families with autistic children, particularly in mothers. Rheumatoid arthritis, systemic lupus erythematosis, and connective tissue disorders were significantly increased, although there were no differences in autoimmune disorders of the central nervous system between groups. The interplay between genetic susceptibility to autoimmune disorders and environmental risk factors, including the intrauterine environment, is an area of active research. Korvatska et al. (2002) have postulated three possible mechanisms by which autoimmunity may be etiologically related to ASD. In a subset of susceptible individuals, an aberrant immune response to developmentally expressed antigens may transiently trigger an inflammatory cascade that produces cytokines limited to specific groups of neurons. Alternatively, an inherent defect in the brain during early development could trigger an immune response, with further effects on brain development through established immunomodulatory mechanisms. A third possibility put forth by Korvatska et al. (2002) is that some individuals with autism have systemic pathology that causes abnormalities in the CNS and immune system separately. Warren (1998) proposed an additional theory, suggesting that immune dysfunction leads to increased episodes of infection of longer duration and chronicity, and to brain damage either directly via the viral antigen or indirectly through an autoimmune process. The immune dysfunction may also reside in the mother, with infections affecting brain development of the fetus during gestation (Warren 1998).

Neurotransmitters and Hormones

Neurotransmitters are known to modulate immunologic activity. The relationship between alterations of neurotransmitters and immune function in ASD has been increasingly studied. Hyperserotonemia is the most consistent finding in samples of children with autism, as well as in their relatives (Korvatska et al. 2002). Chugani et al. (1997) have demonstrated asymmetries of serotonin synthesis in autistic boys, although not in autistic girls or in unaffected siblings, as well as differences in developmental rates of brain serotonin synthesis (Chugani et al. 1999). Serotonin can stimulate T-cell proliferation or exert a suppressive effect, depending on its concentration.

Oxytocin is thought to participate in the development of immune tolerance and act as a promoter of focal adhesion of T-cells. Oxytocin is known to be involved in such affiliative behaviors as nursing, mating, social attachment, bonding, and parental behavior (Insel 1992). A disruption in oxytocin metabolism has been suggested to be related to autism (Insel et al. 1999; Panksepp 1992). Children with autism have been found to have decreased levels of plasma oxytocin (Modahl et al. 1998) and increased levels of oxytocin precursor peptides (Green et al. 2001) compared with control subjects. This suggests a failure in the normal processing of the immature peptide that yields functional oxytocin (Green et al. 2001). This has led some investigators to hypothesize that exposure to high levels of exogenous oxytocin at delivery, via pitocin induction, might make a child vulnerable to the development of autism by causing down-regulation of oxytocin receptors in the immature brain (Hollander et al. 1998). A recent study found that children with autism had significantly higher rates of pitocin induction compared with national norms (Hollander et al. 1998), although later case-control studies failed to confirm this association (Fein et al. 1997; Gale et al. 2003).

Clinical Implications

Many of the studies just reviewed suffered from methodologic limitations, most notably lack of appropriate controls. In addition, predictions of these theories, such as evidence of neurologic damage from autoimmunity and association between findings of immune deficiency and increased infection rates, have not been supported by studies conducted so far. Further research is needed before routine immunologic studies are carried out in all children with autism, unless the child has features of immune dysfunction such as recurrent or difficult-to-treat infections, or infection with organisms that are not usually pathogenic. If these features are present, referral for evaluation by an immunologist or an infectious disease specialist is recommended.

Small studies with poorly defined measures have suggested that interventions using transfer factor, intravenous immunoglobulin, or corticosteroids may have beneficial effects on autistic symptoms (Gupta 2000). Plioplys (1998) reported that 1 of 10 children with autism and immunologic abnormalities on blood tests (primarily increased frequency of activated lymphocytes) appeared to respond to intravenous immunoglobulin (IVIg). The serum abnormalities of the responding child did not differ from the remaining subjects. The author argued that there may be a subgroup of children with autism who respond to IVIg, but that "the use of intravenous immunoglobulin to treat autistic children should be undertaken only with great caution, and only under formal research protocols" (p. 79). DelGiudice-Asch et al. (1999) reported that 6 months of IVIg infusions in seven children with autism had no effect. Since efficacy has not been established to justify the potentially significant side effects of these therapies, which include renal failure, infection, and acute neurologic complications, these treatment approaches are not recommended at the present time and further studies are needed before immunologic approaches to treatment are justified (Krause et al. 2002; Zimmerman 2000).

The most commonly used alternative therapies for ASD are vitamins and dietary supplements (Hyman and Levy 2000). It has been proposed that large doses of vitamin B_6 (often given in conjunction with magnesium to increase absorption) enhance central nervous system function and decrease autistic behavior (Rimland et al. 1978). Most accounts of beneficial effects are anecdotal or case reports (Adams and Conn 1997). The only double-blind, placebo-controlled study conducted to date did not find any differences between groups (Findling et al. 1997), but a meta-analysis of a dozen studies noted improvement in about half of subjects administered high doses of B_6 with magnesium (Pfeiffer et al. 1995). Dimethylglycine (DMG) is a nutritional supplement also suggested to have beneficial effects on behavior by altering neurotransmitter precursors (Rimland 1996). However, two investigations using a double-blind, placebo-control design failed to find any evidence of benefit from DMG (Bolman and Richmond 1999; Kern et al. 2001). Further research on dietary supplements is direly needed, since these treatments are so widely used by families. Parents must be made aware of the potential side effects from excess vitamin exposure, especially if combined with other supplements containing similar ingredients. B_6 toxicity results in a peripheral sensory neuropathy, and magnesium toxicity contributes to cardiac arrythmias (Levy and Hyman 2002). It is important that physicians be aware of the supplements that children are being given and that parents be counseled regarding the complications of exceeding recommended doses.

Toxic Exposure Theories

Another possible biological mechanism proposed to explain the development of autism is exposure to environmental toxins during the prenatal or infancy period (Bernard et al. 2001; Edelson and Cantor 1998; London and Etzel 2000) or metabolic abnormalities that impair the natural detoxification process. It is well established that certain early exogenous exposures (e.g., mercury, lead, ethanol) can have neurotoxic effects and lead to developmental disabilities (Burbacher et al. 1990; Goldman and Koduru 2000; Myers and Davidson 2000; Needleman et al. 1990). Concentrations of lead have been found to be slightly elevated in the blood of children with autism relative to both healthy siblings and nonautistic controls (Accardo et al. 1988; Cohen et al. 1976; Shannon and Graef 1997), although this is thought to be related to increased mouthing of objects by children with autism and not causal of autism. However, this prompted a recommendation by the American Academy of Neurology for periodic lead screening for all children with or at risk for autism (Filipek et al. 2000).

Heavy metal exposure is hypothesized to come from a variety of sources, including air and water pollution, amalgam dental fillings, batteries, residues in foods, and fish and shellfish. One possible source of excessive mercury exposure that has been particularly alarming to both parents and the medical community is thimerosal, an ethylmercury-based preservative included in several vaccines to prevent bacterial contamination. MMR, polio, and varicella vaccines have never contained thimerosal, but it has been included in multiple-use vaccines since the 1930s. Concerns have been raised recently that the cumulative exposure to ethylmercury, via thimerosal, is now far greater than in the past, due to the increased number of vaccines given to children, especially before age 2. This is a controversial theory that has provoked strong reactions on both sides, but current scientific evidence neither proves nor disproves a link between thimerosal and neurodevelopmental disorders (Stratton et al. 2001). Pichichero et al. (2002) studied 61 infants between 2 and 6 months of age who received immunizations containing thimerosal between 1999 and

2000. Blood levels of mercury were measured at various times over 30 days. All levels measured were well below current recommended safety levels. The mercury was cleared within 30 days in the infants tested, primarily through fecal excretion. Although this study is reassuring, replication is needed since thimerosal continues to be used outside the United States, primarily in developing countries that cannot afford the increased cost of single-use vaccines. The American Academy of Pediatrics (AAP), the Advisory Committee on Immunization Practices (ACIP), and the United States Public Health Service (PHS) recommended in 1999 that thimerosal be removed as soon as possible from all vaccines given to infants. At the writing of this book at the end of 2002, thimerosal-free vaccines are currently on the market and routinely used. Influenza vaccine, given annually to susceptible children and adults, is the only vaccine that continues to contain thimerosal in the United States.

Recently, the potential neurodevelopmental effects of pesticides and polychlorinated biphenyls (PCBs) have begun to be explored (Eskenazi et al. 1999; Hsu et al. 1985). Exposure to pesticides has been linked to fetal deaths (Arbuckle and Sever 1998) and childhood cancer (Zahm and Ward 1998), although studies lack exposure information for specific chemicals or classes. The developmental effects of PCBs were described by Hsu et al. (1985) in children born to mothers who consumed contaminated cooking oil. Dermatologic and dental anomalies were noted in infancy, with delays in development, abnormalities in behavior, and increased prevalence of speech problems seen later. A study with lower exposure levels (Jacobson and Jacobson 1996) due to maternal consumption of contaminated fish during pregnancy showed lower IQ scores and poorer reading comprehension at 11-year follow-up, although other studies have failed to find similar effects. Most empirical research conducted to date has not specifically examined social deficits or autism as outcomes of such exposures.

Clinical Implications

Accurate testing for heavy metals exposure requires the use of laboratories with well-maintained, documented quality control measures and established baseline levels of background exposure. Currently, accurate testing for pesticides and other xenobiotic agents is generally limited to academic institutions with toxicology research laboratories. Chelation, a method of chemically binding heavy metals present in the blood to remove them from the body, has increasingly been recommended as a treatment for autism, but without the benefit of controlled studies. Chelation was not shown to improve developmental function in nonautistic children with documented lead intoxication (O'Connor and Rich 1999; Rogan et al.

2001). The chemicals used for chelation have potentially significant side effects of liver and kidney toxicity, severe electrolyte and fluid imbalance, hypersensitivity reactions, and depletion of enzymatically important elements such as copper, lead, and zinc. Children undergoing chelation must be carefully monitored by medical professionals.

Conclusion

The theories and treatment approaches reviewed in this chapter are not yet part of the standard of care for autism spectrum disorders. In many scientific communities and clinical settings, these theories and treatments are dismissed outright. Yet many families are trying these approaches, whether their medical caregivers agree with their decisions or not. Given this situation, practitioners have a responsibility to be aware of and conversant in these approaches. We can be helpful in working *with* families who express the desire to try alternative therapies, rather than let them go at it alone. Practitioners can help in a variety of ways. They can

- Provide a supportive atmosphere for discussing alternatives
- Help families sort out potentially helpful options from those that pose potential danger to the child with ASD, balancing costs/risks with benefits
- Explain the potential mechanism of action and existing research on the treatment
- Monitor potential side effects
- Objectively assess positive treatment effects

We hope that this chapter will help clinicians engaged in such partnerships with their patients.

References

Accardo P, Whitman B, Caul J, et al: Autism and plumbism: a possible association. Clin Pediatr 27:41–44, 1988

Adams L, Conn S: Nutrition and its relationship to autism. Focus on Autism and Other Developmental Disabilities 12:53–58, 1997

Adler HM, Hammett VB: The doctor-patient relationship revisited: an analysis of the placebo effect. Ann Intern Med 78:595–598, 1973

Afzal MA, Minor PD: Vaccines, Crohn's disease and autism. Mol Psychiatry 7 (suppl 2):S49–S50, 2002

Alberti A, Pirrone P, Elia M, et al: Sulphation deficit in "low-functioning" autistic children: a pilot study. Biol Psychiatry 46:420–424, 1999

American Academy of Pediatrics: Report of the Committee of Infectious Diseases, 25th Edition. Elk Grove Village, IL, American Academy of Pediatrics, 2000

Arbuckle TE, Sever LE: Pesticide exposures and fetal death: a review of the epidemiologic literature. Crit Rev Toxicol 28:229–270, 1998

Bauman ML, Kemper TL: The Neurobiology of Autism. Baltimore, MD, Johns Hopkins University Press, 1994

Benitz WE, Tatro DS: The Pediatric Drug Handbook, 3rd Edition. St. Louis, MO, Mosby, 1995

Bernard S, Enayati A, Redwood L, et al: Autism: a novel form of mercury poisoning. Med Hypotheses 56:462–471, 2001

Bishop DV, Edmundson A: Is otitis media a major cause of specific developmental language disorders? Br J Disord Commun 21(3):321–338, 1986

Black C, Kaye JA, Jick H: Relation of childhood gastrointestinal disorders to autism: nested case-control study using data from the UK General Practice Research Database. BMJ 325:419–421, 2002

Bolman WM, Richmond JA: A double-blind, placebo-controlled, crossover pilot trial of low dose dimethylglycine in patients with autistic disorder. J Autism Dev Disord 29:191–194, 1999

Burbacher TM, Rodier PM, Weiss B: Methylmercury developmental neurotoxicity: a comparison of effects in humans and animals. Neurotoxicol Teratol 12:191–202, 1990

Chakrabarti S, Fombonne E: Pervasive developmental disorders in preschool children. JAMA 285:3093–3099, 2001

Chugani DC, Muzik O, Rothermel R, et al: Altered serotonin synthesis in the dentatothalamocortical pathway in autistic boys. Ann Neurol 42:666–669, 1997

Chugani DC, Muzik O, Behen M, et al: Developmental changes in brain serotonin synthesis capacity in autistic and nonautistic children. Ann Neurol 45:287–295, 1999

Cohen DJ, Johnson WT, Caparulo BK: Pica and elevated blood lead level in autistic and atypical children. Am J Dis Child 130:47–48, 1976

Comi AM, Zimmerman AW, Frye VH, et al: Familial clustering of autoimmune disorders and evaluation of medical risk factors in autism. J Child Neurol 14:388–394, 1999

Coniglio S, Lewis J, Lang C, et al: A randomized, double-blind, placebo-controlled trial of single dose intravenous secretin as treatment for children with autism. J Pediatr 138:649–655, 2001

DelGiudice-Asch G, Schmeidler SL, Cunningham-Rundles C, et al: Brief report: a pilot open clinical trial of intravenous immunoglobulin in childhood autism. J Autism Dev Disord 29:157–160, 1999

DeWilde S, Carey IM, Richards N, et al: Do children who become autistic consult more often after MMR vaccination? Br J Gen Pract 51:226–227, 2001

Dunn-Geier J, Ho H, Auersperg E, et al: Effect of secretin on children with autism: a randomized controlled trial. Dev Med Child Neurol 42:796–802, 2000

Edelson SB, Cantor DS: Autism: xenobiotic influences. Toxicol Ind Health 14:553–563, 1998

Eskenazi B, Bradman A, Castorina R: Exposures of children to organophosphate pesticides and their potential adverse health effects. Environ Health Perspect 107 (suppl 3):409–419, 1999

Fein D, Allen D, Dunn M, et al: Pitocin induction and autism. Am J Psychiatry 154:438–439, 1997

Filipek PA, Accardo PJ, Ashwal S, et al: Practice parameter: screening and diagnosis of autism: report of the Quality Standards Subcommittee of the American Academy of Neurology and the Child Neurology Society. Neurology 55:468–479, 2000

Findling RL, Maxwell K, Scotese-Wojtila L, et al: High-dose pyridoxine and magnesium administration in children with autistic disorder: an absence of salutary effects in a double-blind, placebo-controlled study. J Autism Dev Disord 27:467–478, 1997

Fombonne E, Chakrabarti S: No evidence for a new variant of measles-mumps-rubella–induced autism. Pediatrics 108:E58, 2001

Gale S, Ozonoff S, Lainhart J: Pitocin induction in autistic and nonautistic individuals. J Autism Dev Disord 33: 205–208, 2003

Goldman LR, Koduru S: Chemicals in the environment and developmental toxicity to children: a public health and policy perspective. Environ Health Perspect 108 (suppl 3):443–448, 2000

Green L, Fein D, Modahl C, et al: Oxytocin and autistic disorder: alterations in peptide forms. Biol Psychiatry 50:609–613, 2001

Gupta S: Immunological treatments for autism. J Autism Dev Disord 30:475–479, 2000

Hagerman RJ, Falkenstein AR: An association between recurrent otitis media in infancy and later hyperactivity. Clin Pediatr 26:253–257, 1987

Halsey NA, Hyman SL: Measles-mumps-rubella vaccine and autistic spectrum disorder: report from the New Challenges in Childhood Immunizations Conference convened in Oak Brook, Illinois, June 12–13, 2000. Pediatrics 107:E84, 2001

Hollander E, Cartwright C, Wong C, et al: A dimensional approach to the autism spectrum. CNS Spectrum 3:18–39, 1998

Hornig M, Lipkin WI: Infectious and immune factors in the pathogenesis of neurodevelopmental disorders: epidemiology, hypotheses, and animal models. Ment Retard Dev Disabil Res Rev 7:200–210, 2001

Horvath K, Perman J: Autism and gastrointestinal symptoms. Curr Gastroenterol Rep 4:251–258, 2002

Horvath K, Stefanatos G, Sokolski KN, et al: Improved social and language skills after secretin administration in patients with autistic spectrum disorders. J Assoc Acad Minor Phys 9:9–15, 1998

Horvath K, Papadimitriou JC, Rabsztyn A, et al: Gastrointestinal abnormalities in children with autistic disorder. J Pediatr 135:559–563, 1999

Hsu ST, Ma CI, Hsu SK, et al: Discovery and epidemiology of PCB poisoning in Taiwan: a four-year followup. Environ Health Perspect 59:5–10, 1985

Hyman SL, Levy SE: Autistic spectrum disorders: when traditional medicine is not enough. Contemp Pediatr 17:101–116, 2000

Insel TR: Oxytocin—a neuropeptide for affiliation: evidence from behavioral, receptor autoradiographic, and comparative studies. Psychoneuroendocrinology 17:3–35, 1992

Insel TR, O'Brien DJ, Leckman JF: Oxytocin, vasopressin and autism: is there a connection? Biol Psychiatry 45:145–157, 1999

Jacobson JL, Jacobson SW: Intellectual impairment in children exposed to polychlorinated biphenyls in utero. N Engl J Med 335:785–789, 1996

Kaptchuk TJ: The placebo effect in alternative medicine: can the performance of a healing ritual have clinical significance? Ann Intern Med 136:817–825, 2002

Kern JK, Miller VS, Cauller PL, et al: Effectiveness of *N,N*-dimethylglycine in autism and pervasive developmental disorder. J Child Neurol 16:169–173, 2001

Knivsberg AM, Reichelt KL, Nodland M: Reports on dietary intervention in autistic disorders. Nutr Neurosci 4:25–37, 2001

Knivsberg AM, Reichelt KL, Hoien T, et al: A randomized controlled study of dietary intervention in autistic syndromes. Nutr Neurosci 5:251–261, 2002

Konstantareas MM, Homatidis S: Ear infections in autistic and normal children. J Autism Dev Disord 17:585–594, 1987

Korvatska E, Van de Water J, Anders TF, et al: Genetic and immunologic considerations in autism. Neurobiol Dis 9:107–125, 2002

Kozlovskaia GV, Kliushnik TP, Goriunova AV, et al: [Nerve growth factor autoantibodies in children with various forms of mental dysontogenesis and in schizophrenia high-risk group] (Russian). Zh Nevrol Psikhiatr Im S S Korsakova 100:50–52, 2000

Krause I, Xiao-Sond H, Gershwin ME, et al: Brief report: immune factors in autism: a critical review. J Autism Dev Disord 32:337–345, 2002

Le Breton M: Diet Intervention and Autism. London, Jessica Kingsley, 2001

Le Couteur A, Trygstad O, Evered C, et al: Infantile autism and urinary excretion of peptides and protein-associated peptide complexes. J Autism Dev Disord 18:181–190, 1988

Levy SE, Hyman SL: Alternative/complementary approaches to treatment of children with autistic spectrum disorders. Infants Young Child 14:33–42, 2002

London E, Etzel RA: The environment as an etiologic factor in autism: a new direction for research. Environ Health Perspect 108(suppl 3):401–404, 2000

Martin CM, Uhlmann V, Killalea A, et al: Detection of measles virus in children with ileo-colonic lymphoid nodular hyperplasia, enterocolitis and developmental disorder. Mol Psychiatry 7 (suppl 2):S47–S48, 2002

Mason-Brothers A, Ritvo ER, Freeman, BJ, et al: The UCLA–University of Utah Epidemiologic Survey of Autism: Recurrent Infections. Eur Child Adolesc Psychiatry 2:79–90, 1993

Melmed RD, Schneider CK, Sabes RA, et al: Metabolic marker and gastrointestinal symptoms in children with autism and related disorders. J Pediatr Gastroenterol Nutr 31 (suppl 2):S31–S32, 2000

Modahl C, Green L, Fein D, et al: Plasma oxytocin levels in autistic children. Biol Psychiatry 43:270–277, 1998

Myers GJ, Davidson PW: Does methylmercury have a role in causing developmental disabilities in children? Environ Health Perspect 108 (suppl 3):413–420, 2000

Needleman HL, Schell A, Bellinger D, et al: The long-term effects of exposure to low doses of lead in childhood: an 11-year follow-up report. N Engl J Med 322:83–88, 1990

O'Connor ME, Rich D: Children with moderately elevated lead levels: is chelation with DMSA helpful? Clin Pediatr 38:325–331, 1999

Owley T, McMahon W, Cook E, et al: Multisite, double-blind, placebo-controlled trial of porcine secretin in autism. J Am Acad Child Adolesc Psychiatry 40:1293–1299, 2001

Panksepp J: Oxytocin effects on emotional processes: separation distress, social bonding, and relationships to psychiatric disorders. Ann N Y Acad Sci 652:243–252, 1992

Pedersen OS, Liu Y, Reichelt KL: Serotonin uptake stimulating peptide found in plasma of normal individuals and in some autistic urines. J Pept Res 53:641–646, 1999

Pfeiffer SI, Norton J, Nelson L, et al: Efficacy of vitamin B_6 and magnesium in the treatment of autism: a methodology review and summary of outcomes. J Autism Dev Disord 25:481–493, 1995

Pichichero ME, Cernichiari E, Lopreiato J, et al: Mercury concentrations and metabolism in infants receiving vaccines containing thimerosal: a descriptive study. Lancet 360:1737–1741, 2002

Plioplys AV: Intravenous immunoglobulin treatment of children with autism. J Child Neurol 13:79–82, 1998

Rabkin JG, McGrath PJ, Quitkin FM, et al: Effects of pill-giving on maintenance of placebo response in patients with chronic mild depression. Am J Psychiatry 147:1622–1626, 1990

Reichelt KL: Urinary peptide levels and patterns in autistic children from seven countries and the effect of dietary intervention after four years. Developmental Brain Dysfunction 10:44–55, 1997

Rimland B: Dimethylglycine (DMG), a nontoxic metabolite, and autism. Autism Research Review International 4:3, 1996

Rimland B, Callaway E, Dreyfus P: The effect of high doses of vitamin B_6 on autistic children: a double-blind crossover study. Am J Psychiatry 135:472–475, 1978

Roberts W, Weaver L, Brian J, et al: Repeated doses of porcine secretin in the treatment of autism: a randomized, placebo-controlled trial. Pediatrics 107:E71, 2001

Rogan WJ, Dietrich KN, Ware JH et al: The effect of chelation therapy with succimer on neuropsychological development in children exposed to lead. N Engl J Med 344:1421–1426, 2001

Rossi TM, Tjota A: Serologic indicators of celiac disease. J Pediatr Gastroenterol Nutr 26:205–210, 1998

Sandler A, Sutton K, DeWeese J, et al: Lack of benefit of a single dose of synthetic human secretin in the treatment of autism and pervasive developmental disorder. N Engl J Med 341:1801–1806, 1999

Sandler RH, Finegold SM, Bolte ER, et al: Short-term benefit from oral vanco-mycin treatment of regressive-onset autism. J Child Neurol 15:429–435, 2000

Secord GJ, Erickson MT, Bush JP: Neuropsychological sequelae of otitis media in children and adolescents with learning disabilities. J Pediatr Psychol 13:531–542, 1988

Shannon M, Graef JW: Lead intoxication in children with pervasive developmental disorders. J Toxicol Clin Toxicol 34:177–182, 1997

Shaw W, Kassen E, Chaves E: Increased urinary excretion of analogs of Krebs cycle metabolites and arabinose in two brothers with autistic features. Clin Chem 41:1094–1104, 1995

Singh VK, Warren R, Averett R, et al: Circulating autoantibodies to neuronal and glial filament proteins in autism. Pediatr Neurol 17:88–90, 1997

Singh VK, Warren RP, Odell JD, et al: Antibodies to myelin basic protein in children with autistic behavior. Brain Behav Immun 7:97–103, 1993

Smith T, Groen AD, Wynn JW: Randomized trial of intensive early intervention for children with pervasive developmental disorder. Am J Ment Retard 105:269–285, 2000

Stratton K, Gable A, McCormick MC (eds): Immunization Safety Review: Thimerosal-Containing Vaccines and Neurodevelopmental Disorders. Washington, DC, National Academy Press, 2001

Taylor B, Miller E, Farrington CP, et al: Autism and measles, mumps, and rubella vaccine: no epidemiological evidence for a causal association. Lancet 353:2026–2029, 1999

Taylor B, Miller E, Lingam R, et al: Measles, mumps, and rubella vaccination and bowel problems or developmental regression in children with autism: population study. BMJ 324:393–396, 2002

Thomas KB: The placebo in general practice. Lancet 344:1066–1067, 1994

Todd RD, Ciaranello RD: Demonstration of inter- and intraspecies differences in serotonin binding sites by antibodies from an autistic child. Proc Natl Acad Sci U S A 82:612–616, 1985

Vojdani A, Campbell AW, Anyanwu E, et al: Antibodies to neuron-specific antigens in children with autism: possible cross-reaction with encephalitogenic proteins from milk, *Chlamydia pneumoniae* and *Streptococcus* group A. J Neuroimmunol 129:168–177, 2002

Wakefield AJ: Enterocolitis, autism and measles virus. Mol Psychiatry 7(suppl 2):S44–S46, 2002

Wakefield AJ, Murch SH, Anthony A, et al: Ileal-lymphoid-nodular hyperplasia, non-specific colitis, and pervasive developmental disorder in children. Lancet 351:637–641, 1998

Warren R: An immunologic theory for the development of some cases of autism. CNS Spectr 3:71–79, 1998

Whiteley P, Shattock P: Biochemical aspects in autism spectrum disorders: updating the opioid-excess theory and presenting new opportunities for biomedical intervention. Expert Opin Ther Targets 6:175–183, 2002

Whiteley P, Rodgers J, Savery D, et al: A gluten-free diet as an intervention for autism and associated spectrum disorders: preliminary findings. Autism 3:45–
65, 1999

Zahm SH, Ward MH: Pesticide and childhood cancer. Environ Health Perspect
106(suppl):893–908, 1998

Zimmerman AW: Commentary: immunological treatments for autism: in search
of reasons for promising approaches. J Autism Dev Disord 30:481–484, 2000

Chapter 9

Cultural Issues in Autism

John R. Brown, Ph.D.
Sally J. Rogers, Ph.D.

Introduction

Although autism was originally hypothesized to have some association with families of higher levels of education and vocation, we now know that autism appears to occur at equal rates in families of all ethnic and cultural backgrounds (Department of Health and Human Services 2002; Wing 1993). Clinicians involved in the diagnosis and treatment of autism spectrum disorders (ASD) should expect to see families with a wide range of social and cultural characteristics. Most clinicians have faced the challenge, frustration, and feelings of failure involved in trying to provide real help for children and families from cultural backgrounds extremely different from that of the clinician himself or herself. Clinicians familiar with the literature on cultural diversity are aware of its strong and pervasive effects on child development and family functioning. However, when faced with a condition as disabling as autism can be, it is easy to disregard the way a family's cultural experience and history influence the child's functioning, use of available treatments, and long-term outcomes. The purpose of this chapter is to review what is known about the interactions of culture with

209

autism, developmental disabilities, and child development, in order to assist clinicians who work with children with autism and their families within the cultural contexts of their lives.

The themes of cultural relevance and cultural competence are not new to the fields of mental health and education. There has been increasing emphasis on cultural competence and child disability in recent years, with professionals shifting their focus to exploring ways to understand how cultural variables affect disabilities, particularly as they relate to the individual's and family's capacity to cope and progress (Bryan 1999; Lynch and Hanson 1992). These authors have provided helpful descriptions of the normative or modal value systems and cultural themes of various ethnic groups as they relate to disability, with the important caveat that there is no one cultural standard tied to any particular ethnic group. There has been a marked increase in the focus on cultural competence in educational programs as well. The curricula of current training programs for mental health professionals place considerable emphasis on developing cultural awareness and cultural competence. Treatment programs in the fields of mental health and special education are increasingly emphasizing cultural sensitivity.

However, compared with the empirical bases for the other chapters in this book, the research base on the effects of cultural factors in autism is minuscule. At the present time, interest and support for research and intervention programs for ASD have increased dramatically. For example, the U.S. Department of Health and Human Services (2002) reported that funding support for autism research grew from $22 million in FY 1997 to $56 million in FY 2001. The National Institutes of Health (NIH) and other supporters of autism research, aware of the need for cultural representativeness in human studies, require that investigations include research participants who represent the cultural diversity of the geographic locale in which the study takes place. They also require that scientists put forth considerable effort to make research participation accessible to participants from diverse cultural backgrounds. Even so, research involving cultural factors in autism has received little attention (Dyches et al. 2001). Most autism-related studies do not include culture as a significant experimental variable, nor do they include significant numbers of individuals from diverse cultural groups (Mary 1990). Thus, there is little empirical data related specifically to cultural issues in autism available to serve as a framework for the present chapter. There is, however, a body of research in the broader literature involving the interactions between cultural diversity and typical and atypical child development. This literature will provide the basis for raising clinical and research questions concerning the impact of cultural variables on children with ASD and their families.

Culture, the Concept

The term *culture* has been defined as "a learned system of meaning and behavior" that is passed from one generation to the next (Carter and Qureshi 1995; Fairchild 1970; Triandis 1972). The most important concept to hold in mind about culture is that standards and patterns of behavior are culturally derived (Harry 1992). Cultural values determine what is desirable within the individual and the larger society of a given group of people. They are a major factor in contributing to a sense of identity, belonging, and characteristic ways of perceiving, thinking, feeling, and behaving (Gollnick and Chinn 1990). Bryan (1999) noted the following common points of the various definitions:

- Culture is a group orientation; that is, culture consists of behavior, beliefs, attitudes, and values shared by a group of people.
- Culture is behavior, attitudes, beliefs, and values that are learned, not inherited.
- Culture is learned via socialization rather than through a formal teaching process.

Harry (1992) and Thomas (1993) use the term *modal culture* to describe what might be considered typical characteristics of a particular group, but note that individual members may vary considerably in the extent to which they exhibit these modal characteristics. Cultures are seen as changing and adaptable, dynamic rather than static. The dynamic nature of cultural factors and the varying ways in which researchers and practitioners define them have significant implications for both research and clinical practice.

Interaction of Cultural Variables With Autism

If we believe that behavior is culturally determined, then we must assume that the behavior of the individual diagnosed with ASD is also affected by the social context. Do we observe any differences in the phenotypic expression of ASD between an African-American child raised in an African-American family exhibiting modal African-American culture, and an Asian-American child raised within Asian-American modal culture? There are differences in cultural and value orientations that are reflected in the socialization of the child by the family. To the extent that children with autism also are socialized into their respective families, one would expect cultural characteristics to be reflected in the behavior of the child. If cultural differences are observed, what variables are related to the differences in phenotypic expression of the disorder, and what is the relationship between various cultural variables and phenotypic expression? Understanding effects of acculturation in autism could help us understand more about the learning processes that affect phenotypic expression of the disorder. Cultural differences may also interact to influence the manner in which an individual or family responds to various treatments.

The overriding questions being raised here are

- Are the symptoms associated with ASD so pervasive that they obscure the observation of typically observed socialization processes?
- How do socialization processes interact with the severity of the symptoms?
- How does cultural orientation affect choice of treatments and treatment outcomes in ASD?

How will we come to understand the interaction of culture and autism? First, we need to use methodologies in autism research that provide a way of specifying culture as a variable that can be examined. Then we need testable hypotheses that we can examine in clinically relevant studies. Let us begin by considering the issues involved in defining culture as a variable in clinical studies.

The Challenge of Defining Culture for Researchers

In the field of autism, one aspect of the effort to obtain replicable research findings has involved the development of uniform ways of assessing and diagnosing autism spectrum disorders. The Autism Diagnostic Interview–Revised (Le Couteur et al. 1989) and the Autism Diagnostic Observation Schedule (Lord et al. 1989) have been developed as part of this effort and are considered the "gold standard" assessment tools by researchers (Filipek et al. 1999). The development of uniformity in the diagnosis and assessment of ASD through the use of these and other tools will contribute to more meaningful and reliable interpretation of research findings by enabling a clearer understanding of the nature of the participant group from which the findings were derived. However, these tools were not designed to capture cultural variables.

For researchers, exploring the impact of culture or cultural differences presents problems in terms of methodology. There is a lack of uniformity in how terms are used and defined. Most researchers describe their participants in terms of "ethnic cultural groups" (Mason 1994). Minority populations tend to be grouped into broad categories that, in the United States, generally are used as racial designations—typically, African American, Hispanic, American Indian, and Asian Pacific American—despite the fact that the categories jumble geographic, racial, ethnic, and cultural characteristics (Research Exchange 1999). These groups are often contrasted with "mainstream U.S. culture" as if all people in the United States of Caucasian descent share a single set of beliefs, values, and behaviors. Such practices confuse race, culture, language, religious beliefs, and economic and social status, without explicit consideration of their distinction or relative importance.

The concept of race continues to be used as if it were synonymous with "culture" in spite of the awareness that assigning an individual to a group based on physical characteristics such as skin color provides little information about cultural values, beliefs, or behavior. Tatum (1997) and Pfeffer (1998) point out that differences and similarities associated with race may be explained by a shared history and experience, physical proximity, and shared values and beliefs. They also note that race as a concept is a social construction rather than a biological reality. That is, race exists only in the minds of people, not in human biology. Researchers and clinicians must determine the extent to which an individual and family identify with a particular culture rather than relying on assumptions based on physical features. Racial groupings may or may not be important variables, especially when one investigates within-group variations along the many facets of culture and their relationship to various dimensions of autism research.

Socioeconomic level is another variable that confounds attempts to explore cultural variables. Smart and Smart (1992) observe that much of what is thought to be culturally derived is actually the result of economic conditions. Economics play a critical role in coping capacity, and Luft (1995) describes poverty as contributing to a distinctive "sub-cultural lifestyle." While this is an extreme position not endorsed by everyone, it is generally recognized that poverty and minority status interact to contribute significantly to outcomes involving children with disabilities. It is important for researchers and clinicians to differentiate these variables in order to understand how each contributes to treatment outcomes, as well as how each influences the impact of the other.

The cultural aspects of poverty, as well as its economic effects, can serve as barriers to needed services. Bennett (1988) and Harry (1992) point out ways in which poverty may interact with minority status. Parents of children from poor and minority groups are less educated, cut off from information, and tend to experience greater exclusion from educational decisions or services. This exclusion may result from not being able to take time off from work to attend a meeting, not having transportation to get to and from treatment programs, being unable to afford the cost of child care necessary to participate in the child's treatment, and feeling uncomfortable with the size and content of meetings like the Individualized Education Plan (IEP) and team diagnostic processes.

In terms of methodologic issues, there are several ways of capturing economic status. Some researchers use measures of maternal education, which is correlated with parenting and socialization practices. Another common approach is Hollingshead's (1975) rating system, which computes a numerical index based on maternal and paternal education and occupation. Although these variables do not capture culture, they provide a way of quantifying socioeconomic status, which interacts with numerous aspects of child development.

When trying to capture cultural attributes independent of race and socioeconomic status, we face thorny methodologic problems in operationalizing the various factors that contribute to cultural uniqueness. For example, religious beliefs may be a central variable in definitions of culture for some groups (Bailey et al. 1999; Gannoti et al. 2001; Rogers-Dulan and Blacher 1995). How do we reflect this in our research methodology? Do we provide a frequency count of the number of times a person or family attends church, how much they contribute to organized religious groups, or some other form of self-reported measure of the strength of their religious beliefs? Methods must be broad enough to capture the phenomenon in question and yet refined enough to allow for some quantification, so that one can examine how cultural variables interact with other variables of interest. Determining better methods for addressing the range and complexity of cultural variables will facilitate greater clarity, understanding, and interpretation of research findings involving the impact of cultural factors, which in turn may contribute to research findings having greater applicability to the "real world."

One important tool that can be brought to these methodologic challenges is the use of qualitative research methods to generate useful hypotheses for quantitative research. Qualitative methodologies allow the researcher to observe and identify numerous variables that may be related to culture. This enlarges the pool of real-life phenomena to study and quantify.

The lack of cultural diversity of participants in mental health research studies and of research exploring the relationship of cultural factors to psychiatric disorders has not gone unaddressed. Colleagues at the University of California have been particularly involved in studies that seek to understand and counteract the tendency of members of diverse cultural groups to avoid accessing mental health services and to terminate services prematurely (Snowden 2001; Sue and Sue 1990).

A final methodologic issue concerns obtaining research findings that are applicable to real-world settings and generalizable beyond laboratory situations. This has been a major concern of child development researchers over the years (Bronfenbrenner 1977; Vasta 1982). Bronfenbrenner (1977) asserts that emphasis on rigorous research has led to experiments that are elegantly designed but often limited in scope because many of these studies create situations that are unfamiliar or artificial or that call for behavior that has little utility outside the experimental context. Studies that have tried to replicate laboratory findings in clinical or community settings often fail because of the impact of other uncontrolled factors, such as comorbid conditions in the participants from the larger community (Weisz et al. 1992, 1995). This is the issue of efficacy versus effectiveness. Carefully controlled experimental treatment trials may demonstrate positive effects—that is, *treatment efficacy.* Implementing the same experimental treatment in the field raises a host of additional issues—training and competence of the treatment givers, fidelity of the treatment to the original model, nature of the recipients of the treatment, treatment dosage effects, and so forth. These and other variables influence *treatment effectiveness*—that is, the usefulness of a clinical treatment in real-life settings. The methodologic implication is the need to replicate new, efficacious experimental clinical interventions in the field rapidly and to disseminate the findings quickly, so that practitioners can draw from literature that has demonstrated both efficacy and effectiveness.

Research Involving Families, Culture, Child Development, and Child Disability

In addition to facing methodologic challenges, clinicians and researchers will need hypotheses concerning the effects of cultural diversity on development and outcomes in autism. Although research on this topic in autism is sparse, there is considerable research examining the effects of culture on developmental disorders and other types of disability.

Ramirez (1987) has pointed out that much of this research has been devoted to determining why there has been such an overrepresentation of ethnic minority groups in special education programs. This work has focused largely on children with mild disabilities (Harry et al. 1995). Main findings from this work have demonstrated 1) the existence of cultural and linguistic bias in tests, 2) faulty assumptions regarding the universality of the values endorsed by the dominant culture, and 3) erroneous assumptions about the capacity of these groups to learn. The recommendations from this work have direct application to mental health clinicians and include such points as conducting assessments in the child's native or dominant language; including parents in the assessment process; using independent language/cultural interpreters rather than family members or friends; and using alternative assessment approaches when there are questions regarding the appropriateness of formal, standardized tools (Harry et al. 1995).

When clinicians provide care for children with severe disabilities, the magnitude of the disability may overshadow social cultural factors, resulting in a lack of appropriate attention to cultural and linguistic variables in providing evaluations or treatment (Harry et al. 1995). Cultural contexts are formative in a family's responses to the presence of severe physical, intellectual, developmental, or psychiatric disability in their children. Cultural and linguistic variables provide the context within which families decide what goals are important to work toward and the content of treatment activities.

Whether the focus is on mild or severe disabilities or typically developing children, professionals have come to recognize the role that culture plays. A superb example of the helpfulness of including culture as a variable in a study of child development and family patterns comes from work on parenting styles. In a classic study from the 1970s, Baumrind (1971) reported that *authoritarian* parenting, characterized by the imposition of an absolute set of standards, the valuing of obedience and respect for authority, and the discouragement of give-and-take, is detrimental to socialization because it fails to encourage the child's autonomy. In contrast, *authoritative* parenting, characterized by firm control, high demands for maturity, and a willingness to reason and negotiate, was reported to create a much more effective familial environment for transmitting values and promoting autonomy. This finding is well known by clinicians and child developmentalists and has undoubtedly influenced many clinicians in their work with families.

However, an examination of cultural variables illuminates the findings considerably. Dekovic and Janssens (1992) and Grolnick and Ryan (1989) reported that the demonstrated link between authoritative parenting and high levels of internalization of values and autonomy appears to be strongest in a middle-class, Anglo-European context. In other cultural contexts (e.g., African-American, Asian-American, Latino-American), authoritarian parenting appears to be the norm and is less likely to be associated with negative outcomes (Rudy and Grusec 2001). The authors indicate that this apparent discrepancy is explained by the different value orientations observed in the different groups. They point out that middle-class Anglo-Europeans are characterized as valuing individualism, whereas the other groups are described as having a collectivist orientation. In collectivist cultures, self-assertion and independence may be negatively valued, with the promotion of interdependence, cooperation, and compliance more positively valued (Markus and Kitayama 1991). Thus, different parenting styles have very different effects on child outcomes, depending on the cultural background of the family and its peer group.

These findings alert us to the importance of culture in shaping values and behavior and providing the context in which individuals and families determine what is important and the focus of treatment. This is extremely important in establishing individual and family goals and priorities. It may be more important to some families to focus on behaviors that facilitate the capacity to engage in family and community activities than to focus on behaviors that promote individual competence and autonomy. These are not necessarily mutually exclusive goals, but they may lead to different treatment approaches.

Singh-Manoux and Finkenauer (2001) also pointed out that there are cultural variations in the social expression and sharing of emotions. For example, Asians are described as valuing private over public displays of emotion and consequently discourage outward emotional displays in their child-rearing practices. Observations such as these highlight the significance of cultural context in influencing behavior and raise the question of whether a similar pattern might be observed in autism research. That is, might one observe a relationship between individual differences in the recognition and expression of emotions and the extent to which this behavior is emulated within the cultural context within which the individual lives?

Another area of cultural and developmental interaction that has been extensively studied involves modes of communicating and interacting. Young (1970) described African-American children as person oriented, noting that infants were held by someone in the family most of the time and few objects were given to them. Similarly, Lewis (1975) observed extensive interaction among African-American family members and infants involving touching, kissing, and holding the baby's hands. Garcia-Coll (1990) examined developmental skills such as tactile stimulation, verbal and nonverbal interaction, and feeding routines. She observed that minority infants are not only exposed to different patterns of affective and social interactions, but their learning experiences might result in the acquisition of different modes of communication, different means of exploring the environment, and alternative cognitive skills from those characterizing Anglo infants. Early intervention programs for infants with disabilities stress the importance of infant actions on objects and structured language experiences; however, these areas of emphasis may seem culturally inappropriate to some families.

Duarte and Rice (1992) indicated cultural differences in the context in which language is used. These researchers use the term *high context* to refer to a pattern of communication that derives meaning from the style in which information is presented, affective cues, and the language code. This is a pattern that is often observed in African-American families. *Low context* refers to a pattern of communication that is based primarily on the language code itself—the syntax, semantics, and pragmatics of communication—which is more characteristic of Anglo-European, middle-class families. In addition to these stylistic language differences, Boykin (1982) observed that many African-American children are exposed to high-energy, fast-paced home environments. These findings raise questions about current treatment practices in autism that advocate a "one size fits all" teaching style. For example, current educational practices often emphasize isolating the skills to be taught and teaching them in a highly structured manner. Is it possible that mirroring aspects of the child's cultural context in the treatment setting might result in greater achievement?

Research on culture and disability has focused on within- and between-group comparisons of families' capacity to cope and adapt to raising a child with a developmental disability. The findings reported in these studies may illuminate factors to consider when engaged in treatment outcome studies or providing treatment to families from different cultural groups. The unpredictability of the behavior of children diagnosed with autism and the social-interpersonal ramifications experienced by families may accentuate the stress these families experience beyond that experienced by families of children diagnosed with other disabilities (Bristol 1984; Schopler and Mesibov 1984). These two variables—family adaptation and child progress—are linked. Parent characteristics and characteristics of the child's disability form a complex dynamic interaction (Seligman and Darling 1989). The child's characteristics and symptom severity interact with the extent to which the family perceives them as disruptive. This interaction in turn is influenced by a number of factors, including the family's capacity to respond to obstacles and shift its course of action. Other variables, such as gender, religion, child-rearing patterns, and cultural beliefs, interact with symptom severity in complex ways. Religious beliefs, for example, influence the manner in which the family responds to having a child with a disability. Bailey et al. (1999) reported that religious beliefs provide considerable support for Hispanic families. Gannoti et al. (2001) obtained results indicating that religious beliefs can have a positive or negative impact depending on the perspective taken. If having a child with disabilities is perceived as a hex or punishment by God, the impact on the family could be negative. If, on the other hand, having a child with disabilities is perceived as being "chosen" by God, it can have positive influences on the family's capacity to adapt.

Cultural mores may have a direct impact on outcomes for children with disabilities. Modal Hispanic culture is described as placing high value on familialism, allocentrism, and motherhood (Gannoti et al. 2001). Allocentrism and familialism promote supportive attitudes toward the family member with a disability. To a person outside that cultural value system, the expression of these values may be interpreted as overprotectiveness. It may also appear that such values and parenting styles hinder development of personal independence in a child with a disability. Cultural context reminds us that the presence or absence of behavior is a function not only of ability but also of the value placed on it and subsequent opportunities to learn it. Clinicians need to remember that their own values for child outcomes, such as independence, autonomy, and self-assertion, are interpreted differently across cultures. In the case of children with severe disabilities, cultural clashes between professional and parental goals are likely to be exacerbated. For the clinician, developing treatment goals that fit the cultural context in which the child lives enhances acceptance and continued participation by families.

What are the implications of these observations? Observations of the role of culture suggest a complex array of factors operating to influence child development and child learning. Examining cultural variation within studies of child disability provides opportunities to explore development and outcomes at a greater level of specificity. Such knowledge makes research findings more generalizable to real-world questions. This applies to research in general and to disability research, including autism.

Intervention and Treatment

Including cultural variables in the scope of the phenomena to be considered in research places a significant focus on the family. This appears appropriate, as we try to understand the impact of culture on development in autism and other disabilities. Mary (1990) has suggested that the appropriate focal point in a family that has a child with a developmental disability is the family. However, a complex interplay of numerous factors, in addition to cultural variables, determines how well the family copes with the disability, as well as the type of clinical care the child receives. The Surgeon General (Department of Health and Human Services 2001) published a supplement to the 1999 report in which he expressed concern about the existence of striking disparities in mental health care for racial and ethnic minorities compared with Anglo-Americans, noting, "Minorities have less access to, and availability of, mental health services. Minorities are less likely to receive needed mental health services. Minorities in treatment often receive a poorer quality of mental health care. Minorities are underrepresented in mental health research" (p. 35). The Surgeon General painted a bleak picture regarding access and utilization of treatment services by culturally diverse groups. The report noted that cost, fragmentation of service, lack of availability of services, and societal stigma toward mental illness are barriers impeding access and use. It also drew attention to the additional barriers of language and communication, racism and discrimination, and mistrust and fear of treatment.

When one limits the focus to the field of autism, the picture may be even bleaker. Although there has been considerable progress toward developing and disseminating information regarding effective treatments, most of the highly qualified professionals trained in the special skills necessary to develop, organize, and manage programs for individuals diagnosed with autism remain in major university, hospital, and medical center settings in large metropolitan areas. The autism-specific treatment and clinical services in outlying and rural areas, and those available in urban settings to persons of cultural diversity, are often limited, fragmented, costly, or inaccessible.

Although there is no known cure for autism, there are a number of efficacious treatments that enhance the potential for the child to obtain maximum benefit from current therapies (Department of Health and Human Services 2002); see Chapter 6. Given the potentially devastating impact this disorder can have on individuals, their families, health care providers, their teachers, and others, it is imperative that effective treatment services be implemented. If cultural factors in the service delivery system or access to services prevent the family from receiving effective interventions for their child, both the family's capacity to adapt to the exigencies associated with raising the child and the trajectory of the child's progress are likely to be affected.

Clinical Relevance

Many clinical points have already been made in this chapter, but it seems helpful to reiterate the relevant topics here as we reach the concluding pages. When we view children with autism and their families from a cultural perspective, we recognize that they, and everybody else, have a culture, including white Americans. And all people, including those of a dominant culture, vary across a broad spectrum in the extent to which they endorse various values, beliefs, and behaviors associated with their culture (Research Exchange 1999).

Given the relevance of cultural differences to the patterns of child development and disability discussed earlier, clinicians need to determine a family's cultural identity. To what degree does the family endorse values, beliefs, and behavior of the mainstream culture versus the modal culture of the ethnic group of which they are members (Bryan 1999; Harry 1995; Lynch and Hanson 1992)? It is crucial that issues of cultural identity be discussed with families and not merely assumed on the basis of their racial identity and their socioeconomic background. There is no one culture for any particular group; instead, clinicians need to understand where individuals identify themselves along a transcultural continuum (Bryan 1999; Lynch and Hanson 1992).

The style of language usage is an extremely important aspect of effective clinical work. Bailey et al. (1999) demonstrated that language is very salient in affecting outcomes for children diagnosed with developmental disabilities. This effect is especially pronounced in situations in which the family's dominant language is different from the language used in the treatment/school setting and when families are isolated from extended family or other social support. Harry (1995) stresses the importance of providing treatment in the dominant language of the child/family. When language differences are substantial, referral to a clinician who can communicate effectively in the family's language, use of a professional interpreter, or collaboration with another mental health professional who is comfortable in the language is crucial. Family members and friends should not be used as interpreters.

In addition to awareness of a family's cultural identity, values, and beliefs, clinicians need to be aware of the history of the cultural group in the United States. Understanding what has happened to the people of a group in this country can provide some background for cultural understanding of the individual's perception of his or her situation, allowing for greater appreciation of factors contributing to current behavior (Bryan 1999). The clinician needs to be aware of the history and dynamics that may occur between persons of the patient's cultural group and persons of the clinician's cultural group. Such interactions may have significant effects on the quality of the therapeutic relationship.

Bryan (1999) further emphasized the importance of the professional's awareness of his or her own values and the extent to which there may be conflict between these values and the values of the family the clinician is treating. Determine the individual's and family's views of causation and their attitudes toward the helping process. This information allows one to be aware of potential conflicts in values and philosophical beliefs and to take these factors into consideration when engaging the individual and/or family (Bryan 1999).

Clinical services that involve intellectual and academic assessment raise very important issues for children in culturally diverse families.

These issues include test-taking behavior and attitudes, parent reporting of behaviors, standardization norms of the test, and interpretation of the test results within the context of overall adaptive skills in the general environment. All have considerable implications for making educational and intervention decisions and for predicting outcomes for the child. Clinicians need to be very well informed about the interaction of culture and psychological and psychiatric assessment.

In terms of recommending school-based and other intervention programs, the family's cultural background may interact powerfully with many variables in the treatment setting. These may include the location of the program, the staff of the program, the values and beliefs of the intervention approach, the other children and families participating, acceptability of the interaction patterns that mark the intervention approach, and the likelihood of parental follow-through at home. Harry et al. (1995) recommended referral to neighborhood-based programs whenever possible, under the assumption that this will limit linguistic and cultural dissonance for families, facilitate native or dominant language instruction, and maximize the inclusion of culturally syntonic features. Many of the principles of the Head Start program illustrate this recommendation, including location of programs in neighborhoods and strong community and parent representation in the program.

Conclusion

In working with a condition that affects behavior, language, and social interactions as significantly as autism does, it is easy to overlook questions about the contribution of cultural background to the child's presentation and to the kinds of treatment plans and practices that will be implemented. Furthermore, the current state of the science in autism tells us virtually nothing of the interplay between cultural background and autism. Because social learning is significantly affected in autism, some might arrive at the unfounded assumption that cultural background does not affect the functioning or outcome of a child with this disorder. However, everything that we know about the interactions of cultural origins, family interaction patterns, access to education, and child development supports the idea that cultural background should affect the lives of children with autism, as it does in typical development and in other developmental disorders.

With guidance from research in the interaction of culture, child development, and other disabilities, clinicians are encouraged to attend closely to the cultural background of the family of a child with autism, and to the links between the family's cultural background and the values, goals, and norms that they associate with their child. Cultural backgrounds also influence people's access to and usage of mental health, educational, and other types of social services. In many states and locales in this country, access to services for children with autism is won by the knowledge, advocacy, and persistence of individual parents rather than by state mandate or entitlement programs. Clinicians working in the area of autism need to recognize their patients' needs in terms of services and supports, and they need to be knowledgeable about the service delivery system in their region. Autism professionals frequently find themselves in very strong advocacy roles for their patients, and case management time can fill the bulk of professional time. Making calls, attending meetings, and advocating for services is part and parcel of the clinical work needed by families. Professionals may have to offer to provide some of these services, since not all families will know to ask. Services for children with autism come in many shapes and sizes, and there are often many choices for a family to make. Services differ not only in content and philosophy, but also in cultural compatibility. Helping families locate services that feel comfortable and supportive to them is crucial for a good parent-professional relationship and ongoing progress of the child. All these aspects of clinical care require knowledge of the family's cultural background and value system.

This chapter began with the observation that there has been little research regarding cultural issues in autism. To fill this void, research efforts must expand their list of demographic variables to include cultural variables. However, quantification of culture is a daunting task. Pursuing qualitative within- or between-group studies of diverse cultures can provide a "natural" laboratory that may be used to gain greater understanding of ways to capture cultural variables and to identify fruitful lines of future research. The ability to conduct research that is more culturally informative would have an impact in the real world for children and families. Such studies could enhance access to and utilization of mental health services currently available. Numerous authors (e.g., Bryan 1999; Chenn et al. 2002; Franklin 1992; Lynch and Hanson 1992) have recognized the importance of attending to cultural variables as part of the effort to enhance access to and utilization of services, noting that cultural relevance allows interventions to address more directly the social realities of people's lives. Alhough developing ways of capturing cultural variables in research may seem difficult, we cannot afford to forgo the inclusion of these variables for the sake of research rigor. Nor can we afford to offer simplistic linear explanations for complex behavior. Incorporating cultural variables more deeply into both clinical work and research will add to the richness of our understanding of autism and increase the relevance of our work for children with this complex disorder and their families.

References

Bailey DB, Skinner D, Correa V, et al: Needs and supports reported by Latino families of young children with developmental disabilities. Am J Ment Retard 104:437–451, 1999

Baumrind D: Current patterns of parental authority. Developmental Psychology Monographs 4:1–103, 1971

Bennett AT: Gateways to powerlessness: incorporating Hispanic deaf children and families into formal schooling. Disabil Handicap Soc 3:119–151, 1988

Boykin AW: Task variability and the performance of black and white children: vervistic exploration. J Black Stud 12:469–485, 1982

Bristol MM: Family resources and successful adaptation to autistic children, in The Effects of Autism on the Family. Edited by Schopler E, Mesibov GB. New York, Plenum, 1984, pp 289–310

Bronfenbrenner U: Toward an experimental ecology of human development. Am Psychol 32:513–531, 1977

Bryan WV: Multicultural Aspects of Disabilities: A Guide to Understanding and Assisting Minorities in the Rehabilitation Process. Springfield, IL, Charles C Thomas, 1999

Carter RT, Qureshi A: A typology of philosophical assumptions in multicultural counseling and training, in Handbook on Multicultural Counseling. Edited by Ponteratto JG, Casas JM, Suzuki LA, et al. Thousand Oaks, CA, Sage, 1995

Chenn D, Downing JE, Peckham-Hardin KO: Working with families of diverse cultural and linguistic backgrounds: consideration for culturally responsive positive behavior support, in Family, Community, and Disability: Families and Positive Behavior Support. Edited by Lucyshyn JM, Dunlap G, Albin RW. Baltimore, MD, Paul H Brookes, 2002

Dekovic M, Janssens JM: Parents' child rearing style and child's sociometric status. Dev Psychol 28:925–932, 1992

Department of Health and Human Services: Executive Summary—Mental Health: Culture, Race and Ethnicity. Supplement to Mental Health: A Report of the Surgeon General. Washington, DC, Department of Health and Human Services, 2001

Department of Health and Human Services: Report to Congress on Autism. Prepared by the National Institute of Mental Health, National Institutes of Health, and the Department of Health and Human Services. Washington, DC, Department of Health and Human Services, 2002

Duarte JA, Rice BD: Cultural Diversity in Rehabilitation. Nineteenth Institute on Rehabilitation Issues. Fayetteville, Arkansas Research and Training Center in Vocational Rehabilitation, 1992

Dyches TT, Wilder LK, Obiakor FE: Autism: multicultural perspectives, in Autism Spectrum Disorders: Educational and Clinical Interventions. Edited by Wahlberg T, Obiakor FE, Burkhardt S, et al. New York, Elsevier, 2001, pp 151–176

Fairchild HP: Dictionary of Sociology and Related Sciences. Totowa, NJ, Rowan and Allanheld, 1970

Filipek PA, Accardo PJ, Baranek GT: The screening and diagnosis of autism spectrum disorders. J Autism Dev Disord 29:439–484, 1999

Franklin ME: Culturally sensitive instructional practices for African American learners with disabilities. Except Child 59:115–122, 1992

Gannoti ME, Handwerker WP, Grace NE, et al: Sociocultural influences on disability status in Puerto Rican children. Phys Ther 81:1512–1523, 2001

Garcia-Coll CT: Developmental outcome of minority infants: a process-oriented look into our beginnings. Child Dev 61:270–289, 1990

Gollnick DM, Chinn PC (eds): Multicultural Education in a Pluralistic Society. Columbus, OH, Charles E Merrill, 1990

Grolnick WS, Ryan RM: Parent styles associated with children's self-regulation and competence in school. J Educ Psychol 81:143–154, 1989

Harry B: An ethniciographic study of cross-cultural communication with Puerto Rican–American families in the special education system. Am Educ Res J 29:471–494, 1992

Harry B, Grenot-Scheyer M, Smith-Lewis M, et al: Developing culturally inclusive services for individuals with severe disabilities. J Assoc Pers Sev Handicaps 20:99–109, 1995

Hollingshead AB: Four Factor Index of Social Status. New Haven, CT, Yale University Press, 1975

Le Couteur A, Rutter M, Lord C, et al: Autism diagnostic interviews: a standardized investigator-based instrument. J Autism Dev Disord 19:363–387, 1989

Lewis DK: The black family: socialization and sex roles. Phylon 36:221–237, 1975

Lord C, Rutter M, Goode S, et al: Autism diagnostic observation schedule: a standardized observation of communication and social behavior. J Autism Dev Disord 19:185–212, 1989

Luft P: Addressing minority overrepresentation in special education: cultural barriers to effective collaboration. Paper presented at the Annual Convention of the Council for Exceptional Children, Indianapolis, IN, 1995

Lynch EW, Hanson MJ: Developing Cross-Cultural Competence: A Guide for Working With Young Children and Their Families. Baltimore, MD, Paul H Brookes, 1992

Markus HR, Kitayama S: Culture and the self: implications for cognition, emotion, and motivation. Psychol Rev 98:224–253, 1991

Mary NL: Reactions of Black, Hispanic, and White mothers to having a child with handicaps. Ment Retard 28:1–5, 1990

Mason JL: Developing culturally competent organizations focal point. Bulletin of the Research and Training Center on Family Support and Children's Mental Health 8:1–8, 1994

Pfeffer N: Theories of race, ethnicity, and culture. Br Med J 317:1381–1384, 1998

Ramirez BA: Federal policy and the education of American Indian exceptional children and youth: current status and future directions, in American Indian Exceptional Children and Youth. Edited by Johnson MJ, Ramirez BA. Reston, VA, Council for Exceptional Children, 1987, pp 37–54

Research Exchange: Cultural and other considerations that can influence effectiveness within the rehabilitation system. Research Exchange 4, 1999; http://www.ncddr.org/du/researchexchange

Rogers-Dulan J, Blacher J: African American families, religion, and disability: a conceptual framework. Ment Retard 33:226–238, 1995

Rudy D, Grusec JE: Correlates of authoritarian parenting in individualist and collectivist cultures and implications for understanding the transmission of values. J Cross Cult Psychol 32:202–212, 2001

Schopler E, Mesibov GB: The Effects of Autism on the Family. New York, Plenum, 1984

Seligman M, Darling RB: Ordinary Families, Special Children. New York, Guilford, 1989

Singh-Manoux A, Finkenauer C: Cultural variations in social sharing of emotions: an intercultural perspective. J Cross Cult Psychol 32:647–661, 2001

Smart JF, Smart DW: Cultural issues in the rehabilitation of Hispanics. J Rehabil 58:29–37, 1992

Snowden LR: Barriers to effective mental health services for African Americans. Ment Health Serv Res 3:181–187, 2001

Sue DW, Sue D: Counseling the Culturally Different: Theory and Practice. New York, Wiley, 1990

Tatum BD: Why Are All the Black Kids Sitting Together in the Cafeteria? And Other Conversations About Race. New York, Basic Books, 1997

Thomas D: African American families, in Children With Special Needs: Family, Culture and Society. Edited by Paul JL, Simeonsson RJ. Orlando, FL, Harcourt Brace Jovanovich, 1993

Triandis HC: The Analysis of Subjective Culture. New York, Wiley, 1972

Vasta R: Strategies and Techniques of Child Study. New York, Academic Press, 1982

Weisz JR, Weiss B, Donenberg GR: The lab versus the clinic: effects of child and adolescent psychotherapy. Am Psychol 47:1578–1585, 1992

Weisz JR, Donenberg GR, Han SS, et al: Bridging the gap between laboratory and clinic in child and adolescent psychotherapy. J Consult Clin Psychol 63:688–701, 1995

Wing L: Definition and prevalence of autism. Eur Child Adolesc Psychiatry 2:61–74, 1993

Young VH: Family and childhood in a southern Georgia community. Am Anthropol 72:269–288, 1970

Chapter 10

Professional–Parent Collaboration

The M.I.N.D. Institute Model

Thomas F. Anders, M.D.
Charles R. Gardner Jr.
Sarah E. Gardner

In the past several decades, American medicine has recognized the need to include parents as partners in the treatment of their children. This is particularly relevant for children with neurodevelopmental disorders. Moreover, parent advocacy groups have become important political collaborators with professionals in destigmatizing these disorders, in ensuring access to appropriate services, and in securing research funding. This chapter, however,

Dean Emeritus Hibbard Williams, M.D., hosted the first meeting and provided enthusiastic support throughout the formative stages of the M.I.N.D. Institute. Mr. Frank Loge, Medical Center Director, recognized the vision and provided the first matching grant that spurred the M.I.N.D. Institute's endowment. Current School of Medicine Dean Joseph Silva Jr., M.D., and Medical Center Director Robert Chason significantly helped make the M.I.N.D. dream a reality. Without the five founding fathers (Steve Beneto, Chuck Gardner, Rick Hayes, Rick Rollens, and Lou Vismara), their children with autism, and their families, there never would have been a dream or a reality.

focuses on a particularly unique role that parents in Sacramento, California, played in establishing the University of California (UC)–Davis M.I.N.D. Institute and their continuing collaborative role in its governance and growth. The story is worth telling because the M.I.N.D. Institute model may be applicable to other settings.

How does a dream become a vision and then a reality? It happens rarely, and only when the stars are aligned. It takes the coming together of people willing to think outside the box and willing to establish trusting relationships, mixed with burning and unflagging motivation, good humor, patience, and good luck. The relatively short, 5-year history of the UC Davis M.I.N.D. Institute is a good example of these ingredients congealed into a partnership between parents of children with autism and a university.

The story has two beginnings. The first, recounted by one of the authors (T.F.A.), reflects the university's perspective; the second, recounted by the remaining two authors (C.R.G., S.E.G.), reflects the parents' perspective. One beginning occurred when one of us (T.F.A.) arrived at UC Davis. The other occurred when Chas Gardner was born to Chuck and Sarah.

From the university perspective, in 1992 at UC Davis, children who were suspected of having autism or other neurodevelopmental disorders were referred primarily to the Child Development Clinic (Department of Pediatrics) or the Child Neurology Clinic (Department of Neurology) for evaluation. Rarely were children with these conditions referred to the child psychiatry service. In part, this pattern of practice reflected the interests of the respective subspecialists, including significant lack of interest by the child psychiatrists; and in part, it reflected the bias of many parents of children with autism about the appropriateness of psychiatrists as physicians for their children. Some parents remember that it was a psychiatrist who used the term *refrigerator* to describe their interactions with their children, and such characterizations are not easily forgotten or forgiven. Yet in other parts of the country in 1992, children with autism were regularly and routinely diagnosed in child psychiatry clinics. However, it was very rare across the United States for children with autism to be evaluated by an integrated team of medical specialists (pediatricians, child neurologists, child psychiatrists, and child psychologists) effectively working together. From 1992 to 1997, one of us (T.F.A.), newly arrived at UC Davis, attempted to foster collaboration among the three medical specialties in the area of neurodevelopmental disorders, with little success.

From the parents' perspective, the story also began in 1992. If love is the greatest gift to mankind, then surely hope must be the second. In May of that year, Chas, the Gardners' first child, was born to a jubilant father, whose cry "It's a boy!" could be heard throughout the maternity ward. In a single event, life's two greatest gifts were extended, the love of a child and the hope of a family. The Gardners had been given a First Year Book at a baby shower. It was a book dedicated to tracking their child's significant milestones in his first year. In it, on the page titled "Great Expectations," is written: "Dad hopes he will be a major league baseball player and go on to be a successful businessman. Grandma Joan hopes that he will go to Duke and then to Oxford and be fluent in two languages by the time he is twelve. Mom just wants him to be happy and live up to his greatest potential."

At the age of two and a half, the major leaguer who was to go to Oxford was diagnosed with autism. It was a stunningly beautiful day when the family went to see the specialist. The Gardners had done some research on autism prior to the appointment and recognized this diagnosis as a hopeless tragedy for those unfortunate enough to be afflicted. The beauty of the day made it difficult for the Gardners not to be optimistic that they were going to hear that their son had a language delay, and that with some remediation their lives would be back to normal. They said their prayers and walked into the office. After a 3-hour exam, they sat down to hear the pronouncement. No parent could have been prepared for what they heard. They were told that the road would be long for Chas, and that the best they might do was to get on with their lives by finding an appropriate institution for him. In effect, they heard that their son had somehow wandered outside the lines of hope and that, perhaps, they might best call this one a foul and wait for another pitch. The family left the doctor's office and walked back into that perfect day and into the confluence of hope and despair. Nothing that they had ever experienced adequately prepared them for the rushing feeling of having the hopes and dreams for their child ripped from their moorings and swept into the beyond. They could not breathe. William Hazlitt (1778–1830), an English essayist, captured their feelings in his statement "There are none so wretched as those who are without hope." Their son had ventured to that place beyond hope, and his parents had discovered a place beyond pain.

The ride home was quiet. It was as if the family were waiting for an awakening from somebody else's dream. This could not be their life. It was other people who had children with disabilities. Somehow, some way, there must have been a mistake. This was a burden that did not belong to them. Prior to that day, although they had not recognized it, their lives had been perfect. They wanted that back.

But there was no awakening. To the contrary, there was no sleeping in their house. Chas did not sleep, not even nap. Not ever. The Gardners slept in shifts to stand watch. To make matters worse, he was beyond hyperactive. He ran through the house unable to attend to anything for more than a few seconds. He had no interest in toys other than to turn them on their sides and spin their wheels. He preferred spinning twigs, placing his hands under running water, and watching Disney sing-along videos. In general, he preferred to engage in all manners of behavior that were inappropriate. His parents could not take him to stores for the most basic of errands. Tantrums were the norm.

For Christmas they bought a variety of toys, wrapped them, and carefully placed them under the tree. On Christmas Day, they learned that the joy of Christmas is truly in the giving. Chas had been up all night, so his parents finally led him to the tree to open presents. They were so excited. They put the theme music from *A Charlie Brown Christmas* on the stereo to set the mood. They remembered the Christmases of their own childhood and could not wait to share their experiences with their son. Chas looked blankly at the presents and walked over to the tree, more interested in the ornaments. He was oblivious to the traditions of Christmas, the stocking filled with everything he should love, and the mystery of what was inside his carefully wrapped presents. He was not unappreciative, just indifferent. His parents wanted so desperately to give him something. They wanted a smile and perhaps some small validation that they were okay as parents. They didn't expect "great"; they just wanted to be okay. They tried to laugh off the pain while *A Charlie Brown Christmas* played in the background. When they tried to assist him in opening a present, Chas slammed his head on the floor and went into an hour-long tantrum. They walked outside and sat on the patio looking through the glass at the tree and the neatly wrapped presents. Later that evening they sat quietly and opened the presents themselves while Chas pulled twigs off the tree and twirled them. The Autism Grinch had stolen Christmas. They did not comprehend this at the time, but it was a scene that would be replayed not only every holiday, but every birthday and other special day as well. As often as the Autism Grinch came, the Gardners never got used to the emptiness that he left behind.

During the long nights of sleeping in shifts, Chas's parents began to search for answers on the Internet. Autism had been recognized for 50 years, and although some gains had been reported from behavioral interventions, the Gardners hoped that the medical community of researchers had been doing something more, something that might provide a spark of hope. They were dismayed to discover that there was no nationally organized research effort. The experts had declared that although autism was ostensibly treatable, it was not, nor could it ever be, curable. Some went further to say that it was irresponsible to give parents false hope. Apparently few of the experts had read Victor Frankel. They did not understand that sometimes hope in any form is sustaining.

The Gardners read all of the autism books and noticed that none of them mentioned the chronic gastrointestinal distress and sleep disturbance that plagued their son. Other parents of children with autism reported similar problems. It seemed to them impossible that a person could go without sleep for such an extended period of time and there not be a biological mechanism involved. In fact, it seemed irresponsible not to be looking at autism as a medical disorder with an associated medical treatment.

They took Chas to see their pediatrician. They told her that they had noticed that when Chas was up at night screaming, it appeared that he was holding his stomach. They went on to say that he had always had diarrhea and that they were concerned he might have celiac disease. They asked if there was something that could be done for his symptoms. They were told that there was no medical treatment for autism and were sent home. It occurred to them that had Chas just had a fever with the same set of symptoms, a multitude of specialists would have been engaged to relieve his suffering. Somehow his label of autism seemed to prejudice the medical community against considering any treatment options.

This response ran contrary to the Gardners' concept of science. They continued their search, determined to find something to help their son. What they found were a few bright spots of research being done in relative isolation, without significant interdisciplinary collaboration or coordination. They called individual researchers to learn about their studies. As the Gardners began to create their own inventory of research findings, they asked individual scientists if they were aware of the work being done by other scientists. Invariably, the answer was negative. They noticed some overlap in several studies under way. Given the limited amount of funding available for autism research, it seemed extremely inefficient not to support a coordinated effort. In addition to the lack of coordination between researchers, there were clinicians scattered across the country working with individual families. They were trying a variety of treatments, and some were trying to develop clinical research protocols, but their trials were poorly funded and in some cases poorly designed. Some trials employed questionable ethical standards.

The Gardners also identified groups of educators utilizing a variety of behavioral techniques. The educators, in a similar state as the scientists and clinicians, were employing multiple strategies derived from a variety of theories with little collaboration, communication, or evaluation. They also found a number of opportunists making claims about untested treatments and cures by leveraging the Internet. As desperate parents, they found it daunting to understand the science, manage their difficult child, and keep the driving force of hope from steering the family to irrational, possibly dangerous, treatments.

Sadly they came to realize that the basic scientists and clinicians were not communicating within their respective disciplines, let alone across disciplines. Furthermore, no one was talking to the educators. Everyone was working toward a common goal, but there was no coordination of effort. It was equivalent to constructing a building without plans. The concrete, steel, and drywall contractors were at the building site, just building.

The more scientists that the Gardners spoke to, the more they became convinced that autism was a disease process and that it could be treated and cured. An idea was forming that if research could be coordinated in one central location, getting the basic scientists, clinicians, and educators to communicate and collaborate, one might reach the Holy Grail of understanding autism, providing better treatments, and even, perhaps, preventing or curing it.

One evening Chuck Gardner met with another parent and M.I.N.D. cofounder, Rick Hayes, to discuss this concept. The two parents refined the idea and put it down on paper as a business plan. The idea of an organization with a three-pronged approach was formalized. The organization should have an interdisciplinary model and should mandate collaboration among the researchers. The three-legged stool should be made up of educational, clinical, and basic science components. The treatments would begin in the laboratory. They would then be exported to the clinic, where they would be refined and moved into clinical trials. By having an educational component, the trials could be tested in the real-life setting of the school and their effectiveness assessed by evaluation researchers. They called their plan *Project Hope*. There was one obstacle: the parents did not know any researchers to help them implement it. However, they had friends who knew the Dean Emeritus of the UC Davis School of Medicine. These friends agreed to set up a dinner. Dr. Anders, Chair of the Psychiatry Department and a board-certified child and adolescent psychiatrist with clinical and research experience with children with autism, was also invited.

Several weeks later, during the drive to that dinner at the dean's house, the radio announcer noted that it was the first day of the Age of Aquarius. The Gardners had heard for years about the dawning of the Age of Aquarius but had always thought it to be just a line in a song. They never realized that it had an actual start date. The radio announcer went on to explain that it was a point in time when people would set aside their notions of war and begin to work together for the higher calling of the common good. Thus, on that first day of Aquarius in 1997, these separate and distinct beginnings came together as the three authors of this chapter first met at a dinner hosted by the Dean Emeritus of the School of Medicine, Hibbard Williams, M.D.

Characteristic of his persona as a building contractor, Mr. Gardner had not come to dinner for idle, social chitchat. He passionately discussed his dream, and what's more, he brought his "set of drawings," the formal plan called *Project Hope*. As parents of a young child with autism, the Gardners also came pressed for time. They wanted action in a time frame that would benefit Chas. That evening, the Gardners told the unfortunately all-too-familiar story of the uncertainties in diagnosis, the confusion in the minds of professionals about etiology, the false reassurances, the delays in treatment, the fragmented services, and the prophesies of a grim prognosis. They described their overwhelming feelings of hopelessness, frustration, and abandonment.

The Gardners had become convinced that no appropriate, integrated, sensitive medical treatment programs existed anywhere in the country and that, moreover, research in the field of autism was similarly fragmented and underfunded. Their dream, their passion, their *Project Hope,* was to establish the "solution" at UC Davis Medical Center, situated in their home city of Sacramento, California, the capital of the largest state in the union.

The dinner ended on a positive note, despite significant skepticism and reserve expressed by Dr. Anders. His concerns were twofold. First, other medical centers with a focus on comprehensive autism research and treatment already existed in the United States; in fact, several very distinguished ones existed in California. Second, Dr. Anders was skeptical that a major research university such as UC Davis, with much on its plate at that time, could be moved to prioritize a new comprehensive program in autism. Nonetheless, Dr. Anders agreed to organize a meeting of UC Davis scientists with Mr. Gardner.

The meeting of UC Davis neuroscientists, immunologists, geneticists, biochemists, and clinicians was held within the month. At the meeting, there was lively discussion among the scientists, clinicians, and parents, who rarely, if ever, had communicated with each other before. The scientists expressed some interest in focusing their research on autism but guessed that funding of $10 million would be necessary to get the project under way. During the month in which the meeting was being arranged, Mr. Gardner had turned his vision, *Project Hope,* into a research proposal for an integrated medical research program focused on autism, which he submitted in response to a call for applications from the California Department of Developmental Services. Four parent members of Families for Early Autism Treatment (FEAT), the Sacramento-based national parent advocacy and support group, none of whom had ever prepared a grant application before, had come together to write the final proposal over a long weekend. It certainly did not hurt that the proposal was accompanied by a cover letter of strong endorsement signed by California's then-Governor Pete Wilson. The FEAT authors may have been neophyte grant writers, but their cover letter indicated that they were not naïve politically. Shortly after the meeting of UC Davis scientists, the grant was rated first by the selection committee, and UC Davis received $250,000 from the State of California to begin the pilot project as a partner with FEAT.

Still dubious that UC Davis could or should become a "dream" clinical and research center for children with autism, Dr. Anders convened a second meeting of scientists. The first meeting had been composed of scientists from UC Davis who had never worked in the field of autism. The second meeting included only scientists who were already established leaders in the field of autism research. Again, Chuck Gardner and other parents who by then had joined the parent team attended. When the scientist visitors heard about the resources at UC Davis, including its Neuroscience Center, Division of Biological Sciences, School of Veterinary Medicine, and Primate Center, and when they experienced firsthand the excitement, optimism, and commitment of the parent team, they unanimously and enthusiastically endorsed the development of *Project Hope* at UC Davis. All concurred with Chuck Gardner's initial assessment that at the time "there was no place for integrated, multi-specialty autism research and practice like the one envisioned in *Project Hope,* anywhere in the country."

Six months had passed since the initial dinner. Dr. Anders, slow to warm up, was still skeptical. He had become convinced that the idea was sound, and that UC Davis might well be the place, but where would the projected $10 million come from? Again, the parents had the answer. A group of parents (the "four dads," as they came to be called[1]) had organized themselves. They had independently met with the Medical Center Director and extracted a promise to match their fundraising to a total hospital commitment of $1.5 million. Within 60 days, the dads had met their target and gained the Medical Center's match. Within 4 months, *Project Hope* had pledges of $4.0 million for the university's endowment pool. Two newly endowed chairs were part of this package. Clearly, the School of Medicine's dean, and the campus's provost and chancellor, were now aware of *Project Hope*. But the four dads were not content. In the spring of 1998, they approached the California State Legislature and were successful in having a bill introduced authorizing the establishment of the M.I.N.D. Institute. The bill also provided an annually recurring appropriation of $2.0 million for operations. The acronym M.I.N.D. had been proposed by one of the dads. It stands for Medical Investigation of Neu-

---

[1]The five fathers mentioned in the acknowledgments worked together and supported each other from the outset. Four of them continued the process through to the end and came to be known as the "four dads."

rodevelopmental Disorders and reflects two guiding principles that have governed the institute ever since. First, the M.I.N.D. Institute is a medical enterprise focused on investigation. Second, the focus on neurodevelopmental disorders goes beyond autism per se, although autism research and treatment is a high priority. A liberal Democrat, Senator Diane Watson, had introduced the bill, and Pete Wilson, the conservative Republican governor, signed it. Never before had the two collaborated in this way. The entrepreneurism of the parents and the State's perceived need for neurodevelopmental research and services in a university setting had been an unbeatable combination. As one of the dads first observed, "The stars were aligned in the heavens." This has become one of the M.I.N.D. Institute's principal mottos. When the bill became a statute, the University of California assigned responsibility for the M.I.N.D. Institute to the Davis campus and its School of Medicine.

The annual appropriation, which was doubled in the subsequent legislative session and approved by Governor Gray Davis, a Democrat, proved the bipartisan attraction of the cause and the bipartisan energy of the four dads. In addition to the increased annual appropriation that year, the legislature and the governor authorized a one-time appropriation of $25 million for recruitment and start-up costs. In 1999, only 2½ years after the initial dinner, the M.I.N.D. Institute dream had become a reality. The M.I.N.D. Institute had succeeded in capturing the attention of not only the entire University of California system, but also the nation.

From another perspective, accruing such fame and fortune so rapidly has presented challenges. In an era of fledgling start-up companies that begin with a flash and end just as quickly, financed by large dowries from venture capitalists interested only in the return on their investment, the M.I.N.D. Institute did not want to flash and burn. In its rapid rise, the institute had accrued many stakeholders, all with high hopes and expectations, and often with conflicting strategic directions, timetables, and degrees of realism. However, the university was committed to making the M.I.N.D. Institute unique, and the M.I.N.D. leadership was committed to keeping parents and academics as partners within the constraints of university governance.

An Executive Board composed of equal numbers of members from the university, the founding parents, and relevant community agencies was established. Retreats, strategic planning, and recruitment of new leadership were accomplished. For each of the major leadership recruitments and initiatives, parents and faculty engaged in the university's processes jointly as partners. A table of organization with four operational committees was established: a Clinical Services Committee, a Research Committee, an Education Committee, and a Development Committee. M.I.N.D. Institute faculty or staff members chaired the committees, but representation on each included parents and community members as well. Academic representation on the committees and on the Executive Board reflects the makeup of the UC Davis campus. Thus, the Executive Board consists of deans and chairs from both medical and nonmedical departments and schools. Faculty on the research committee come from the Division of Biological Sciences and the Primate Center; on the Education Committee, from the School of Education and the Department of Human and Community Development; and on the Clinical Services Committee, from the three primary medical departments, Pediatrics, Neurology, and Psychiatry. Parents and relevant community agency and school district members round out each committee.

What have the last several years been like? Some have likened it to a long and scary ride on a roller coaster. There have been highs and lows, but never a dull moment. Parent-community-university partnerships are not always easy, but they are essential. The university as a governing body can be painfully slow and methodical; the parents' timetable is urgent. In fact, the greatest area of conflict has been "timing." It is obvious why parents want crises resolved urgently and answers immediately: the well-being of their children is at stake. It is also apparent why the university needs to be cautious. Regulatory oversight, institutional priorities, and academic freedom are determinants not to be taken lightly.

Another area of controversy has been research direction. Parents, as nonscientists, are potentially vulnerable to fads, especially as avid consumers of the Internet. In contrast, scientists are not always sufficiently sensitive to the latest "hot" areas in the clinical arena, as discussed in Chapter 8. The M.I.N.D. Institute has been successful in stimulating areas of innovative research that, while scientifically sound, may not be ready for customary federal funding. However, the line between innovation and fad may become fuzzy. And often parents and more traditional scientists have not agreed at first about research priorities and directions. Having parents as voting members of all operational committees and participating in setting research, clinical, and educational priorities has been an enlightening experience for all participants. It has been essential for building the trust between parents, scientists, educators, and clinicians that is essential for the long-term success and continued growth of the M.I.N.D. Institute.

A third area of conflict has been in the distribution of resources between missions and between disorders. How much of the resources should be devoted to clinical activities versus research and educational activities? How much of the resources should be devoted to autism versus the broader neurodevelopmental spectrum? In this area, all participants have strong opinions; and, of course, as new, distinguished scientists have been recruited to the M.I.N.D. Institute, the numbers of opinions related to these questions has multiplied.

But differences of opinion are not new to organizations, and conflicts, especially in young, rapidly expanding organizations, are healthy. All constituencies need to continually educate each other. Three basic constructs guide this effort: open communication, mutual education, and building trust. Parents meet with staff and leadership regularly and often, both formally through their assignments on committees, and informally by picking up the telephone or sending e-mails. List servers, newsletters, and the M.I.N.D. web site provide additional opportunities for communication. Minutes of all meetings are distributed widely.

From the perspective of mutual education, parents are always invited to scientific seminars, recruitment seminars, and community educational events sponsored by the M.I.N.D. Institute. Similarly, academic faculty attend FEAT meetings and participate actively in events sponsored by community agencies. Finally, trust is something that can only be built over time. Parents need to experience, firsthand, that M.I.N.D. professionals indeed have their child's and family's best interests at heart and are responsive to their needs and respectful of their values. And M.I.N.D. faculty and staff need to recognize that impatience, indefatigable hope, and constructive criticism from parents are not attacks to be taken personally, but benefits that accrue from the partnership and the trusting relationship. The parent-academic-community partnership in integrating the delivery of service, the support of research, and the advance of education is what makes the M.I.N.D. Institute unique, and it is the energy, enthusiasm, and commitment of all parties that continue to result in its success. There is no doubt that any one party alone could not succeed.

How successful have the first 4 years been? State funding in FY 2003 has been continued despite serious budget deficits in California. Private contributions and federal research grant support also have increased dramatically. Recruitment of highly qualified research and clinical faculty and staff has been steady. M.I.N.D. funding has supported innovative research on neurodevelopmental disorders throughout the UC system and the nation. A competitive grants program has been in operation for 4 years and funded 52 research projects. Local community agencies and school districts have profited from M.I.N.D. Institute funding and from its telemedicine school-focused interactive videoconferencing program, TeleMIND. And children and families have benefited from a comprehensive, interdisciplinary team evaluation in the M.I.N.D. Clinic where developmental pediatricians, child neurologists, child psychiatrists, and child psychologists work in the same physical facility specially designed (by Mr. Gardner) to meet the needs of children with neurodevelopmental disorders and their parents.

Our greatest sign of success, however, is that we have rapidly outgrown the initially assigned quarters and will soon be moving into a newly constructed M.I.N.D. Institute (see Figure 10–1). This construction project, again under the direction of Chuck Gardner, is the most rapidly conceived and completed building project in UC Davis history, with only 28 months from initial planning to occupancy. Ground was broken on September 8, 2001, and programs will open in April 2003. The building design has two primary organizing concepts. First, spaces are designed to be a haven for families who may have traveled from afar. Second, the design fosters collaboration among scientists, clinicians, and families. Eating and resource areas, such as community rooms and library facilities, are shared. Specific attention has been given to creating an atmosphere that promotes chance interaction between researchers, doctors, and parents.

The new M.I.N.D. Institute campus will consist of two buildings, totaling 102,000 square feet, located on 11 acres of the UC Davis Medical Center campus (see Figure 10–1). A research building, with space for both wet and dry laboratories, will be connected to a clinical-academic building. Pediatrics, genetics, child neurology, child/adolescent psychiatry, and child psychology will be its academic occupants. Researchers from multiple fields will occupy the research building. Finally, the publication of this volume attests to the success of the M.I.N.D. Institute.

In summary, the parent-academic-community partnership makes the M.I.N.D. Institute unique, infused with energy, optimism, and innovation. The partnership has been, and must continue to be, more than mere rhetoric. A meaningful, long-term collaborative relationship between parents, the university, and the greater community is essential to the continued growth, progress, and success of our collective efforts. The founding motto can be restated: "When the partnership flourishes, the stars remain aligned."

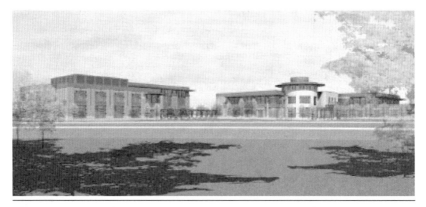

Figure 10–1. The new M.I.N.D. Institute campus (architect's rendition).

Appendix

Resources

General Information on Autism Spectrum Disorders

Books

Bashe PR, Kirby B: The OASIS Guide to Asperger Syndrome: Advice, Support, Insights, and Inspiration. New York, Crown, 2001

Cohen DJ, Volkmar FR: Handbook of Autism and Pervasive Developmental Disorders, 2nd Edition. New York, Wiley, 1997

Klin A, Volkmar F, Sparrow S (eds): Asperger's Syndrome. New York, Guilford, 2000

Mesibov GB, Adams LW, Klinger L: Autism: Understanding the Disorder. New York, Plenum, 1998

Ratey J, Johnson C: Shadow Syndromes: The Mild Forms of Major Mental Disorders That Sabotage Us. New York, Bantam Doubleday Dell, 1998

Schopler E, Mesibov G, Kunce L (eds): Asperger Syndrome or High-Functioning Autism? New York, Plenum, 1998

Siegel B: The World of the Autistic Child: Understanding and Treating Autistic Spectrum Disorders. Oxford, UK, Oxford University Press, 1998

Sigman M, Capps L: Children With Autism: A Developmental Perspective. Cambridge, MA, Harvard University Press, 1997

Waltz M: Pervasive Developmental Disorders: Finding a Diagnosis and Getting Help for Parents and Patients With PDDNOS and Atypical PDD. Cambridge, MA, O'Reilly, 1999

Practice Parameters

American Academy of Child and Adolescent Psychiatry

Volkmar FR, Pomeroy JCE, Realmuto G, et al: Practice parameters for the assessment and treatment of children, adolescents, and adults with autism and other pervasive developmental disorders. J Am Acad Child Adolesc Psychiatry 38 (suppl 12):32S–54S, 1999

American Academy of Neurology

Filipek PA, Accardo PJ, Ashwal S, et al: Practice parameter: screening and diagnosis of autism. Neurology 55:468–479, 2000

California Department of Developmental Services

Autistic spectrum disorders: best practice guidelines for screening, diagnosis, and assessment, 2002. Available at: www.ddhealthinfo.org/asd.asp

Multidisciplinary Consensus Panel

Filipek PA, Accardo PJ, Baranek GT, et al: The screening and diagnosis of autistic spectrum disorders. J Autism Dev Disord 29:439–484, 1999

Web Sites

http://www.asperger.org
http://www.autism.com/ari
http://www.autism-society.org
http://www.canfoundation.org
http://www.udel.edu/bkirby/asperger
http://www.firstsigns.org
http://www.autismtoday.com
http://www.aspennj.org
http://www.autism.org
http://www.unc.edu/~cory/autism-info
http://www.naar.org

Internet Bookstores With ASD Specialty

http://www.SpecialNeeds.com
http://www.autismbooks.com
http://www.autismsociety-nc.org

Parent Resources and Support

Books

Andron L: Our Journey Through High-Functioning Autism and Asperger Syndrome: A Roadmap. London, Kingsley, 2001

Attwood T: Asperger's Syndrome: A Guide for Parents and Professionals. London, Kingsley, 1998

Fling E: Eating an Artichoke: A Mother's Perspective on Asperger Syndrome. London, Kingsley, 2000

Grandin T: Thinking in Pictures and Other Reports From My Life With Autism. New York, Vintage Books, 1996

Harris S: Siblings of Children With Autism: A Guide for Families. Bethesda, MD, Woodbine House, 1994

Hart C: Without Reason: A Family Copes With Two Generations of Autism. Arlington, VA, Future Horizons, 1989

Hart C: A Parent's Guide to Autism: Answers to the Most Common Questions. Riverside, NJ, Pocket Books, 1993

Ozonoff S, Dawson G, McPartland J: A Parent's Guide to Asperger Syndrome and High-Functioning Autism: How to Meet the Challenges and Help Your Child Thrive. New York, Guilford, 2002

Park C: Exiting Nirvana: My Daughter's Life With Autism. Boston, MA, Back Bay Books, 2002

Powers M: Children With Autism: A Parent's Guide, 2nd Edition. Bethesda, MD, Woodbine House, 2000

Willey L: Pretending to Be Normal: Living With Asperger's Syndrome. London, Kingsley, 1999

Willey L: Asperger Syndrome in the Family: Redefining Normal. London, Kingsley, 2001

Support Groups

Autism Society of America (ASA)
  (800) 328-8476
  http://www.autism-society.org
Families for Early Autism Treatment (FEAT)
  http://www.feat.org
Asperger Syndrome Education Network (ASPEN)
  (732) 321-0880
  http://www.aspennj.org

Web Sites

http://www.maapservices.org
http://www.patientcenters.com/autism/news/stress_family.html
http://www.faaas.org
http://www.our-kids.org

Autism Screening and Diagnostic Instruments

Autism Diagnostic Interview–Revised
  Western Psychological Services
  (800) 648-8857
Autism Diagnostic Observation Schedule
  Western Psychological Services
  (800) 648-8857
Checklist for Autism in Toddlers
  In appendix of: Baron-Cohen S, Allen J, Gillberg C: "Can Autism Be Detected at 18 Months? The Needle, the Haystack, and the CHAT." British Journal of Psychiatry 161:839–843, 1992
  Also available from First Signs, Inc., at http://www.firstsigns.org
Childhood Autism Rating Scale (CARS)
  Western Psychological Services
  (800) 648-8857
Modified Checklist for Autism in Toddlers
  In appendix of: Robins DL, Fein D, Barton M, et al: "The Modified Checklist for Autism in Toddlers: An Initial Study Investigating the Early Detection of Autism and Pervasive Developmental Disorders. Journal of Autism and Developmental Disorders 31:131–144, 2001
  Also available from First Signs, Inc., at http://www.firstsigns.org
Pervasive Developmental Disorders Screening Test (PDDST)
  Available from the author, Bryna Siegel, Ph.D.
  (415) 476-7385
Screening Tool for Autism in Two-Year-Olds (STAT)
  Available from the author, Wendy Stone, Ph.D.
  (615) 936-0249

Training

Autism Diagnostic Interview and Autism Diagnostic Observation Schedule
Contact:
Center Administrator
University of Michigan Autism and Communication Disorders Center
1111 East Catherine
Ann Arbor, MI 48109-2054
Phone: (734) 936-8600
Fax: (734) 936-0068

Intervention Resources for Autism Spectrum Disorders

Education

Books

Bender M, Valletutti PJ, Baglin CA: A Functional Curriculum for Teaching Students With Disabilities, 3rd Edition, Vol 1: Self-Care, Motor Skills, Household Management, and Living Skills. Austin, TX, Pro-Ed, 1996

Bender M, Valletutti PJ, Baglin CA: A Functional Curriculum for Teaching Students With Disabilities, Vol 4: Interpersonal, Competitive Job-Finding, and Leisure-Time Skills. Austin, TX, Pro-Ed, 1998

Blenk K, Fine D: Making School Inclusion Work: A Guide to Everyday Practices. Cambridge, MA, Brookline Books, 1997

Bricker D, Woods-Cripe JJ: An Activity-Based Approach to Early Intervention. Baltimore, MD, Brookes, 1992

Cumine V, Leach J, Stevenson G: Asperger Syndrome: A Practical Guide for Teachers. London, Fulton, 1998

Downing JE: Including Students With Severe and Multiple Disabilities in Typical Classrooms: Practical Strategies for Teachers. Baltimore, MD, Brookes, 1996

Fouse B: Creating a Win-Win IEP for Students With Autism: A How-to Manual for Parents and Educators. Arlington, VA, Future Horizons, 1999

Fullerton A: Higher Functioning Adolescents and Young Adults With Autism: A Teacher's Guide. Austin, TX, Pro-Ed, 1996

Gibb G, Dyches TT: Guide to Writing Quality Individualized Education Programs (IEPs): What's Best for Students. Boston, MA, Allyn & Bacon, 1999

Greenspan S, Wieder S: The Child With Special Needs: Encouraging Intellectual and Emotional Growth: The Comprehensive Approach to Developmental Challenges Including Autism, PDD, Language and Speech Problems, and Other Related Disorders. Cambridge, MA, Perseus, 1998

Harris S, Handleman J: Preschool Education Programs for Children With Autism. Austin, TX, Pro-Ed, 2001

Hodgdon LA: Visual Strategies for Improving Communication: Practical Supports for School and Home. Troy, MI, QuickRoberts, 1995

Leaf R, McEachin J: A Work in Progress: Behavior Management Strategies and a Curriculum for Intensive Behavioral Treatment. New York, DRL Books, 1999

Maurice C, Green G, Luce S: Behavioral Intervention for Young Children With Autism: A Manual for Parents and Professionals. Austin, TX, Pro-Ed, 1996

McClannahan, LE, Krantz PJ: Activity Schedules for Children With Autism: Teaching Independent Behavior. Bethesda, MD, Woodbine House, 1999

Moyes R, Moreno S: Incorporating Social Goals in the Classroom: A Guide for Teachers and Parents of Children With High-Functioning Autism and Asperger Syndrome. London, Kingsley, 2001

Myles B, Adreon D: Asperger Syndrome and Adolescence: Practical Solutions for School Success. Shawnee Mission, KS, Autism Asperger, 2001

National Research Council: Educating Children With Autism. Washington, DC, National Academy Press, 2001

Schopler E, Mesibov GB: Learning and Cognition in Autism. New York, Plenum, 1995

Schopler E, Lansing M, Waters L: Teaching Activities for Autistic Children: Individualized Assessment and Treatment for Autistic Children and Developmentally Disabled Children. Austin, TX, Pro-Ed, 1983

Siegel L: The Complete IEP Guide: How to Advocate for Your Special Education Child, 2nd Edition. Berkeley, CA, Nolo Press, 2001

Smith M, Belcher R, Johrs P: A Guide to Successful Employment for People with Autism. Baltimore, MD, Brookes, 1997

Valletutti PJ, Bender M, Hoffnung A: A Functional Curriculum for Teaching Students With Disabilities, 3rd Edition, Vol 2: Nonverbal and Oral Communication. Austin, TX, Pro-Ed, 1996

Valletutti PJ, Bender M, Sims-Tucker B: A Functional Curriculum for Teaching Students With Disabilities, 3rd Edition, Vol 3: Functional Academics. Austin, TX, Pro-Ed, 1996

Wagner S: Inclusive Programming for Elementary Students With Autism. Arlington, VA, Future Horizons, 1999

Web Sites and Software

http://www.wrightslaw.com (special education laws)
http://www.do2learn.com
http://www.mayer-johnson.com
http://www.ldonline.org
http://www.difflearn.com
http://www.inspiration.org

Social Interventions

Books

Antonello S: Social Skills Development: Practical Strategies for Adolescents and Adults With Developmental Disabilities. Boston, MA, Allyn & Bacon, 1996

Bloomquist ML: Skills Training for Children With Behavior Disorders. New York, Guilford, 1996

Duke M, Nowicki S, Martin E: Teaching Your Child the Language of Social Success. Atlanta, Peachtree, 1996

Faherty C: Asperger's . . . What Does It Mean to Me? A Workbook Explaining Self Awareness and Life Lessons to the Child or Youth With High Functioning Autism or Asperger's. Arlington, VA, Future Horizons, 2000

Frankel F: Good Friends Are Hard to Find: Help Your Child Find, Make and Keep Friends. Los Angeles, CA, Perspective, 1996

Freeman S, Dake L: Teach Me Language: A Social-Language Manual for Children With Autism, Asperger's Syndrome and Related Disorders. Langley, BC, SKF Books, 1997

Garcia-Winner M: Inside Out: What Makes a Person with Social Cognitive Deficits Tick? San Jose, CA, Winner, 2000

Garrity C, Baris M, Porter W: Bully Proofing Your Child: A Parent's Guide. Longmont, CO, Sopris West, 2000

Gray C: Taming the Recess Jungle. Arlington, VA, Future Horizons, 1993

Gray C: The New Social Story Book, Illustrated Edition. Arlington, VA, Future Horizons, 2000

Gutstein S: Autism/Asperger's: Solving the Relationship Puzzle. Arlington, VA, Future Horizons, 2001

Gutstein SG, Sheely RK: Relationship Development Intervention With Young Children: Social and Emotional Development Activities for Asperger Syndrome, Autism, PDD, and NLD. London, Jessica Kingsley, 2002

McAfee J: Navigating the Social World: A Curriculum for Individuals With Asperger's Syndrome, High Functioning Autism and Related Disorders. Arlington, VA, Future Horizons, 2001

Moyes RA: Incorporating Social Goals in the Classroom: A Guide for Teachers and Parents of Children With High-Functioning Autism and Asperger Syndrome. London, Jessica Kingsley, 2001

Nowicki S, Duke M: Helping the Child Who Doesn't Fit In. Atlanta, GA, Peachtree, 1992

Quill KA: Teaching Children With Autism: Strategies to Enhance Communication and Socialization. San Diego, CA, Singular, 1995

Quill KA: Do-Watch-Listen-Say: Social and Communication Intervention for Children With Autism. Baltimore, MD, Brookes, 2000

Sargent LR: Social Skills for School and Community: Systematic Instruction for Children and Youth With Cognitive Delays. Colorado Springs, CO, Division on Mental Retardation and Developmental Disabilities of the Council for Exceptional Children, 1998

Sheridan S: Why Don't They Like Me? Helping Your Child Make and Keep Friends. Longmont, CO, Sopris West, 1998

Vermeulen P: I Am Special: Introducing Children and Young People to Their Autism Spectrum Disorder. London, Jessica Kingsley, 2001

Behavioral and Sensory Issues

Books

Anderson E, Emmons P: Unlocking the Mysteries of Sensory Dysfunction. Arlington, VA, Future Horizons, 1996

Durand VM: Sleep Better! A Guide to Improving Sleep for Children With Special Needs. Baltimore, MD, Brookes, 1997

Kranowitz CS: The Out of Sync Child: Recognizing and Coping With Sensory Integration Dysfunction. Bellevue, WA, Perigee, 1998

Myles BS, Southwick J: Asperger Syndrome and Difficult Moments: Practical Solutions for Tantrums, Rage, and Meltdowns. Shawnee Mission, KS, Autism Asperger, 1999

Myles BS, Cook K, Miller L, et al: Asperger Syndrome and Sensory Issues: Practical Solutions for Making Sense of the World. Shawnee Mission, KS, Autism Asperger, 2000

Newport J, Newport M: Autism, Asperger's, and Sexuality. Arlington, VA, Future Horizons, 2002

Schopler E: Parent Survival Manual: A Guide to Crisis Resolution in Autism and Related Developmental Disorders. New York, Plenum, 1995

Alternative Treatments

Books

LeBreton M: Diet Interventions and Autism. London, Jessica Kingsley, 2001

Marohn S: The Natural Medicine Guide to Autism. Charlottesville, VA, Hampton Roads, 2002

McCandless J: Children with Starving Brains: A Medical Treatment Guide for Autism Spectrum Disorder. New York, Bramble Books, 2002

Seroussi K, Rimland B: Unraveling the Mystery of Autism and Pervasive Developmental Disorder. New York, Simon & Schuster, 2000

Shaw W: Biological Treatments for Autism and PDD. Lenexa, KS, Great Plains Laboratory, 2002

Web Sites

http://www.AutismNDI.com (Autism Network for Dietary Intervention)
http://www.gfcfdiet.com
http://www.aap.org/bpi/Alternative.html
http://nccam.nih.gov/nccam

Information on Related Disorders

Books

Greene RW: The Explosive Child: A New Approach for Understanding and Parenting Easily Frustrated, "Chronically Inflexible" Children. New York, HarperCollins, 2001

Hagerman RJ, Hagerman PJ: Fragile X Syndrome: Diagnosis, Treatment, Research, 3rd Edition. Baltimore, MD, Johns Hopkins University Press, 2002

Papolos DF, Papolos J: The Bipolar Child: The Definitive and Reassuring Guide to Childhood's Most Misunderstood Disorder. New York, Broadway Books, 2002

Stewart K: Helping a Child With Nonverbal Learning Disorder or Asperger Syndrome: A Parent's Guide. Oakland, CA, New Harbinger, 2002

Tanguay P, Rourke B: Nonverbal Learning Disabilities at Home: A Parent's Guide. London, Jessica Kingsley, 2001

Turecki S, Tonner L: The Difficult Child. New York, Bantam Doubleday Dell, 2000

Web Sites

http://www.nldline.com (Nonverbal Learning Disabilities)
http://www.chadd.org (Children and Adults With Attention Deficit Disorder)
http://www.ldanatl.org (Learning Disabilities Association of America)
http://www.thearc.org (Association for Retarded Citizens, ARC)
http://www.fragilex.org (Fragile X syndrome)

Medical Centers/Universities/Clinics With ASD Specialization

Alabama

Center for Autism Resources and Education, Inc. (C.A.R.E.)
PO Box 2673
Tuscaloosa, AL 35403
Phone: (205) 349-2774
Fax: (205) 349-2774

Pervasive Developmental Disorders Clinic
University of Alabama Department of Psychology
PO Box 870348
Tuscaloosa, AL 35487
(205) 348-5000

Alaska

Center for Human Development
University of Alaska
2330 Nichols Street
Anchorage, AK 99508
(907) 272-8270
http://www.alaskachd.org

Arizona

Melmed Center
  5020 East Shea Boulevard, Suite 100
  Scottsdale, AZ 85254
  (480) 443-0050
  http://www.melmedcenter.com
Southwest Autism Research Center
  1002 East McDowell, Suite A
  Phoenix, AZ 85006
  (602) 340-8717
  http://www.autismcenter.org

California

Autism Intervention Center
  Children's Hospital and Health Center, San Diego
  3020 Children's Way, MC 5042
  San Diego, CA 92123
  (858) 966-7453
Autism Research Center
  University of California, Santa Barbara
  1163A Phelps Hall
  Santa Barbara, CA
  (805) 893-2176
Center for Asperger's Assessment and Intervention
  The HELP Group
  13130 Burbank Boulevard
  Sherman Oaks, CA
  (818) 779-5175
Children's Hospital Oakland
  Child Development Center and Communication Clinic
  5220 Claremont Avenue
  Oakland, CA 94609
  (510) 428-3351
For OC Kids
  University of California, Irvine
  1915 West Orangewood Avenue, Suite 200
  Orange, CA 92868-2045
  (888) 962-5437

M.I.N.D. Institute
  University of California, Davis
  2825 50th Street
  Sacramento, CA 95817
  M.I.N.D. Clinic: (888) 883-0961
  General questions: (916) 734-6495
  http://www.mindinstitute.org
Pervasive Developmental Disorders Clinic
  Stanford University
  401 Quarry Road
  Palo Alto, CA 94304-1419
  (650) 498-9111
Pervasive Developmental Disorders Clinic
  University of California, San Francisco
  401 Parnassus Avenue
  San Francisco, CA 94143
  (415) 476-7385
UCLA Autism Clinic
  300 Medical Plaza, Suite 1100
  Los Angeles, CA 90024
  (310) 825-0458
UCLA Neuropsychiatric Institute
  760 Westwood Plaza
  PO Box 956967
  Los Angeles, CA 90024
  (310) 825-0511

Colorado

University of Colorado Health Sciences Center
  JFK Partners: Autism and Developmental Disability Clinic
  4200 E. 9th Avenue
  Denver, CO 80262
  (303) 315-6511

Connecticut

Center for Children With Special Needs
  359-A Merrow Road
  Tolland, CT 06084
  (860) 870-5313

Yale Child Study Center Developmental Disabilities Clinic
230 South Frontage Road
New Haven, CT 06519
(203) 737-4337
http://info.med.Yale.edu/chldstdy/autism

Delaware

Delaware Autism Program
144 Brennen Drive
Newark, DE 19713
Phone: (302) 454-2202 ext. 101
Fax: (302) 454-5427

Florida

Center for Autism and Related Disabilities (CARD)
1500 Monza Avenue
Coral Gables, FL 33146-3004
Phone: (305) 284-6564 or (800) 9-AUTISM ext. 2
http://www.psy.miami.edu/card (this website will link to all CARD
centers across the state)

Georgia

Emory Autism Resource Center
Emory University
718 Gatewood Road
Atlanta, GA 30322
(404) 727-8350

Illinois

University of Chicago Department of Psychiatry
5841 S. Maryland Avenue
Chicago, IL 60637
Phone: (773) 702-0621

Illinois Center for Autism
  548 South Ruby Lane
  Fairview Heights, IL 62208-2614
  (618) 398-7500
  http://www.illinoiscenterforautism.org

Indiana

Indiana Resource Center for Autism
  Indiana Institute on Disability and Community
  2853 E. Tenth Street
  Bloomington, IN 47408
  Phone: (812) 855-6508
  Fax: (812) 855-9630

Iowa

Regional Autism Services Program
  Child Health Specialty Clinic
  100 Hawkins Drive
  Iowa City, IA 52242-1011
  (319) 356-4619
  http://www.medicine.uiowa.edu/autismservices

Kansas

Autism-Asperger Resource Center
  4001 HC Miller Building
  3901 Rainbow Boulevard
  Kansas City, KS 66160
  Phone: (913) 588-5988
  Fax: (913) 588-5942
  http://www.kumc.edu/aarc

Kentucky

Kentucky Autism Training Center
  Weisskopf Center for the Evaluation of Children
  911 S. Brook Street
  Louisville, KY 40203
  Phone: (502) 852-4631 or (800) 334-8635 ext. 4631
  Fax: (502) 852-7148

Louisiana

Louisiana State University Health Sciences Center
  Human Development Center
  1100 Florida Avenue
  New Orleans, LA 70119-2799
  (504) 942-8380
  http://www.laautism.org

Maryland

Kennedy Krieger Institute
  707 North Broadway
  Baltimore, MD 21205
  (888) 554-2080

Massachusetts

Eunice Kennedy Shriver Center
  University of Massachusetts Medical School
  55 Lake Avenue North
  Worcester, MA 01655
  (781) 642-0001
  http://www.umassmed.edu/shriver
McLean Center for Neurointegrative Services
  115 Mill Street
  Belmont, MA 02178
  (617) 855-2847
The May Institute, Inc.
  220 Norwood Park South, Suite 204
  Norwood, MA 02062
  (800) 778-7601
  http://www.mayinstitute.org

Michigan

University of Michigan Autism and Communication Disorders Center
  1111 East Catherine
  Ann Arbor, MI 48109-2054
  (734) 936-8600

Missouri

Judevine Center for Autism
    9455 Rott Road
    St. Louis, MO 63127
    Phone: (314) 849-4440
    Fax: (314) 849-2721

Nevada

Department of Psychology/296
    University of Nevada, Reno
    Reno, NV 89557
    (775) 784-6828 ext. 2034
    http://www.psyc.unr.edu/autism/index.html

New Jersey

Douglass Developmental Disabilities Center
    Rutgers, The State University
    25 Gibbons Circle
    New Brunswick, NJ 08901-8528
    (732) 932-9137
    http://gsappweb.rutgers.edu/dddc
UMDNJ Autism Center
    University of Medicine and Dentistry of New Jersey
    185 South Orange Avenue
    Newark, NJ 07103
    (973) 972-8930

New Mexico

University of New Mexico
    Center for Development and Disability
    Department of Pediatrics
    2300 Menaul Boulevard, NE
    Albuquerque, NM 87107
    (505) 272-3000
    http://cdd.unm.edu

New York

Institute for Child Development
  State University of New York
  Binghamton, NY 13902-6000
  (607) 777-2829
  http://128.226.8.112/icdext
Schneider Children's Hospital
  Developmental and Behavioral Pediatrics
  Schneider Children's Hospital
  269-01 76th Avenue
  New Hyde Park, NY 11040
  (718) 470-3540
Strong Center for Developmental Disabilities
  University of Rochester School of Medicine and Dentistry
  601 Elmwood Avenue
  Rochester, NY 14642
  (800) 462-4344
  http://www.urmc.rochester.edu/strong/scdd/welcome.html
The Institute for Basic Research in Developmental Disabilities
  George A. Jervis Clinic
  1050 Forest Hill Road
  Staten Island, NY 10314
  (718) 494-5127 or (718) 494-5284

North Carolina

Treatment and Education of Autistic and Related
    Communication-Handicapped Children (TEACCH)
  CB #6305
  Chapel Hill, NC 27599
  Phone: (919) 966-5156
  Fax: (919) 966-4003
  http://www.teacch.com

North Dakota

Child Evaluation and Treatment Program
  University of North Dakota, School of Medicine
  PO Box 9013
  Grand Forks, ND 58020
  (701) 780-2477

Ohio

Kelly O'Leary Center for Pervasive Developmental Disorders
  Cincinnati Children's Hospital Medical Center
  3333 Burnet Avenue
  Cincinnati, OH 45229-3039
  (513) 636-4688
  http://www.cincinnatichildrens.org
Nisonger Center UAP
  The Ohio State University
  1581 Dodd Drive
  McCampbell Hall
  Columbus, OH 43210-1296
  (614) 292-8365
  http://www.osu.edu/units/osunc

Oregon

Center on Human Development
  University of Oregon
  College of Education
  5252 University of Oregon
  Eugene, OR 97403-5252
  (541) 346-3591
  http://darkwing.uoregon.edu/~uap/index.html
Child Development and Rehabilitation Center
  PO Box 574
  Portland, OR 97207-0574
  (503) 494-8095 or (800) 452-3563
  http://cdrc.ohsu.edu/index.php

Pennsylvania

Autism Center of Children's Hospital of Pittsburgh
  3705 Fifth Avenue
  Pittsburgh, PA 15668
  Phone: (412) 692-6538
  Fax: (412) 692-5679
  http://www.uclid.org:8080/uclid/index.html

Autism Research Program and Social Disabilities Clinic
    University of Pittsburgh School of Medicine
    3811 O'Hara Street
    430 Bellefield Towers
    Pittsburgh, PA 15213
    (412) 624-0818
Autism Spectrum Resource Center
    14 South State Street
    Newtown, PA 18940
    Phone: (215) 860-3743
    Fax: (215) 860-3745
    http://www.autismsrc.org
Institute on Disabilities
    Temple University
    423 Ritter Annex 13th and Cecil B. Moore Avenue
    Philadelphia, PA 19122
    Phone: (215) 204-1356
    Fax: (215) 204-6336
    http://www.temple.edu/inst_disabilities

Rhode Island

Bradley Hospital Developmental Disabilities Program
    1011 Veteran's Memorial Parkway
    East Providence, RI 02915
    (401) 434-3400

South Carolina

Carolina Autism Resource and Evaluation (CARE) Center
    Fairfield Office Park
    1064 Gardner Road, Suite 301
    Charleston, SC 29407
    (843) 852-4172
    http://www.state.sc.us/ddsn/pubs/care/care.htm
South Carolina Early Autism Project
    2630B Hardee Cove
    Sumter, SC 29150
    Phone: (803) 905-4427 or (803) 775-1249

South Dakota

South Dakota University Affiliated Program
   Health Science Center
   1400 West 22nd Street
   Sioux Falls, SD 57105
   (605) 357-1439
   http://www.usd.edu/sduap

Tennessee

Child Development Center
   Vanderbilt University
   2100 Pierce Avenue
   Nashville, TN 37232
   (615) 322-2709

Texas

Connections Center
   4120 Bellaire Boulevard
   Houston, TX 77025
   (713) 838-1362
   http://www.connectionscenter.com

Utah

University of Utah Autism Program
   546 Chipeta Way, Suite 458
   Salt Lake City, UT 84108
   Clinic: (801) 585-1212
   Research: (801) 585-9098

Vermont

Center on Disability and Community Inclusion
   University Affiliated Program of Vermont
   University of Vermont/College of Education
   Burlington Square, Suite 450
   Burlington, VT 05401
   (802) 656-4031
   http://www.uvm.edu/~cdci

Virginia

Virginia Commonwealth University
  Virginia Institute for Developmental Disabilities
  PO Box 843020
  700 E. Franklin Street, 10th Floor
  Richmond, VA 23284-3020
  (804) 828-3876
  http://www.vcu.edu/partnership/index.html
The Autism Program of Virginia (TAP Virginia)
  1400 Westwood Avenue, Suite 106
  Richmond, VA 23227
  (800) 649-8481 or (804) 355-0300
  http://www.autismva.org

Washington

University of Washington Autism Center
  Center on Human Development and Disability
  Box 357920
  University of Washington
  Seattle, WA 98195
  (206) 221-6806
  http://depts.washington.edu/uwautism/index.html

West Virginia

The West Virginia Autism Training Center
  Marshall University College of Education and Human Services
  400 Hal Greer Boulevard, Suite 316
  Huntington, WV 25755
  (304) 696-2332 or (800) 344-5115 (WV Only)
  http://www.marshall.edu/coe/atc
West Virginia University
  Center for Excellence in Disabilities
  955 Hartman Run Road
  Morgantown, WV 26505
  (304) 293-4692
  http://www.ced.wvu.edu

Wisconsin

Waisman Center
   1500 Highland Avenue
   Madison, WI 53705-2280
   (608) 263-5776
   http://www.waisman.wisc.edu
Wisconsin Early Autism Project
   6402 Odana Road
   Madison, WI 53719
   (608) 288-9040
   http://www.wiautism.com

Index

*Page numbers printed in **boldface type** refer to tables.*